Carcinogenesis and Mutagenesis Testing

T0321187

Contemporary Biomedicine

CARCINOGENESIS AND MUTAGENESIS TESTING

Edited by

J. F. Douglas

Scientific Services Inc.
Front Royal, Virginia

Humana Press · Clifton, New Jersey

Library of Congress Cataloging in Publication Data
Main entry under title:

Carcinogenesis and mutagenesis testing.

   (Contemporary medicine)
   Includes bibliographies.
   1. Carcinogenicity testing.   2. Mutagenicity testing.
I. Douglas, J. F.   II. Series.   [DNLM: 1. Carcinogens—
analysis.   2. Mutagens—analysis.   3. Mutagenicity tests
—methods.   QZ 202 C2644]
RC268.65.C367   1984   616.99'4071   84-12820
ISBN 0-89603-042-3

© 1984 The HUMANA Press Inc.
Crescent Manor
PO Box 2148
Clifton, NJ 07015

All rights reserved·

No part of this book may be reproduced, stored in a retrieval system,
or transmitted, in any form or by any means, electronic, mechanical, photo-
copying, microfilming, recording, or otherwise without written
permission from the Publisher.

Printed in the United States of America.

Preface

Cancer has become the most critical health problem in the United States. It is expected that 25% of the people will develop this dread disease, and many of these will die from the malady. The causes of cancer are varied, but the best estimate available is that 70–90% arise from environmental factors. These statistics have triggered widespread governmental action along two lines: (1) An effort to identify those chemicals and conditions that give rise to malignant processes has been mounted by the Carcinogenesis Testing Program, the National Cancer Program, and subsequently, the National Toxicology Program. (2) Regulatory laws have been enacted that are administered by agencies such as TSCA, FIFRA, EPA, FDA, OSHA, and so on, whose mission is to minimize public exposure to carcinogens.

Since direct verification that specific chemicals induce cancer in humans is necessarily limited to known incidences of unanticipated exposure and is therefore rare, most chemicals are identified as carcinogens only by laboratory experiments. At present, the only accepted procedure is long-term animal bioassay, and not only are these studies expensive and time-consuming, but current worldwide resources permit the evaluation of only 300–400 chemicals per year, a miniscule amount compared to what is available in the commercial world: 30,000 existing chemicals, with approximately 700 new such materials being introduced every year. The known synergistic effects of chemical mixtures compound the problem to the point that it becomes almost insoluble, and the future resolution of its staggering complexities undoubtedly must lie in the development of reliable short-term tests for carcinogenicity and mutagenicity that correlate with the results of actual bioassays.

Federal regulations—through TSCA, FIFRA, the clean air and water acts, the occupational health laws, and the drug acts—now require that industrial and commercial establishments ensure public safety through proof that their operations will not constitute a human health hazard. The implementation of these requirements is a tremendous task that can be accomplished only with the understanding and by the considerable efforts of those individuals and organizations involved.

The purpose of this book then, is twofold: first, to provide industry, government, and commerce with the wide range of conceptual and practical information necessary to understand the fields of carcinogenicity and the short-term tests for it that are fundamental to the identification of carcinogenic materials. And second, to stimulate thinking and research in those areas that will provide effective means for reducing exposure to specific chemicals and, hence, the incidence of that modern scourge, cancer.

To fulfill these purposes, the book is organized along two broad lines: first, the basic scientific principles that underlie our present concepts of carcinogenicity and mutagenicity are introduced, and secondly, the assay procedures for carcinogenicity and mutagenicity currently employed are discussed, including their merits, deficiencies, and the practical details of the techniques necessary to successfully carry out these assays.

CONTENTS

CHAPTER 4

John O. Rundell

CHAPTER 5

R. J. M. Fry and H. P. Witschi

CHAPTER 6

D. J. Koropatnick and J. J. Berman

Section B: Carcinogenesis

CHAPTER 7

J. M. Ward

CHAPTER 8

J. M. Ward

CHAPTER 9

J. F. Douglas

CHAPTER 10

Cipriano Cueto, Jr.

Part II: Practical Carcinogenesis and Mutagenesis Assay Methodology

Section A: Gene Mutation Assays

CHAPTER 13

Mouse Lymphoma Cell Assays........................ 207
Paul E. Kirby

CHAPTER 14

Chinese Hamster Ovary Mutation Assays 227
David J. Brusick

CHAPTER 15

David J. Brusick

Section B: DNA Damage and Repair Assays

Section C: Cytogenetic Assays

Section D: Transformation Assays

CHAPTER 19

In Vitro Transformation Assays Using Mouse Embryo Cell
John O. Rundell

CHAPTER 20

In Vitro Transformation Assays Using Mouse Embryo Cell
John O. Rundell

CHAPTER 21

In Vitro Transformation Assays Using Diploid Syrian Ham-
John O. Rundell and Judith A. Poiley

Section E: Short-Term In Vivo Carcinogenesis Assays

CHAPTER 22

L. H. Smith and H. P. Witschi

Section F: Conduct of Carcinogen Bioassays

Contributors

JULES J. BERMAN • *National Cancer Institute, Frederick Cancer Research Facility, Frederick, Maryland*

DAVID J. BRUSICK • *Department of Molecular Toxicology, Litton Bionetics Incorporated, Kensington, Maryland*

CIPRIANO CUETO, JR. • *Dynamac Corporation, Rockville, Maryland*

J. FIELDING DOUGLAS • *Scientific Services Incorporated, Front Royal, Virginia*

R. J. M. FRY • *Biology Division, Oak Ridge National Laboratory, Oak Ridge, Tennessee*

STEVE R. HAWORTH • *Microbiological Associates, Bethesda, Maryland*

PAUL E. KIRBY • *Microbiological Associates, Bethesda, Maryland*

D. JAMES KOROPATNICK • *University of Calgary, Calgary, Canada*

JUDITH A. POILEY • *Litton Bionetics, Incorporated, Kensington, Maryland*

JOHN O. RUNDELL • *Litton Bionetics, Incorporated, Kensington, Maryland*

L. H. SMITH • *Biology Division, Oak Ridge National Laboratory, Oak Ridge, Tennessee*

JERROLD WARD • *National Cancer Institute, Frederick Cancer Research Facility, Frederick, Maryland*

HANSPETER WITSCHI • *Biology Division, Oak Ridge National Laboratory, Oak Ridge, Tennessee*

Part I

The Fundamental Biology

Section A

Mutagenesis and Other Short-Term Tests

Chapter 1

An Overview of Short-Term Testing

S. R. Haworth

During the last decade, the utilization of short-term tests for genetic activity has increased dramatically. This demand for short-term tests has arisen for a complex variety of scientific, social, and economic factors.

The tremendous development and industrial use of new chemicals since the second World War has seen over 50,000 synthetic compounds introduced into the environment with perhaps another 1000 being introduced each year. Since certain of these chemicals have been shown to have adverse effects on human health, a proper concern for safety has lead to intensive testing and regulation of human exposure to these materials. There is clear evidence that chemicals do in fact cause cancer in man. Approximately 20 individual chemicals have been convincingly identified as carcinogens, and the US Government now prints a yearly list of human carcinogens. How many other human carcinogens are among the thousands of chemicals that already exist and among the hundreds of new ones that are synthesized each year is unknown. Clearly, society needs to know which of these chemicals are potential hazards so that their production and human exposure can be carefully controlled. The currently standard test for carcinogenicity—the rodent lifetime bioassay—is too expensive and lengthy to evaluate each of the thousands of chemicals already in our environment. Therefore, great effort has been devoted to the development of less expensive and faster tests. These short-term tests are employed as predictors of carcinogenicity and they permit prioritization of the many chemicals that cannot be tested by longer and more costly procedures. The growing data base for a complex of short-term tests suggests that these tests have demonstrable merit as predictors of animal carcinogenicity. However, much work remains in test development, evaluation, and validation before a definitive conclusion can be reached regarding the correlation of short-term test results and human carcinogenicity. The five classes of in vitro short-term tests are:

1. Primary DNA damage and repair.
2. Bacterial gene mutation.
3. Mammalian cell gene mutation.
4. Mammalian cell chromosome damage.
5. Mammalian cell transformation.

Most of the short-term tests do not measure carcinogenicity directly. Instead, they evaluate the genetic activity of chemicals by assessing their ability to cause gene mutations, chromosome loss or damage, or primary structural damage to DNA, the genetic material. That mutations in somatic cells are critical to cancer development has been proposed and discussed for several years. Existing data from short-term tests indicate that there is indeed a correlation between mutagenicity and carcinogenicity. Thus, of the hundreds of known animal carcinogens evaluated in short-term tests, a significantly high percentage of them have also been found to be mutagenic. It has also been shown that short-term tests function equally as well as animal bioassays in detecting human carcinogens (Table 1, courtesy of David J. Brusick, Litton Bionetics). The responses summarized in this table were obtained from the IARC Monographs.

The average animal carcinogen is an electron-deficient chemical that attacks the electron-rich nucleic acid bases of DNA. Not all carcinogens are mutagens however. Some materials, such as asbestos or certain hormones, are thought to cause cancer through epigenetic mechanisms in which the interruption of normal cell physiology may lead to the cancerous state. Immune suppression may also be a critical factor in chemical carcinogenesis.

Carcinogen detection is not the only reason that the genetic activity of chemicals should be determined. Many geneticists feel that the greatest risk to the human race is not a chemical's carcinogenicity, but its mutagenicity. Although somatic mutations may lead to cancer and death, quite beyond the economic impact and the great emotional trauma caused by cancer, the genetic impact on future generations might ultimately prove the most serious effect, and it may also be avoidable. It is known that mutations that occur in germ cells can have dramatic effects on the

Table 1
Comparison of In Vitro and In Vivo Test Results of Known or Suspected
Human Carcinogens

Chemical	IARC status[a]	Short-term test results	Rodent bioassay results
4-Aminobiphenyl	HC	+	+
Arsenic	HC	+	−
Asbestos	HC	Limited	−
Benzene	HC	+	Limited
Benzidine	HC	+	+
BCME	HC	+	+
Chromium	HC	Limited	+
DES	HC	+	+
Melphalan	HC		+
Mustard gas	HC	+	+
2-Naphthylamine	HC	+	+
Vinyl chloride	HC	+	+
Aflatoxin	PHC	+	+
Dimethylsulfate	PHC	+	+
Cadmium	PHC	Limited	+
Chlorambucil	PHC	+	Limited
Acrylonitrile	PHC	+	+
Amitrole	PHC	Limited	+
Auramine	PHC	+	Limited
Beryllium	PHC	+	+
Carbon tetrachloride	PHC	−	+
Cyclophosphamide	PHC	+	+
Dimethylcarbamoyl chloride	PHC		+
Ethylene oxide	PHC	+	Limited

[a]HC = human carcinogen, PHC = probable human carcinogen.

gene pool of an organism. Deleterious mutations in human germ cells could accumulate undetected for generations before being expressed as structural malformations, emotional abnormalities, or other genetic dysfunctions. Animal models for detecting mutations are subject to the same criticisms as are animal models for carcinogenicity. Clearly then, short-term genetic tests may in fact be identifying potential human mutagens, as well as potential human carcinogens.

From an economic standpoint, the rapidly escalating costs of conducting time-consuming long-term in vivo studies make it almost inevitable that the use of short-term genetic tests will continue to increase. In addition, short-term tests have applicability where rodent studies do not, for example, to evaluate some biomedical devices and drug residues in food animals. The regulatory agencies responsible in these two areas are currently placing greater emphasis on these short-term evaluations.

Aside from their lower cost and short duration, short-term in vitro tests systems for genetic activity offer flexibility in protocol design and in the kinds of materials that can be tested. Although all of the test systems are aqueous systems, the test materials do not have to be water soluble, nor is there an absolute requirement for solubility in any solvent. Uniform suspensions can often be successfully dispersed into the test systems. Test materials do not have to be pure substances. Complex mixtures of substances have been successfully evaluated in these test systems. In fact, a test system such as that of Ames can be used to monitor production lots of a chemical for small quantities of mutagenic impurities. In the same manner, one can use the Ames test to evaluate chemical lots from different suppliers to select the "cleanest" supply of the chemical when mutagenic impurities are known to be possibly present. Test materials need not be only solids or liquids. Many of the test systems have been successfully modified to test gases or highly volatile materials.

Since many chemicals are not mutagenic or carcinogenic until after they have been metabolized by human tissue or human intestinal microflora, it can be of value to monitor various body fluids for the presence of mutagenic activity after exposure to the test materials. This approach can even be applied to humans who are suspected victims of exposure to known mutagens or carcinogens. Monitoring human urine for mutagenic activity and peripheral lymphocytes for genetic damage can now be conducted in a rather routine fashion, and a number of industrial firms are evaluating personnel exposure through short-term cytogenetic screens.

The use of short-term tests to monitor environmental pollution sources has been successfully applied to many situations. These include the analysis of automobile exhaust, of stack emissions, of industrial water effluents, and of drainage from chemical waste storage areas.

The phrase "short-term tests" covers a number of different laboratory evaluations, including bacterial and mammalian mutagenesis, mammalian cell transformation, chromosome aberration, bacterial and mammalian DNA repairs, insect systems, and tissue experiments.

Although an individual test may not be sufficiently reliable as a predictor of effect in humans, a battery of well-thought-out procedures can show a good correlation with long-term rodent tests. Careful selection of what test combinations to employ, i.e., testing strategy, is an important component of the short-term test approach to chemical evaluation.

Chapter 2

Genetic Toxicology

Applications and Testing Strategies

David J. Brusick

Application and Testing Strategies

Application of short-term tests to chemical safety evaluation requires tailoring the tests to specific situations and needs. Screening for mutagenicity usually involves the application of a broad range of tests measuring numerous genotoxic endpoints such as point (gene) mutation, chromosome damage, and somatic recombination events (3, 9). The adaptation of short-term tests to carcinogenicity prediction requires a slightly different array of tests from those employed in mutagenicity screening.

Testing for genetic effects as a primary objective requires the use of short-term tests that measure definitive mutational damage. The type of test organism employed is not critical since DNA functions similarly in all organisms, permitting reasonably accurate extrapolation of DNA damage over many phylogenetic levels. The ultimate test for genetic toxicity is one in which the demonstration of chemically induced heritable genetic alterations can be measured. Thus, the reproductive system of the test organism is the critical target site in this type of assessment.

Short-term test strategies for carcinogenic potential do not necessarily require that the applied tests measure well-defined genetic alterations, but rather that they employ tests measuring endpoints whose results cor-

7

relate well with the carcinogenic profiles of the same chemicals in vivo. These tests may include those that detect mutation or chromosomal damage, but more often they involve processes such as cell transformation and the stimulation of enzymatic DNA repair (2, 8, 18, 21). Somatic cells are the critical targets for genotoxic events leading to tumor production and, thus, the induced events need not be of the heritable classes measured in genetic toxicology.

The application of in vitro and in vivo tests as they apply to mutagen and carcinogen testing is shown in Table 1.

It is important in carcinogenicity screening to broaden the nature of the assays so that phenomena such as tumor promotion and altered immunocompetence can be evaluated. These parameters are more likely to influence the degree of in vivo activity for tumor induction than they are for heritable genetic damage. Figure 1 illustrates the hypothetical role

TABLE 1
The Application of Genetic Testing Methods to Carcinogen and Mutation Assessment

Primary type identification obtained	Genetic testing[a]			
	In vitro detection of mutation induction and chromosome damage	In vivo detection of mutation induction and chromosome damage		In vitro/in vivo detection of genotoxic damage not leading to somatic or gonadal heritable alterations
		Somatic	Gonadal	
Identification of presumptive animal carcinogens	A	A	NA	A
Identification of presumptive animal mutagens	A	A	A	(NA)
Risk analysis for heritable genetic effects	NA	NA	A	NA
Risk analysis for carcinogenic effects	NA	(A)	NA	NA
Identification of animal mutagens	NA	A	A	NA

[a]A = applicable; NA = not applicable; ( ) = implies special circumstances of explanation.

HYPOTHESIZED FACTORS AFFECTING TUMOR POTENCY

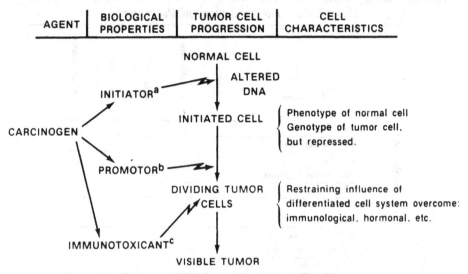

Fig. 1. Proposed interaction of initiation, promotion, and immunological factors in the etiology of tumor development in mammals.

that genetic (initiation) and ancillary (promotion and immunotoxicity) play in the development of malignancy in vivo (5, 11).

If a chemical possessed the capacity to induce all three of the phenomena identified in Fig. 1 it presumably would be a more potent animal carcinogen than a chemical possessing only one or two of the three characteristics. A limited survey of the published literature appears to support this assumption (Table 2). At the present time, however, only a small number of known carcinogens have been subjected to such an extensive in vitro evaluation.

An estimate of carcinogenic potency based only on the degree of mutagenicity seems to work for some classes of chemicals but not others. It might well be that the failure of these analyses to take into account other bioactivity modifying factors, such as promotion and immunotoxicity, is the missing element that would have permitted greater utilization of the results of short-term assays in estimating in vivo carcinogenic potency. Although some preliminary correlations of mutagenic activity and carcinogenic potency appear to be encouraging, these comparisons using the Ames test (7) and Mouse Lymphoma Assay (6) have not yet been extended beyond a small group of reference carcinogens. Application of such potency comparisons to a wider range of chem-

TABLE 2

A Comparison of Carcinogenic Potency with the Frequency of Unequivocal Positive Activity Responses in a Battery of Short-Term Assays Including Measures of Immunofunction and Promotion[a]

	Compound	Mutation	Transformation	UDS	Promotion	Immunofunction
Non-Carcinogens	Cholesterol	-	-	-		
	Dimethylsulfoxide	-	-	-		
	Acetone	-	-	-		
	Tetramethyl benzidine	-	-	-		
	TPA [phorbol ester]	-	-	-	+	
Carcinogens +	saccharin	+ / -	+ / -	-		
	Diphenyl nitrosamine	+ / -	+ / -			
	4-acetylaminoflourene	+ / -	+ / -	-		
	UV irradiation	+	+	+		
++	Benzo[e]pyrene	+ / -	+ / -	+		
	Urethan	+ / -	+	+		
	Methylmethane sulfonate	+	+	+		
	Beta-naphthylamine	+	+	+		
	TRIS	+	+			+
	Diethylnitrosamine	+	+	+		+
	3-methylcholanthrene	+	+	+		+
	Cyclophosphamide	+	+	+		+
+++	Diethylstibestrol	+	+	+		+
	Bis-chloromethylether	+	+	+		
	Aflatoxin B1	+	+	+		
	Gamma irradiation	+	+	+		
	Formaldehyde	+	+	+	+	+

IN VIVO CARCINOGENIC POTENCY

Symbols in table are: [-], inactive; [+], active; [+/-], weakly active.

[a]Source of Information: refs. 6, 7, 10, 12–15, 17–19.

icals has not resulted in correlations that support the hypothesis mentioned above; possibly, too, this merely emphasizes the unavailability of good carcinogenesis potency data for most in vivo studies.

The assignment of specific short-term tests to carcinogenic assessments is not based on the results of rigorous validation efforts. At the

TABLE 3
Examples of Chemicals Requiring Assessment in Multitest Battery Covering
Different Genetic Endpoints and Phylogenetic Levels[a]

Compound	Suspected animal carcinogen	Characteristic
Benzene	+	Detected *only* in cytogenetic tests
Formaldehyde	+	Not detected in standard bacterial tests
Urethan (ethylcarbamate)	+	Not detected in most *in vitro* assays; is positive in animal cytogenetics and *Drosophila*
Hexamethylphosphoramide	+	Not detected in standard bacterial tests
Procarbazine	+	Not detected in standard bacterial tests
DES	+	Detected in mammalian cell mutagenesis and transformation but is not active in other in vitro tests
Acrylonitrile	+	Not detected in standard bacterial tests
Saccharin	+	Detected best in cytogenetic assays; weak or negative in all others
Lead acetate	+	Detected *only* in cell transformation assays
Aminotriazole	+	Detected *only* in cell transformation assays
p,p'-DDE	+	Detected in mammalian cell mutation but not bacteria

[a]Many of these chemicals would be missed if testing were limited to microbial and/or cytogenetic tests. The application of three to five short-term tests to each chemical is necessary to provide adequate coverage in general testing. If more than five tests are applied, the possibility of generating false positives increases.

present time, validation studies for many short-term tests are in progress, but it will be some time before the results are available to assist in making assignment of the tests to specific testing roles. However, as demonstrated in Table 3, a number of important chemical mutagens might not have been detected if only simple microbial or cytogenetic test procedures had been used in isolation.

The most promising attempt to evaluate critically each of the short-term assays and assess their applicability in various safety evaluation roles is the current GeneTox program developed by the Environmental Protection Agency (20). This undertaking involves the selection of expert panels to systematically review all published literature for an assay, prepare a written report discussing the strengths and weaknesses of the test, and develop a table showing the test's performance with chemicals that have been evaluated by the test.

Once all of the expert panels have reviewed their respective assay systems, an Assessment Panel will prepare an overview of all tests and will make recommendations for testing strategies and assignment of assays to specific roles in genetic testing.

The first portion of the GeneTox program is almost complete and was reported in the open literature. The second phase involving the Assessment Panel will require extensive data analysis and interpretation and may not be completed until the end of 1984. In the interim, development of testing strategies must rely upon published reviews of test performance (1, 3, 4, 9, 18) and proposed testing schemes (3). Neither of these approaches, however, will have the advantage of a comprehensive data review equal to the GeneTox effort.

Although most of the regulatory aims of the Federal Government have prepared schemes or recommendations regarding test batteries or strategies, there has been a concerted effort to devise a unified scheme that approaches both mutagenic and carcinogenic phenomena. A test strategy recently described by the Office of Toxic Substances appears to be the most comprehensive agency approach to this end. The basic outline of this system is shown in Figure 2. The plan suggests that a minimum group of tests, including gene mutation, UDS, and cytogenetics, is sufficient to screen for both mutagens and carcinogens. Positives in this basic battery would push chemicals into higher level tests. Large-scale in vivo bioassays will still represent the ultimate assessments. A minimal test battery for the evaluation of new chemicals has been defined by the OECD (16). This battery consists of point mutation tests in bacteria (the Ames *Salmonella* assay and the *E. coli* WP$_2$ reverse mutation assay) and chromosome analysis by either in vitro or in vivo techniques. Positive responses in either the microbial or cytogenic assays would require additional testing in eukaryotic systems, much like the scheme shown in Fig. 2.

Table 4 is an attempt to summarize twenty short-term assays according to their perceived roles in chemical hazard assessment. This summary is for general recommendations and is based on review articles and the

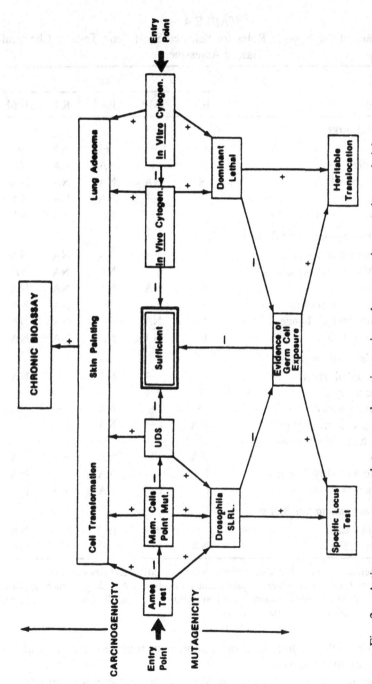

Fig. 2.   A tier system approach to general carcinogenic and mutagenic screening and risk assessment. The tests are only recommendations and in some cases may be substituted by other more relevant test systems.

TABLE 4

A Summary of the Possible Roles for Selected Short-Term Tests in Chemical Hazard Assessment

General assay type	Roles[a]				
	ICP	IMP	EA	RA	HPM
Microbial Assays					
Ames test	+ +	+	+	NA	(+)
WP$_2$ and derivations	+	+	NA	NA	NA
Bacterial repair tests	+	NA	NA	NA	NA
Yeast mutation	+	+ +	NA	NA	NA
Yeast mitotic recombination	+	+	NA	NA	NA
In Vitro Mammaliam Cell Assays					
Mouse lymphoma assay	+	+ +	NA	NA	NA
CHO or V79 mutation assays	+	+ +	NA	NA	NA
UDS assays	+ +	NA	NA	NA	NA
Chromosome abberations	+	+ +	+	NA	NA
Sister chromatid exchange	+ +	NA	+	NA	NA
Cell transformation	+ +	NA	NA	NA	NA
In Vivo Mammalian Assays					
Dominant lethal assay	NA	+ +	NA	+	NA
Cytogenic analysis	+	+ +	+	+ +	+ + +
Micronucleus assay	+	+	NA	(+)	NA
Spermhead abnormality assay	NA	(+)	NA	(+)	+
Heritable translocation assay in mice	NA	+	NA	+ +	NA
Specific locus assay in mice	NA	+ +	NA	+ +	NA
DNA adherent formation	(+)	(+)	NA	+ +	(+)
In Vivo Submammalian Assays					
Drosophila assays	+	+ +	(+)	(+)	NA
Plant cytogenetics	NA	(+)	+	NA	NA

[a]ICP, identifies mammalian carcinogenic potential; IMP, identifies mammalian mutagenic potential; EA, environmental assessment application; RA, risk assessment application; HPM, human population monitoring application: + = applicable, + = < ; (+), possible application under some conditions.

experience of the author. It is not intended to represent any official assignment of those tests.

In summary, one must conclude that no consensus regarding an overall generalized testing approach or strategy exists. Testing approaches are most successful when tailored to a specific situation or chemical class. For general purposes, the scheme shown in Fig. 2 appears to be adequate, assuming that some information concerning the metabolism, promotion, or cocarcinogenic effects as well as immunotoxicity could be developed along with the genotoxicity data. This scheme includes the analysis of DNA from exposed animals for the presence of macromelecular binding. DNA binding under such conditions strongly implies that genotoxic material as a suspect carcinogen. The results of the EPA GeneTox program as well as the ongoing validation efforts supported primarily by the Federal Government may generate significant alternatives to this testing strategy in the future.

References

1. Ames, B. N., *Science* **204,** 587 (1979).
2. Brusick, D. J., *Chemosphere* **5,** 403 (1978).
3. Brusick, D. J., Utility of Short-Term Genetic Tests in Chemical Safety Evaluation; evolving issues, in *Proceedings of the 4th Toxic Control Conference,* Miller, M. L., ed., Government Institutes Inc., Washington, DC, **4,** 40 (1979).
4. Brusick, D. J., *Principles of Genetic Toxicology,* Plenum, New York, 1980.
5. Burnet, F. M., *Immunological Surveillance,* Pergamon Press, Oxford, England, 1970.
6. Clive, D., Johnson, K. O., Spector, J. F. S., Batson, A. G., and Brown, M. M. , *Mutation Res.* **59,** 61 (1979).
7. Fox, J. L., *Chem. Eng. News,* 34 (1977).
8. Heidelberger, C., and Mondal, S., In Vitro Chemical Carcinogenesis, in *Carcinogens: Identification and Mechanisms of Action,* Griffin, A. C., and Shaw, C. R., eds., Raven Press, New York, 1979, pp. 83–92.
9. Hollstein, M., McCann, J., Angelosanto, F., and Nicholas, W., *Mutation Res.* **65,** 133 (1979).
10. Kakunaga, T., *Int. J. Cancer* **12,** 463 (1973).
11. Kopelivich, L., Bias, N. E., and Helson, L., *Nature* **282,** 619 (1979).
12. Luster, M. I., Faith, R. E., and McLachlan, J. A., *Bull. Environ. Contam. Toxicol.* **20,** 433 (1978).
13. Malmgren, R. A., Bennison, B. E., and McKinley, T. W., *Proc. Soc. Exp. Biol. Med.* **79,** 484 (1952).
14. Martin, C. N., McDermid, A. C., and Garner, R. C., *Cancer Res.* **38,** 2621 (1978).
15. Mondal, S., Brankow, D. W., and Heidelberger, *Cancer Res.* **36,** 2254 (1976).

16. Organization for Economic Cooperation and Development (OECD), *Mutagenicity Tests and Their Role in Identifying Mutagens and Carcinogens,* Ottowa, Canada, March, 1980.

17. Padarathsingh, M. L., Dean, J. H., and Keys, L., Effects of Alkylating Agents on the Immune Response, in *Biological Relevance of Immune Suppression:* Alterations by Genetic, Environmental, and Therapeutic Factors. Dean, J. H., and Padarathsingh, M., eds., Van Nostrand Reinhold Co., New York, 1981, pp. 176–189.

18. Pienta, R. J., A Hamster Embryo Cell Model System for Identifying Carcinogens, in *Carcinogens: Identification and Mechanisms of Action,* Griffin, A. C., and Shaw, C. R., eds., Raven Press, New York, 1979, pp. 121–141.

19. Thor, D. E., Reichert, D. F., and Flippen, J. H., *J. Reticulendothelial Soc.* **22,** 243 (1977).

20. Waters, M. D., The Gene-Tox Program, in *Banbury Report, Vol. 2, Mammalian Cell Mutagenisis: The Maturation of Test Systems,* Hsie, A. W., O'Neill, J. P., and McEthney, V. K., eds., Cold Spring Harbor Laboratory, Cold Spring Harbor, NY, 1979, pp. 449–457.

21. Williams, G. M., The Detection of Chemical Mutagens/Carcinogens by DNA Repair and Mutagenesis in Liver Cultures, in *Chemical Mutagens,* vol. VI, deServes, F. J., and Hollaender, A., eds., Plenum Press, New York, 1980, pp. 61–79.

Chapter 3

Consequences of Genotoxic Effects

David J. Brusick

Categories of Genotoxic Alterations

Genotoxic effects can be categorized into those that lead directly to transmissable alterations (gene mutation and certain classes of chromosomal damage) and those that are secondary to the production of heritable changes (DNA strand breakage and DNA repair processes). Both types are related and in most instances are induced by the same agents; however, as far as defining their impact on genetic disease and/or cancer initiation, the group of effects defined as "direct" measures of DNA damage is most critical to detect.

Gene Mutation

Definition

Mutation at the gene level (also referred to as specific locus mutation) is a consequence of DNA nucleotide changes that occur spontaneously or are induced by chemical and physical agents. These nucleotide changes result in new, stable DNA configurations that, after fixation, are capable of replicating in DNA during cell division. The consequences of these changes depend on several variables that will be discussed later.

17

Effects of Gene Mutation

Exposure of a test organism to a broad range of concentrations of a typical mutagen produces a spectrum of damage to the DNA as well as to other cellular macromolecules (Fig. 1). A substantial portion of this damage results in cytotoxic effects and eventual death to the cell and/or organism. A limited portion of the damage is reversible via enzymatic DNA repair phenomena and increased intracellular turnover of new macromolecules. The remainder of the DNA damage is of a stable nature and will be transmitted linearly to all progeny of the affected cell. A portion of this stable damage can consist of chromosome damage, but a majority will exist as gene mutation.

The consequences of gene mutation depend, to a large extent, on the cellular role of the gene involved as well as the location within the gene of the molecular changes associated with the specific mutagenic lesion. The cellular roles for genes ranges from regulatory activities to the production of structural products and enzymes. The typical types of mutations detected in screening programs are those associated with structural genes. This is related to the ease of detection of this class of events. The relation-

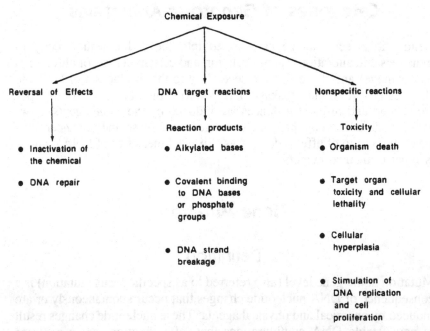

Fig. 1.   The types of intracellular reactions to chemical exposure. The DNA target reactions are those of primary interest to genetic toxicology. From Brusick (4).

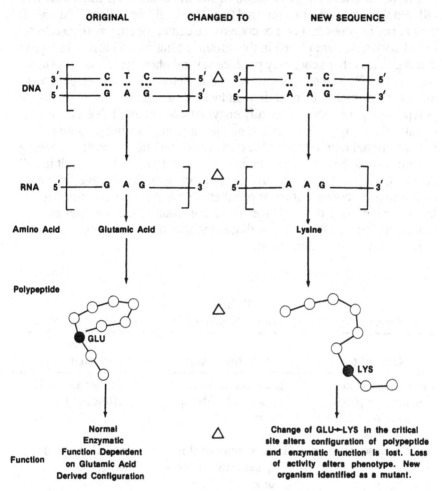

Fig. 2. An example of the DNA, RNA, and polypeptide relationships involved in mutation induction. A single base-pair altered by a mutagenic event results in a changed amino acid in the polypeptide. The single amino acid change produces a nonfunctional "mutant" polypeptide. From Brusick (4).

ship between the DNA change and the polypeptide gene product is shown in Fig. 2. The example depicted in the figure indicates that, as a result of the change in the amino acid, a nonfunctional gene product is formed. If the amino acid substitution induced by the mutagenic alteration occurs at a site in the polypeptide that is not critical for normal structural or enzymatic activity, the genetic lesion will not be detected. For example, nu-

merous amino acid substitutions are known in human hemoglobin protein
that have no effect on the function of the molecule (13). Mutations that
fall into this class are often referred to as "neutral" or "silent." Mutation
may occur in genes that do not code for structural or enzymatic products.
Regulatory genes are placed in this group. Mutations occurring in a gene
that regulates other genes may produce several phenotypic changes simultaneously (21). The common tests used to detect mutagens employ techniques that measure mutation induction in genes that produce a
polypeptide gene product, usually enzymatic in nature (Table 1). This facilitates the design of the test and simply involves looking for gain or loss
in a nutritional requirement. One other characteristic of genetic screening
systems is that the loss of the sentinel gene function must not result in cell
death. In other words, assays screen for genetic damage in genes
controlling functions that are supplementable and are not intrinsically going to lead to cell death. Under these constraints, the question of how
representative of all genes are those few that have been selected for in
vitro bioassays continues to arise.

TABLE 1

A Survey of the Types of Genes Employed in Genetic Testing Batteries

Name of test	Selective system	Gene involved ( )[a]
Gene mutation in mouse lymphoma (L5178Y), CHO or V-79 Cells	Resistance to toxic nucleotide DNA pre-cursors	Thymidine kinase (S); HGPRT (S)
Ames reverse mutation	Loss of nutritional re-quirements for histi-dine	*His* G; C or D (S)
E. coli. WP$_2$ reverse mutation	Loss of nutritional re-quirements for tryp-tophan	*Try* (S)
Gene mutation in mam-malian cells (general)	Resistance to ouabain, a membrane transport antagonist for Na$^+$ and K$^+$	Membrane transport (S)
Drosophila forward mu-tation	X-linked recessive le-thality in F$_2$ progeny	Multiple types (S or R)

[a](S) = structural genes; (R) = regulatory genes.

Mechanisms of Mutation Induction

The molecular processes acting to generate a stable mutation in DNA have been derived from studies using microorganisms, primarily prokaryotic bacteria (3). Again, the question of how well these mechanisms represent the events that occur during mutation induction in mammalian cells has not been satisfactorily answered. Most of the mechanisms identified in bacteria appear consistent for eukaryotic microorganisms such as yeast (2, 5) and *Neurospora crassa* (14). The structure of mammalian chromosomes, however, is considerably more complex than bacteria and yeast and basic information on mutagenic mechanisms at the molecular level in mammalian cells is needed.

Models that have been elucidated for bacterial mutagenesis consist of two general classes of changes:

Nucleotide Substitution or Base-Pair Substitution (BPS) Changes

This class involves mechanisms leading to a qualitative change in the nucleotide sequence in a single codon. This change may (as shown in Fig. 2) result in a critical amino acid shift producing a defective gene product and thus inducing a mutant phenotype; or the change, if induced in a noncritical portion of the polypeptide product, may not be expressed as a mutation.

Nucleotide or Base-Pair Additions and Deletion Mutations

This class is also designated as frameshift (FS), since a reading frameshift is the operational consequence of addition or deletion of single base pairs to the DNA content of a gene. In prokaryotic cells, the transcription and translation of DNA encoded information into gene products occurs via the reading of triplet codons from the initiating end of a gene (or transcriptional subunit) to the termination. A single nucleotide insertion (or deletion) would put the reading sequence out of phase by one base-pair. The consequence is assumed to be similar to that shown in Fig. 3, in which all amino acids following the insertion are nonsensical when compared to the original nonmutant sequence.

It has been generally assumed that both mechanisms operate in mammalian cells as well as bacteria, although the amount of confirming data in mammalian DNA is very small.

MECHANISM OF FRAMESHIFT MUTATION INDUCTION

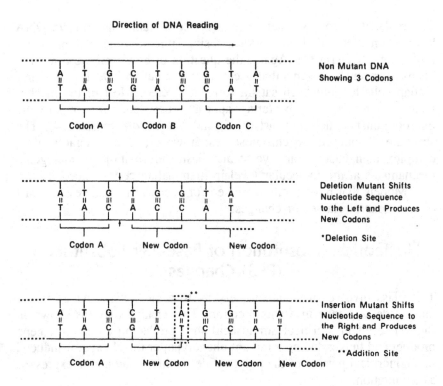

The production of new codons by deletion or insertion of base pairs will shift the sequence frame of nucleotide pairs. All codons subsequent to the mutant site will be incorrectly translated and the gene product defective.

Fig. 3. The mechanisms of frameshift mutation induction. The production of new codons by deletion or insertion of base pairs will shift the sequence frame of nucleotide pairs. All codons subsequent to the mutant site will be incorrectly translated and the gene produce defective. From Brusick (4).

Operational Aspects Mutation Detection

Gene mutation can be detected in most microbial, insect, and in vitro mammalian cell tests. Detection of gene mutation in vivo with mammals is technically very difficult because of the limited number of gene loci assessable by current techniques. Large animal populations must be employed to detect even moderate increases in mutant frequencies with in vivo techniques. The most widely accepted in vivo assay presently available is the Mouse Specific Locus Assay (MSLA) and its somatic cell version, the Mouse Somatic Mutation Spot Assay (MSMSA). Both of these tests are limited to the analysis of only a few structural genes (4) and the former, which measures heritable lesions, requires rather large animal populations in order to perform an analysis (15).

Two types of selective systems are used to measure mutation. Mutations can be detected in a forward mutation system by the identification of a new varient phenotype among a population of exposed test organisms. Forward mutation systems theoretically permit testing at all genes; however, as indicated earlier, only those genes whose function is not essential to basic cell survival can be used in mutation detection. Most forward mutation systems operate by selecting for mutation at a single gene rather than a sampling of all genes. The system used in the Mouse Lymphoma Assay is a good example of how such a selective system operates (Fig. 4). Forward mutation assays for detection of point mutations have been developed for most types of test organisms (Table 2).

SELECTION OF MUTAGEN-INDUCED TK-/- PHENOTYPES

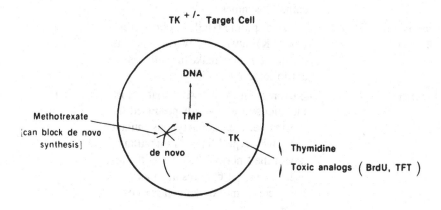

Mutant TK-/- cells are resistant to the toxic analogs BrdU or TFT and synthesize their DNA by de novo pathways. Nonmutant TK + /- cells will die in the presence of these analogs.

Fig. 4. Selection system for forward mutation at the thymidine kinase (TK) locus in mouse lymphoma L5178Y cells. Populations of Tk + / − cells are exposed to the test agent and these placed in growth medium supplemented with toxic nucleotide precursors. Mutant TK + / − cells are resistant to the toxic analogs BrdU or TFT and synthesize their DNA by *de novo* pathways. Nonmutant TK + / − cells will die in the presence of these analogs.

TABLE 2
Examples of Forward Mutation Systems in Tests Employed in
Genetic Toxicology

Target organism	Forward mutation selection system	Reference
Bacteria	6-Thioguanine (6-TG) resistance in *Salmonella typhimurium*. Mutants are detected by growth in 6-TG when it is incorporated into the plating medium	19
Yeast	Resistance to canavanine sulfate. Mutants are defective in a membrane transport enzyme necessary for the incorporation of this toxic amino acid analog into cellular proteins.	1, 4
Mold	Forward mutation at the adenine-3 (*ad*-3) gene of *Neurospora crassa*. Mutants are identified by their purple color. This pigment results from the loss of the *ad*-3 allele that involved adenine biosynthesis	1, 14
Mammalian cells in vitro	The loss of purine (HGPRT) or pyrimidine (TK) salvage pathways. Mutants in these gene loci make the cells resistant to toxic nucleotides	8
Mammals	The expression of recessive coat color mutations in F_1 hybrids produced in crosses between homozygous mutant and "wild-type" lines. A mutation at any of the "normal" alleles in the respective parent may result in an F_1 complete or mosaic animal for coat color	15
Insects	Recessive lethality carried on the X-chromosome. The lethal trait is expressed in the hemizygous state in the male F_2 progeny	20

The second method of analysis for gene mutation is one that measures reverse mutation induction. In such a system one starts with a population of test organisms carrying a gene mutation, most commonly one producing a nutritional requirement inhibiting the organisms from growing in their normal culture medium. Selection of mutants is accomplished by placing a large population of treated mutant organisms in the unsupplemented selective medium and screening for those which grow. The only growth observable should be from mutant genes undergoing reverse (back) mutation to the nonmutant genotype. The Ames test is a good example of a reverse mutation system (3). Reverse mutation assays have been developed in other test organisms, but it is a technique primarily applied to microbial test systems.

There is no reason to believe that different phenomena are measured in forward and reverse mutation assays and responses should correspond in most cases. The primary reason for the development of reverse mutation systems is their simplicity and high level of resolution (large population sampled).

Effect of DNA Repair on Mutation

During the evolution of complex biological systems, enzyme systems capable of maintaining the integrity of DNA appeared. Repair systems are unique to DNA and their development emphasizes the importance of preventing damage to this macromolecule.

Multiple repair systems evolved in organisms providing the potential for a multifaceted response to genotoxic agents by exposed organisms. The primary repair mechanism is referred to as excision repair (10). This process involves localization of the damaged DNA segment followed by enzymatic removal of a single-stranded DNA segment and resynthesis (Fig. 5). Excision repair is rapid and generally error-free; however, for it to be effective the repair of damage must occur prior to the next round of DNA replication. Because the damage remains in the nuclei during the next round of DNA replication, there is a significantly higher probability for the induction of mutation or cell death. Loss of excision repair by an organism increases its mutagenic sensitivity to many mutagens, but not all. Chemicals that tend to act on DNA by forming inter- and intrastrand linkages (e.g., bifunctional alkylating agents) will not be more mutagenic in excision repair-deficient organisms. Because crosslinks are not repaired, they produce cell death by inhibiting DNA replication rather than by inducing mutation. Thus, lack of repair does not automatically result in enhanced mutagenesis. Post-replication repair is another repair phenomenon that facilitates repair in replicating DNA by a gap-filling process that may involve recombination mechanisms (10). This process supplements excision repair in overall DNA protection.

The excision repair pathway is considered to be a highly accurate system; however, other repair processes such as SOS repair or post-

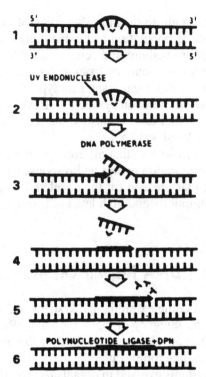

Fig. 5. A model for excision-repair. 1. A UV-irradiated double helix of DNA is represented containing one pyrimidine dimer. 2. The region adjacent and on the 5' side of the dimer is attacked by an endonuclease specific for UV-irradiated DNA. 3. DNA polymerase binds to DNA at the nicked site and, by addition of 5' nucleotide triphosphates, starts repair polymerization of the damaged strand using the template of the complementary strand. The dimer region becomes displaced. 4. When the 5' to 3' exonuclease site of the polymerase reaches the next hydrogen bonded base pair, the phosphodiester bond is hydrolyzed, releasing the dimer in a short oligonucleotide. 5. The polymerizing and hydrolytic activities may continue in the 5' to 3' direction until 6. 6. The polymerase displaced by polynucleotide ligase, together with DPN, restores the integrity of the phosphodiester backbone of DNA. From Kelly et al., *Nature* **224:** 495, 1969.

replication repair contain biochemical pathways that may actually introduce errors during the repair processes. The phenomenon of repair-induced mutation may well be a natural byproduct of secondary repair systems, such as SOS repair whose primary goals are to protect the linear integrity of the DNA molecule (prevent cell death) even at the expense of introducing new mutations. This may be best shown in Fig. 6. The dose–response curve in this figure illustrates the response of three bacte-

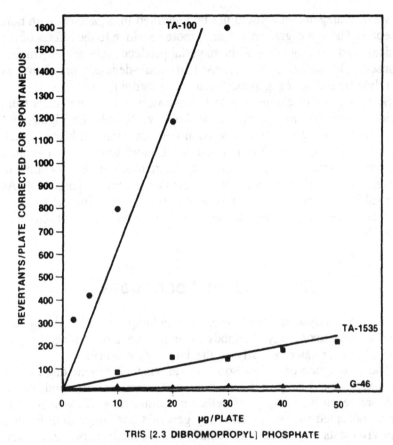

Fig. 6. Differential strain sensitivity to Tris-(2,3-dibromopropyl) phosphate. On each of the three mutant strains is carried the same site of chemical activity. The differential response is a result of the repair characteristics. From Brusick (4).

ria strains to Tris-2,3-(dibromopropyl) phosphate. Strain G-46 has normal excision repair, but no plasmid pKM101; strain TA1535 lacks the excision repair system but has no plasmid; and strain TA100 has no excision repair, and also contains the plasmid pKM101, which is believed to affect the SOS error-prone repair pathway, and introduces additional genetic alterations into the DNA. The dose–response curves fit the description of the strain repair modifications.

It should be noted that by removing excision repair capacity from an organism, chemicals that are not genotoxic do not become mutagenic. Rather, the detectable effect level (minimum detectable concentration) is lowered by one or two orders of magnitude. This permits detection of very weak mutagens that would not be identified in organisms with normal repair. The test organism becomes more sensitive to the effects of the chemical, and therefore less of the material produces substantially higher responses. The meaning of responses in repair-deficient organisms as they relate to predicting genetic hazard is uncertain (3).

Similar types of chemical effects are observed in human cells from individuals affected by the genetic deficiency, Xeroderma Pigmentosa (XP), which is analogous to the excision-deficient strain of bacteria such as TA1535 (16). Cells of XP individuals are more sensitive to mutation induction, and interestingly, XP individuals are much more susceptible to environmentally induced cancer than their normal counterparts (16). As described in another section of this book, assays measuring the stimulation of DNA repair are useful techniques to evaluate the genotoxicity of chemicals.

Chromosome Aberrations

Chromosome analysis is one of the earliest techniques employed in genetics and genetic toxicology. Methods for preparing and staining chromosomes were originated as early as the late 19th century.

The association of chromosome alterations with genetic disease and other toxicological endpoints was established early in this century.

More recently, analysis of cells for chromosome damage has become an accepted method of assessing genetic toxicology. Both in vitro and in vivo tests are used for screening, and the analysis of human lymphocytes is an established method for monitoring human exposure to potential mutagenic and clastogenic agents (12, 17).

The cells used in somatic cell cytogenetic evaluations may be derived from any proliferating source, such as continuously growing cell lines in culture, circulating lymphocytes, or bone marrow cells in mammals; even plant and insect cells may be employed. A compound such as colchicine is employed to arrest the cells in metaphase of mitosis, where chromosomes can be stained and visualized. Cytological evaluation consists of examining cell preparations for the frequency of cells in mitosis (mitotic index), the number of chromosomes per cell, and the structural integrity of chromosomes in the metaphase set. Occasionally, analysis of chromosomal association or disassociation within pairs will be made.

After a sufficient sample of cells in metaphase has been examined, the results are analyzed for any deviation from the normal background values. This same set of procedures is followed regardless of whether the cells are from in vitro cell culture or from mammalian bone marrow.

Reasonably standard nomenclature exists to describe the types of chromosome alterations that can be scored. A set of these, along with brief descriptions is given in Table 3. Even so, cytogenetic analysis is subjective and it is not uncommon for two investigators to score the same aberration differently. This can be largely avoided through preliminary scoring standardization procedures employing a single set of slides.

Specific types of aberrations such as reciprocal translocations cannot be visualized in normal staining (Giemsa) procedures, and special strains that produce banding must be used (Fig. 7). Banding procedures facilitate the detection of chromosome damage otherwise missed since chromosomes have reasonably unique banding sequences. Therefore, a karyotype constructed from banded chromosomes may show variable banding patterns in two chromosomes that would have been identified as homologous and normal.

Although metaphase analysis is probably the most widely used cytogenetic method, other types of tests have been developed for general screening (11):

Anaphase Analysis

Occasionally chemicals produce effects in chromatin that alter the dispersal of chromosomes in cell division (i.e., chromosome bridges, nonsymmetrical segration, nondisjunction, and so on). Standard metaphase analysis cannot detect segregational damage. The anaphase method scores cells during the anaphase stage of mitosis when chromosomes are separating at the metaphase plate. Anaphase arrest follows the investigation to detect increases in segregational errors or serious effects to the spindle fiber system. This technique is not widely used and requires an experienced cytogeneticist to accurately interpret the findings.

Sister Chromatid Exchange (SCE)

SCE analysis is a cytological technique, but the consequence of the event is not equivalent to a chromosomal aberration. SCE occurs in all normal leukocytic cells and no toxicological damage has been attributed to these events.

Sister chromatid exchange appears to be reciprocal exchange of chromosomal material between sister chromatids (Fig. 8). Because sister chromatids are genotypically identical, there should be no changes in genetic material regardless of the number of exchanges. Therefore, chemicals that induce only SCE cannot *per se* be classified as mutagenic.

TABLE 3

Definitions of Aberrations

Symbol	Definition
tg	Chromatid gap: An achromatic region in one chromatid, the size of which is equal to or smaller than the width of the chromatid
tb	Chromatid break: An achromatic region in one chromatid larger than the width of the chromatid. It may be aligned or unaligned
sq	Chromosome gap: Same as tg only in both chromatids
sb	Chromosome break: Same as tb only in both chromatids
td	Chromatid deletion: Deletion material at the end of one chromatid.
f	Fragment: A single chromatid without an evident centromere
af	Acentric fragment: Two aligned (parallel) chromatids without an evident centromere.
t	Translocation: Obvious transfer of material between two or more chromosomes
tr	Triradial: An abnormal arrangement of paired chromatids resulting in a triarmed configuration
qr	Quadridradial: An abnormal arrangement of paired chromatids resulting in a four-armed configuration
pu	Pulverized chromosome: A spread containing one fragmented or pulverized chromosome
pu+	Pulverized chromosomes: A spread containing two or more fragmented or pulverized chromosomes, but with some intact chromosomes still remaining
puc	Pulverized cell: A cell in which all the chromosomes are totally fragmented
cr	Complex rearrangement: An abnormal translocation figure that involves many chromosomes and is the result of several of breaks and mispairing chromatids
r	Ring: A chromosome that is a result of telomeric deletions at both ends of the chromosome and the subsequent joining of the ends of the two chromosome arms
min	Minute: A small chromosome that contains a centromere and does not belong in the karyotype.
pp	Polyploid: A cell in which the chromosome number is an even multiple of the haploid number, or n, and is greater than $2n$
h	Hyperdiploid: A cell in which the chromosome number is greater than $2n + 1$, but is not an even multiple of n
d	Dicentric: A chromosome containing two centromeres
<	Greater than 10 aberrations: A cell that contains more than 10 aberrations

30

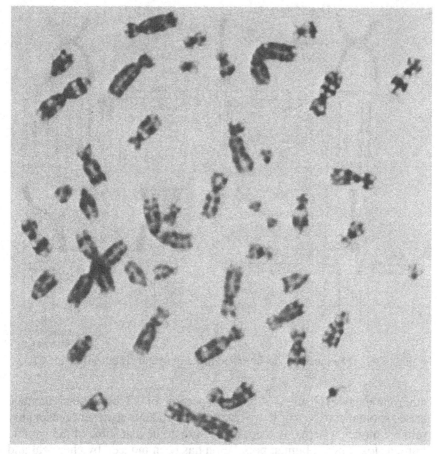

Fig. 7. Banded chromosome.

The precise mechanism of SCE is not known and considerable effort is being expended to relate these events to a biological response such as gene mutation or chromosome breakage. The only relationship that seems to be consistent is a concordance between point mutation induction and SCE induction (7).

Association of Genetic Effects with Human Disease

The present disease burden in humans directly associated with heritable alterations is by most standards substantial. The origin of this burden is not known and it is not possible to assign any specific portion of it to

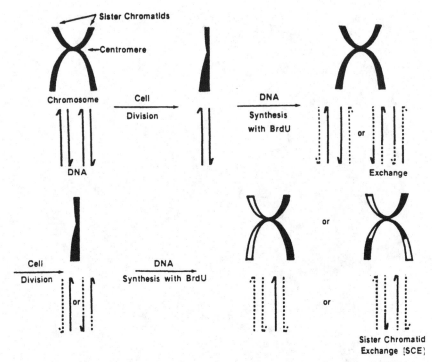

Fig. 8A.   The mechanisms involved in staining and visualization of SCEs.

environmental exposures. A certain portion of all mutational damage arises spontaneously, but if we assume that rodents represent reasonably reliable model systems, it is not difficult to argue that some of the genetic burden (load) in the human population has been induced by chemical and physical mutagens.

In addition to heritable genetic damage, chemicals with mutagenic and/or clastogenic properties are also believed to contribute to the human cancer and birth defect burdens (9, 18). A genotoxic lesion is hypothesized as the irreversible initiating event in malignant cell transformation in chemical carcinogens, and a substantial number of spontaneous abortions, stillbirths, and fetal abnormalities are associated with abnormal chromosome configurations (12).

Types of Mutations Found in Humans

Genetic disease in humans can be categorized according to the type of inheritance patterns emerging from family pedigree analysis:

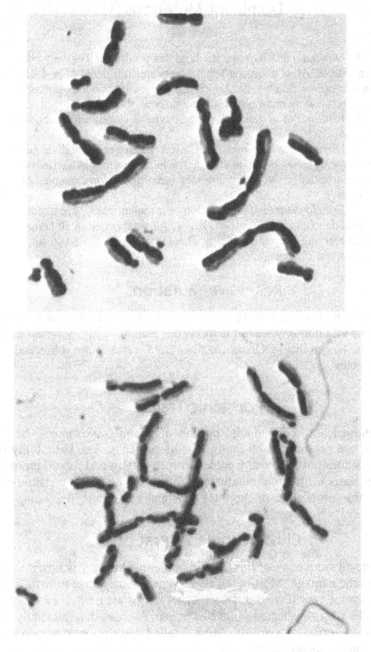

Fig. 8B.   Actual photos of SCEs in cells are shown above. Controls are on the top and treated on the bottom [diagram adapted from Brusick (4)].

Dominant Mutations

1. *Dominant lethal* events are those that result in cell or early embryonic death. Most dominant lethal events are considered to be aberrations or numerical alterations in chromosomes. It has been estimated that approximately one-third of all spontaneous abortions occurring in the first trimester of gestation have some type of chromosomal abnormality (6).

2. *Dominant viable* mutations affect heterozygous individuals (carrying only a single mutant allele). The mutations may be carried on either autosomal or sex chromosomes (see Fig. 9 for examples of heritability).

3. *Semidominant mutations* exhibit the mutant phenotype to only a limited degree in heterozygotes, but are fully expressed in all homozygotes carrying the mutant alleles. These too may be located on autosomes or sex chromosomes.

Recessive Mutations

Recessive mutations are expressed only in individuals carrying the mutant alleles in a homozygous or hemizygous state (see Fig. 9 for an illustration of heritability). Occassionally, mild effects are observed in heterozygotes.

Polygenic Traits

It is believed that a substantial portion of "family-associated" health problems are determined by multiple pairs of genes. The heritability of such traits does not follow any predetermined pattern and formal proof of a genetic basis is often not obtainable. This group of effects constitutes a considerable proportion of the total genetically determined conditions.

Chromosome Alterations

A significant frequency of the genetic burden of humans is observed as chromosome damage. Most of the affected individuals arise from *de novo* changes, since very few chromosomal aberrations are heritable in nature.

Table 4 lists a selected sample of human diseases determined by the mutations described previously. More detailed description of human mutations can be found in ref. (13).

The probability of any single mutation becoming fixed in the human gene pool is very low. For example, a new mutation induced in a sperma-

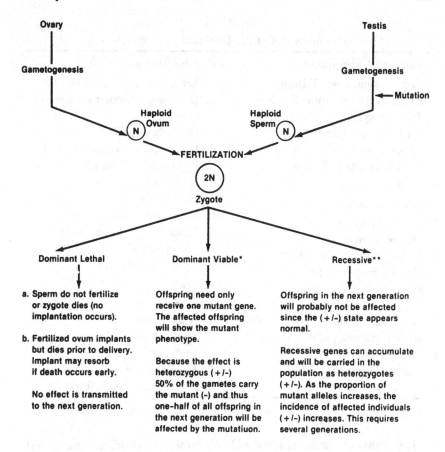

Fig. 9. Consequences of different types of germ cell mutations in mammals.

togonial cell of a man must first be able to pass through the meiotic process; if it survives meiosis, there is still a very small chance that a sperm carrying that specific mutation will be involved in fertilization. If the mutant is involved in fertilization and the embryo proceeds to parturition, the new mutation must still be disseminated into the general gene pool and this process will be influenced by factors involved in subsequent repro-

TABLE 4
Examples of Genetic Disorders in Humans[a]

Chromosomal Abnormalities	Recessive Mutations
1. Down's syndrome (Trisomy 21)	1. *Xeroderma pigmentosum* (AR)
2. Klinefelter's syndrome (XXX)	2. Duchenne muscular dystrophy (XR)
3. Turner's syndrome (XO)	3. Hemophilia (XR)
4. Cri Du Chat (deletion of chromosome)	4. Lesch-Nyhan syndrome (XR)
5. Numerous other trisomies	5. Sickle cell disease (AR)
6. XYY	6. Galactosemia (AR)
	7. PKU (AR)
Dominant Mutations	8. Diabetes mellitus (AR?)
1. Familial polyposis (AD)	9. Fanconi's syndrome (AR)
2. Neurofibromatosis (AD)	10. Albinism (AR)
3. Huntington's chorea (AD)	11. Cystic fibrosis (AR)
4. Hepatic prophyria (AD)	*Polygenic*
5. Crouzon's craniofacial dysostosis (AD)	1. Cleft lip
6. Anchondroplasia dwarfism (AD)	2. Anencephaly
7. Retinoblastoma (AD)	3. Spina bifida
8. Aniridia (AD)	4. Clubfoot
9. Chondrodystrophy (AD)	5. Idiopathic epilepsy
	6. Congenital heart defects

[a]AD, autosomal dominant; AR, autosomal recessive; XR, X-linked recessive.

ductive efforts of the mutant individual (number of children, and so on). Therefore, mutant fixation is a complex process and in the final analysis selective pressures (for or against a new mutant) must also be considered.

However, because of the serious physical, emotional, and financial consequences of increases in human mutational burden, attempts to reduce exposure to environmental mutagens are essential.

Until reliable quantitation of the current genetic load in the human population is calculated, attempts to assess the impact of mutagen exposure directly in human populations will be meaningless. Even if a reliable estimate of the current load existed, extremely large numbers of individuals must be examined to detect significant increases in mutations. For example, a study employing all current methodology for human monitoring would need 25,000 subjects to detect a 50% increase in the mutation rate (*12*).

It has been recommended by human geneticists that a series of steps be taken in order to detect a general increase in human mutation rates:

1. Newborns and spontaneous abortions should be systematically karyotyped.

2. Newborns should be screened for variant proteins that might have resulted from mutations (this would also require examination of both parents).

3. Sentinal dominant mutations in newborns should be registered.

4. Individuals involved in chemical exposures likely to introduce mutations should be carefully monitored as well as all offspring.

References

1. Brown, M. M., Wassom, J. S., Malling, H. V., Shelby, M. D., and Von Halle, E. S., *J. Natl. Cancer Inst.* **62,** 841 (1979).

2. Brusick, D. J., *J. Bacteriol.* **108,** 1134 (1972).

3. Brusick, D. J., Bacterial Mutagenesis and Its Role in Identification of Potential Animal Carcinogens, in *Carcinogens: Identification and Mechanisms of Action,* Griffin, A. C., and Shaw, C. R., eds., Raven Press, New York, pp. 93–105.

4. Brusick, D. J., *Principles of Genetic Toxicology,* Plenum Press, New York, 1980.

5. Brusick, D. J., and Mayer, V. W., *Environ. Health Perspect.* **6,** 83 (1973).

6. Carr, D. H., *Ann. Rev. Genet.* **5,** 65 (1971).

7. Carrano, A. J., Thompson, L. H., Lindl, P. A., and Minkler, J. L., *Nature* **271,** 551 (1978).

8. Chu, E. H. Y., and Powell, S. S., *Adv. Hum. Genet.* **7,** 189 (1976).

9. Magee, P. N., The Relationship Between Mutagenesis, Carcinogenesis and Teratogenesis, in *Progress in Genetic Toxicology,* Scott, D., Bridges, B. A., and Sobels, F. H., eds., Elsevier/North-Holland Biomedical Press, Amsterdam, 1977, pp. 15–27.

10. Beers, R. F., Jr., Harriott, R. M., and Tilghnon, R. C., eds., *Molecular and Cellular Repair Processes,* The Johns Hopkins University Press, Baltimore, Maryland, 1971.

11. *Methods for Chromosome Analysis, Toxicol. Appl. Pharmacol.* **22,** 269 (1972).

12. Monitoring of Human Populations, in *Evaluation of Genetic Risks of Environmental Chemicals,* Ramel, C., ed., Royal Swedish Academy of Sciences, Göteborgs Offsettryckeri AB, Stockhold, Sweden, 1973, pp. 17–21.

13. Novitski, E., *Human Genetics,* Macmillan, New York, 1977.

14. Ong, T. M., *Mutation Res.* **53,** 297 (1978).

15. Russell, L. B., *Arch. Toxicol.* **38,** 75 (1977).

16. Setlow, R. B., *Nature* **271,** 713 (1978).

17. Shaw, M. W., Chromosome Mutations in Man, in *Mutagenic Effects of Environmental Contaminants,* Sutton, H. E., and Harris, M. I., eds., Academic Press, New York, 1972, p. 81.
18. *Testing for Mutagens/Carcinogens,* Butterworth, B. E., ed., CRS Press, West Palm Beach, Florida, 1977, pp. 13–38.
19. Thilly, W. G., and Liber, H. L., A Discussion of Gene Locus Mutation Assays in Bacterial, Rodent, and Human Cells, in *Strategies for Short-Term for Mutagens/Carcinogens,* Butterworth, B. E., ed., CRC Press, West Palm Beach, FL, 1977, pp. 39–54.
20. Vogel, E., The Relationship Between Mutation Pattern and Concentration by Chemical Mutagens in *Drosophila,* in *Screening Tests in Chemical Carcinogenesis,* Montesano, R., Bartsch, H., and Tomatis, L., eds., Lyon (IARC Scientific Publications No. 12), 1976.
21. Watson, J., *Molecular Biology of the Gene,* Benjamin, New York, 1970.

Chapter 4

In Vitro Cell Transformation

An Overview

John O. Rundell

Introduction

Cell transformation assays are presently in wide use in academic, government, and industrial research laboratories and have been applied to studies on the mechanisms of carcinogenesis as well as on the problem of screening chemicals for their carcinogenic potential. The potential importance of these assays, in the context of chemical carcinogen screening, lies in their postulated phenomonological relation to the process of carcinogenesis. Because of this relationship, analyses of the results of certain of these tests may not be wholly dependent upon activity correlations, as are the results of tests that measure the mutagenic, clastogenic, or DNA damaging potentials of test chemicals. Cell transformation assays have been described that measure the chemical induction of malignant properties, and since the acquisition of malignancy is the biological property measured in rodent bioassay, these tests are of particular interest. The purpose, then, of the sections that follow is to describe briefly the development of these tests, to analyze some of the data supporting their relevance to carcinogenesis studies, and to identify those factors that require further development.

39

Test Origins and System Diversity

The initial observations of chemical carcinogen induction of in vitro cell transformation were reported by Earle in 1943 (*28*). Carcinogen-treated C3H mouse fibroblast cultures developed time-related alterations in growth patterns and cellular morphology and, after serial subcultivation, were found to be tumorigenic (i.e., were transplantable into C3H mice). Control (untreated) cells, similarly subcultivated, also developed tumorigenic potential and thus were described as having spontaneously transformed. After a hiatus of nearly 20 yr, Berwald and Sachs, using hamster embryo cells, were able conclusively to demonstrate that carcinogenic hydrocarbons could induce in vitro neoplastic transformation (*10*). Also using cultured Syrian hamster embryo cells, Kuroki and Sato found that treatments with the chemical carcinogen, 4NQO, induced morphological transformation and these transformed cells formed fibrosarcomas upon transplantation into the syngeneic hosts (*42*). In contrast to the findings of Earle (*28*), Berwald and Sachs (*10*) and Kuroki (*42*) did not observe morphological transformation or transplantability among control (untreated) hamster cell cultures. However, tumorigenic Syrian hamster embryo cell lines have been established without known viral involvement or carcinogen treatment, demonstrating that spontaneous transformation of cultured hamster cells can occur (e.g., see ref. *32*). The observations of Berwald and Sachs and Kuroki et al. have been confirmed and extended by DiPaolo (*22*), whose use of Syrian hamster embryo cell cultures in studies of in vitro carcinogenesis have been of major significance to the development of the field (*20–24*).

These studies formed the empirical basis for the currently recognized field of in vitro transformation and were conducted using treatments of mass cultures of mouse fibroblasts or Syrian hamster embryo cells with culture maintenance and serial subcultivation through periods as long as approximately 300 d. The mass culture method has been reported to have been successfully applied to cells derived from Syrian hamster embryos (*15*), rat embryos (*31*), guinea pig embryos (*29*), and a variety of human cells (*40, 45*), among others. However, this method suffers from several disadvantages, including the requirement for serial subcultivation over a timeframe ranging from a few months to nearly a year. In addition, such systems are nonquantitative, and it was this limitation that led to the development of quantitative or semiquantitative assay systems using colony or focus cellular morphology as the measured endpoint. The earliest report of the use of a quantitative endpoint (colony morphology) was published by Huberman and Sachs in 1966 (*35*) and confirmed by DiPaolo in 1969 (*22*). However, though these authors showed that the number of morphologically altered Syrian hamster embryo (SHE) cell colonies increased with increasing concentration of B(a)P, they did not address the question of the connection between altered morphology and malignancy. The correlation between SHE cell morphological and neoplastic transformation was established later by DiPaolo and his coworkers. Using a quantitative SHE cell colony transformation assay, these authors isolated polycyclic hydrocarbon-induced morphological transformants, serially subcultured them to large numbers, and injected them into irradiated or unirradiated newborn hamsters with the result that approximately 50% of the isolates were found to produce progressively growing fibrosarcomas in the transplant hosts (24). The importance of these observations is that they form the basis for the working hypothesis that the process of chemical induction of in vitro morphological transformation of SHE cells represents the first observable stage in the process of malignant transformation.

Support for the conclusion that morphological transformation is related to the process of carcinogenesis has evolved through continuing studies using the SHE-colony assay and the development of two important cell line transformation systems. These two mouse cell assay systems, the Balb/c-3T3 cell assay developed by Kakunaga (39) and the C3H/10T½ cell assay developed in Heidelberger's laboratory (56), have been successfully applied to carcinogen screening studies. Both assay systems exhibit significant technical advantages over the SHE cell-colony assay. Principal among these advantages is that these assays measure the development of foci of transformed cells that are readily distinguishable from a background of normal cells. Thus, the scoring of these assays does not require the considerable technical expertise needed to recognize the morphologically transformed colonies in the SHE-colony assay. In addition, establishment of appropriate test conditions for the Balb/C-3T3 cell and C3H/10T½ cell assays is greatly simplified and less rigorous compared to the SHE-colony assay.

The aforementioned transformation assay systems, employing embryonic cell strains or established cell lines, measure the chemical induction of altered cellular morphologies using either colony or focal transformation as the measured endpoints. Alternative approaches to the use of cellular morphology in the evaluation of chemical induction of cell transformation have been described. These approaches exploit a general in vitro characteristic of cultured tumor cells—the ability to form colonies in soft agar (30). The first of these systems utilized BHK-21 cells and was initially described by di Mayorca in 1973 (19). The BHK-21 assay measures the ability of carcinogen-treated cells to form colonies in soft agar and has been widely used for carcinogen screening in Europe (54, 60).

The use of the anchorage-independent phenotype (growth in soft agar) is of considerable interest and has recently been applied by Colburn for the detection of tumor promoters using mouse epidermal cell lines in vitro (17).

Two additional types of transformation assays have been described: assays measuring chemical–virus interactions and assays using epithelial cells. In the first group, the Syrian hamster embryo cell–simian adenovirus enhancement assay described by Casto (14) and the Fischer rat embryo cell–Rauscher leukemia virus assay described by Freeman et al. (31) have been best characterized. Traul (63) has recently established a similar Rauscher leukemia virus-infected cell line that is also suitable for transformation studies. The basis for these two assays lies in the observation that pretreatments of cells with chemical carcinogens result in enhancements of viral-induced cell transformation. Although the mechanism of chemical enhancement of viral transformation is unknown, it has been postulated that carcinogen activity in these assays may be virus-directed or related to chemical induction of an increase in the number of host cell DNA viral genome attachment sites (see ref. 16).

The several cell transformation assay systems described thus far all utilize fibroblast or fibroblast-like target cell populations. In the case of studies involving SHE, Balb/C-3T3, or C3H/10T½ cells, transplantations of chemically induced transformants into syngeneic hosts or athymic mice have generally resulted in the formation of poorly differentiated firbrosarcomas (23, 39, 56). From a teleological point of view, this is a problem, because the majority of in situ human and rodent tumors are carcinomas rather than sarcomas. For this reason, in vitro transformation assays using fibroblastic target cells have been criticized as possibly irrelevant in relation to the predominant tumor form. Accordingly, several workers have investigated malignant transformation systems utilizing differentiated (epithelial) target cells. Among the target cells utilized were those derived from mouse and hamster dermal or epidermal cells (18, 61). In general, however, morphological alterations were not observed in these studies, and transformation was evaluated by transplantations of the cells into appropriate hosts or by assay for the anchorage-independent phenotype among the progeny of the carcinogen-treated populations (17, 18). Systems such as these, using epithelial-like cell strains, may provide important new tools for studies of the mechanisms of carcinogenesis, but their present usefulness for routine screening is limited by their nonquantitative nature.

Nearly 40 yr have now elapsed since Earle's original observations on cellular transformation. Over this time period, a variety of transformation assay systems have been described and new approaches (e.g., epithelial cell transformation) are still being developed. The field of in vitro transformation is, then, an emergent one, so there is currently no consensus of opinion on an ideal system for use in routine screening. Nevertheless, from among the many assay systems described, only a few are in general use for mechanistic studies as well as for the screening for carcinogens. In the United States, these assay systems are the Balb/c-3T3, the C3H/10T½, and the Syrian hamster embryo (SHE) cell transformation assays. Several factors have contributed to the application of these tests in lieu of the available spectrum of systems. These factors, which are briefly analyzed in the following chapters, include demonstrations of their relevance to studies of the mechanisms of carcinogenesis, their technical feasibility, their sensitivity, and their predictive accuracy.

The Transformed Morphology

Most in vitro cell transformation assays measure the appearance of morphologically altered cells. These altered morphologies are recognized in relation to a normal phenotype(s) that is typical of the target cell population used. In general, recognition of the transformed phenotype(s) is relatively unambiguous for assay systems using established cell lines (e.g., Balb/c-3T3 and C3H/10T½ c18 cells), but is technically more difficult in assays using embryonic cell strains (e.g., SHE cells). The basis for this difference lies in the morphological uniformity of the cloned cell lines vs the marked heterogeneity of morphologies typical of cell strains derived from whole embryos. Balb/c-3T3 and C3H/10T½ cells exhibit distinct morphologies, but each is nonetheless characterized by marked morphological uniformity. In contrast, SHE cell populations exhibit a variety of cellular morphologies representative of the complexity of the embryos from which they were derived. The range of the morphological alterations arising as a consequence of chemical treatments of these target cell types is, in part, a reflection of the morphological characteristics observed in the untreated cell populations. Accordingly, evaluations of the transformed phenotype in the relatively homogeneous murine cell line assays using Balb/c-3T3 or C3H/10½ cells are straightforward in comparison to analyses of transformation in heterogeneous SHE cell populations, and this consideration has been of major importance in the application of these target cell types in carcinogen screening assays.

An important operational difference also distinguishes the Balb/c-3T3 and C3H/10T½ transformation assays from the SHE cell system. The Balb/c-3T3 and the C3H/10T½ assays, as normally conducted, utilize a focal transformation endpoint (*39, 56*), whereas the SHE assay measures the appearance of morphologically transformed colonies (22). A focus assay has been described for the SHE cell assay (15), and a colony assay has been described for Balb/c-3T3 cells (25), but since these modifications have not been widely employed, the present discussion will consider only the SHE colony assays originally described by DiPaolo (15, see also 48–50) and the Balb/c-3T3 focus assay developed by Kakanaga (39). The conduct of focal transformation assays, whether using Balb/c-3T3 or C3H/10T½ cells, involves test chemical treatments of cultured target cells plated and maintained as mass cultures. Discrete cell colonies are not observed in assays using these cells. Instead, a monolayer of contact-inhibited cells develops and morphological transformants are recognized as foci of altered cells superimposed upon this normal-appearing monolayer. In contrast, SHE cell transformation assays are conducted so that discrete cell colonies develop, i.e., SHE target cells are plated at low densities so that mass cultures, consisting of cellular monolayers, do not develop. Recognition of the transformed phenotype in SHE cell assays is then dependent upon evaluations of each surviving colony. Accordingly, preliminary scoring of the Balb/c-3T3 and C3H/10T½ assays can be rapidly accomplished by macroscopic examination of the stained culture dishes, whereas analysis of the SHE assay is greatly more labor intensive.

Although the assay designs just described for the Balb/c-3T3, C3H/10T½, and SHE cell transformation assays differ, the scored phenotypes are remarkably similar. The morphological criteria described by Kakunaga for Balb/c-3T3 cells (39), by Reznikoff et al. for C3H/10T½ cells (56), and by DiPaolo (22) and Pienta (49, 50) for SHE cells contain certain important common features. In essence, the morphologically transformed phenotype is characterized by release from contact inhibition (density-dependent inhibition of cellular growth) and loss of cellular order (disorientation). For transformed foci of Balb/c-3T3 cells, two principal morphological types have been described (39). These were transformed cellular foci of fibroblastic or epithelial-like morphologies exhibiting evidence of random orientation (crisscrossing) characterized by the overlapping of cell processes and the nuclei of adjacent cells or sublayers of cells (loss of contact inhibition). These characteristics of transformed foci of Balb/c-3T3 cells are illustrated in Fig. 1A. The focal transformed morphologies described for C3H/10T½ cells were quite similar except that three principal morphologies were observed (56). These included foci of condensed or closely packed cells (Type 1), foci exhibiting pronounced piling up but little evidence of disorientation (Type II), and foci consisting of multilayered, highly disoriented polar fibroblastic cells (Type III). A representative C3H/10T½ cell focus is illustrated in

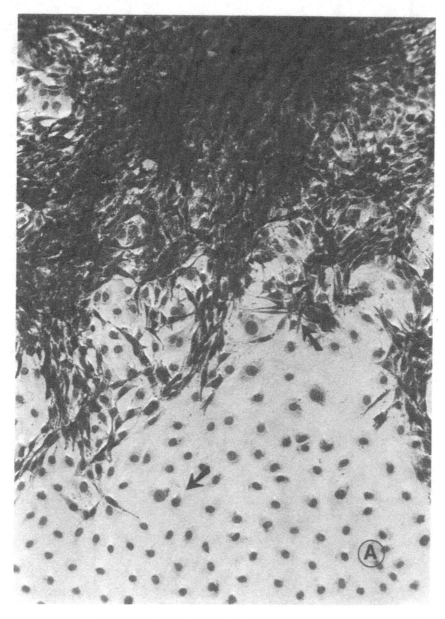

Fig. 1A. Photomicrographs showing cellular organization at the periphery of transformed foci of Balb/c-3T3 and C3H/10T½ Cl 8 cells and transformed and normal SHE cell colonies: a Balb/c-3T3 transformed focus showing an area of the normal monolayer (lower arrow) and evidence of extensive cellular disorientation and piling up at the focus edge (upper arrow and superior area).

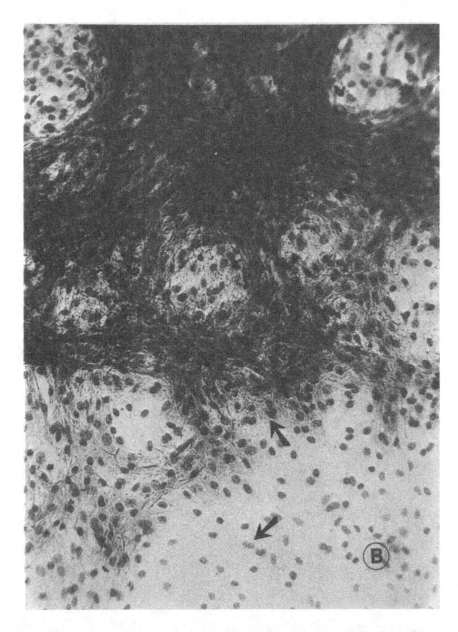

Fig. 1B. Photomicrograph of a typical C3H/10T½ Cl 8 focus (Type II) showing the continguous monolayer of normal cells and an aspect of the multilayered and densely stained focus (upper area and superior area).

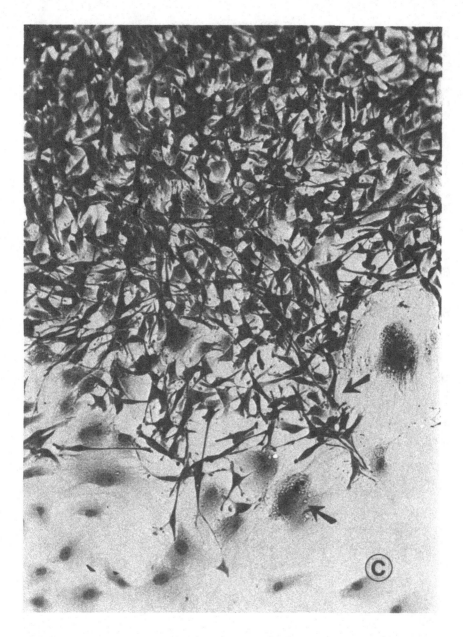

Fig. 1C. Photomicrograph showing an aspect of the edge of a transformed SHE cell colony. The lower arrow identifies an irradiated SHE feeder cell. The area adjacent to and superior to the upper arrow shows the abundant criss-crossing and cellular disorientation typical of the SHE cell transformed phenotype.

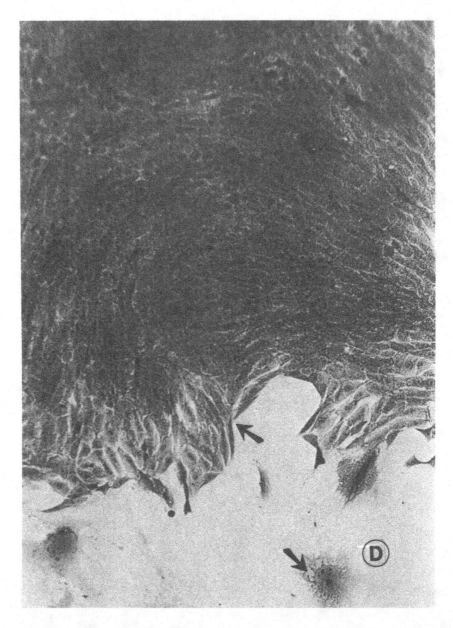

Fig. 1D.   An edge detail of a normal SHE cell colony. Note the irradiated
feeder cell (lower arrow), and the highly ordered cells exhibiting a swirled pattern at and above the upper arrow.

Fig. 1B. Transformed SHE cell colonies exhibit morphological qualities that are quite similar to those described for Balb/c-3T3 and Type III C3H/10T½ cl 8 foci. These colonies are characterized by random cellular orientation at or near the edge of the colony (*21, 22, 24, 50*). A typical fibroblast-like transformed SHE cell colony is shown in Fig. 1C, which may be contrasted with the normal colony depicted in Fig. 1D.

These descriptions and illustrations are not intended to definitively identify the several kinds of transformed phenotypes, but they will nonetheless serve to emphasize the fact that the altered morphologies scored in Balb/c-3T3, C3H/10T½, and SHE cell transformation assays share the central features of uncontrolled growth and loss of cellular orientation. These characteristics have also been observed in cultured tumor cells, but are not characteristic of cultured cell populations derived from normal tissues. The significance of this observation is that the in vitro induction of morphologically altered cells has an in vivo corrollary, which supports the idea that there are mechanistic similarities between *in situ* tumorigenesis and in vitro cell transformation.

The Relation Between In Vitro Transformed Morphology and Cellular Malignancy

Additional support for the concept that in vitro cell transformation and in vivo carcinogenesis are allied processes has been obtained through the conduct of transplantation and agar growth experiments. Similar experiments have been conducted using morphological transformants isolated from carcinogen-treated Balb/c-3T3, C3H/10T½, and SHE cell populations. In each case, the isolated transformants were identified by phase-contrast microscopy in assays employing the same designs as those conducted for evaluations using stained preparations. In general, isolations were performed by use of cloning cylinders (*53*) or by scraping away the colonies or foci (*13*), and the transformed cells thus obtained were cultured until the cell populations expanded sufficiently for the testing of their expression of the secondary phenotype. Representative data describing the relationships between morphological transformation, anchorage independence, and malignant phenotypes for Balb/c-3T3, C3H/10T½, and SHE cells are summarized in Table 1.

The number of cell generations that elapsed between tranformant isolation and the testing for the expression of the anchorage independent and tumorigenic phenotypes was generally not determined, but several important conclusions can still be formulated from the data summarized

TABLE 1

Summary of Data Describing the Relationship Between Morphological Transformation and the Acquisition of Malignant Properties among Transformed Balb/C-3T3, C3H/10T½, and Syrian Hamster Embryo Cells Isolated from In Vitro Transformation Assays

Target cell	Clone	Total No. of isolated morphological transformants tested	ar^+ Incidence[a]	Transplantability incidence[b]	Phenotypic coincidence[c]	Author (ref.)
Balb/c-3T3	A31-714	13	0.75	0.88	0.77	Kakunaga (39)
	A31-113	7	1.0	0.29	0.29	Sivak (58)
	A31-113 (c14)	26	0.91	(0.88)	0.89	Rundell et al. (57)
	A31 (recloned)	23	NT[a]	0.10–0.50 (0.50–1.0)	NA[c]	DiPaolo et al. (25)
	A31 (recloned)	6	0.83	0.60	0.75	Quarles and Tennant (55)
C3H/10T½	C1 8[f]	12	NT	0.67	NA	Reznikoff et al. (56)
		5	NT	0.60	NA	Jones et al. (37)
		21	0.71	NT	NA	Bertram (8)
		7	NT	1.0	NA	Benedict (6)

50

4	NT	1.0	NA	Terzaghi and Little (62)
4	1.0	1.0	1.0	Jones et al. (38)
SHE	N/A			
8	NT	0.86	NA	DiPaolo (21)
6	1.0	1.0	1.0	Borek (11)
5	NT	1.0	NA	Doniger et al. (26)
9[g]	NT	1.0	NA	Pienta et al. (50)

[a] Calculated as the ratio of morphologically transformed isolate–derived cell populations exhibiting the ability to grow in soft agar to the total number of isolate populations tested. See references cited for the experimental conditions and criteria used to determine the ar^+ phenotype.

[b] The ratio of the number of isolates forming tumors after injection into host animals to the total number of isolates tested. Experimental conditions, host species and inoculum sizes are given in the cited references. Values were for transplantation experiments using unirradiated animals. Tumor incidence in irradiated animals are given in parentheses.

[c] The phenotypic coincidence was calculated as the proportion of morphologically transformed isolates tested that expressed both the ar^+ and tumorigenic phenotypes.

[d] NT = not tested.

[e] NA = not applicable (both phenotypes were not tested).

[f] Pooled date from studies of Type III and Type II foci.

[g] Isolates were obtained from colony assay cultures containing one or more transformed colonies.

in Table 1. The first of these conclusions is that the majority of the morphologically transformed isolates also expressed the anchorage independence phenotype. This latter phenotype has been shown by several investigators (e.g., see ref. *30*), to be highly correlated with malignancy and, therefore, its expression by in vitro transformants is consistent with the postulated relation between the in vitro and the in vivo observations cited earlier. The transplantation data shown in Table 1 also supports this relationship. In fact, most of the studies reported in this summary showed excellent correlation between the scored transformants and the acquisition of malignancy. Transplantation incidences ranging from 10% (0.10) for a Balb/c-3T3 A31 experiment using unirradiated host animals (*25*) to 100% (1.0) for several experiments using Balb/c-3T3 (*25*), C3H/10T½ (*6, 38, 62,*) and SHE (*26, 50, 62,*) tranformants have been reported. Another important point to be made from these data is that when the incidences of the anchorage independence and tumorigenic phenotypes were compared, these phenotypes were highly coincident with the scored morphologies. Thus, phenotypic coincidences of 1.0 were obtained by Jones et al. for four transformed C3H/10T½ isolates (*38*) and by Borek for six SHE cell morphological transformants (*50*), whereas a mean concidence of 0.68 was found for the 52 Balb/c-3T3 isolates reported in Table 1. These data support the relevance of the Balb/c-3T3, C3H/10T½, and SHE cell transformation assays to studies of chemical carcinogenic potential; that is, a significant proportion of the scored endpoints of these in vitro cell transformation assays were malignantly transformed cells. One may conclude from these results that such assay systems measure a process that is in fact allied to the process of carcinogenesis *per se*.

The Response Charactertistics of Balb/c-3T3, C3H/10T½, and SHE Cells Toward Chemical Carcinogen Treatment

Another line of evidence bearing on questions of the usefulness of cell transformation assays in the process of carcinogen screening can be derived from an analysis of the responses of Balb/c-3T3, C3H/10T½, and SHE cells toward treatments with known carcinogens and noncarcinogens. Such an analysis is shown in Table 2. These data were compiled from the published results of studies using protocols similar in design to those described elsewhere in this volume (Chapters 19 and 20 for Balb/c-3T3 and C3H/10T½ and Chapter 21 for SHE cells). The qualitative analyses listed were those of the cited authors. Approximately 55 chemicals have been tested in Balb/c-3T3 cells; more than 150 have been

TABLE 2

Summary of Transformation Assay Results for Chemicals Tested in the Balb/C-3T3, C3H/10T½, and SHE-Cell Transformation Assays

Chemical[a]	In vivo carcino-genicity[b]	Balb/c-3T3			C3H/10T½			SHE		
		Dose[c]	Activity	Ref.	Dose[c]	Activity	Ref.	Dose[e]	Activity	Ref.
AAAF	U	0.02	+	Sivak et al. (58)	~6.8	+	Landolph (44)	10.0	+	Pienta et al. (48)
		2.0	+	Rundell et al. (57)				4.0	+	Huberman et al. (33)
ARA-C	U	0.08	+	Rundell et al. (57)	~0.24	+	Jones et al. (59)	~0.024[d]	+	Kouri et al. (41)
B(a)P	R, M	12.0	+	Rundell et al. (57)	0.25	+	Mondal et al. (46)	5.0	+	DiPaolo et al. (41)
		5.0	+	Dunkel et al. (27)				10.0	+	Barrett et al. (20)
		10.0	+	Kakunaga (39)				20.0	+	Dunkel (27)
CP	R, M	2.600	+	Rundell et al. (57)	500.0	−	Benedict et al. (4,5)	50.0	±	Dunkel et al. (27)

(continued)

53

TABLE 2 (continued)

Chemical[a]	In vivo carcino-genicity[b]	Balb/c-3T3 Dose[c]	Activity	Ref.	C3H/10T½ Dose[c]	Activity	Ref.	SHE Dose[e]	Activity	Ref.
DBA	R, M	100	−	Dunkel et al. (27)	40.0	+	Reznikoff et al. (56)	10.0	+	DiPaolo et al. (22)
		300.0	+	Rundell et al. (57)				15.0	+	Pienta et al. (48)
		0.5	+	Sivak et al. (58)						
DMBA	0	0.02	+	Dunkel et al. (27)	3.0	+	Reznikoff et al. (56)	5.0	+	Huberman et al. (33)
		0.25	+	Rundell et al. (57)	0.25	+	Mondal et al. (46)	0.1	+	Dunkel et al. (27)
3-MCA	U	10.0	+	Kukunga (39)	37.0	+	Nesnow (47)	1.0	+	Dunkel et al. (27)
		100.0	+	Dunkel et al. (27)	5.0	+	Bertram (8)	7.5	+	Huberman et al. (33)

Agent	Species[b]	Dose		Reference	Dose		Reference	Dose		Reference
MNNG	R, M	40.0	+	Reznikoff et al. (56)	40.0	+	Reznikoff et al. (56)	5.0	+	Rundell et al. (57)
		1.0	+	Dunkel et al. (27)	1.0	+	Mondal et al. (46)	1.0	+	Rundell et al. (57)
		0.5	+	DiPaolo et al. (20)	2.0	+	Reznikoff et al. (56)	0.5	+	Dunkel et al. (27)
					4.0	+	Bertram (9)	4.0	−	Rundell et al. (57)
TPA	U	0.1	−	Dunkel et al. (27)	0.1	−	Mondal et al. (47)	0.01	−	Sivak et al. (58)

[a]The abbreviations used are acetoxy-2-acetylaminofluorene (AAAF), cytosine arabinoside (ARA-C), benzo(a)pyrene (B(a)P), cyclophosphamide (CP), dibenz(a,h)anthracene (DBA), 7,12-dimethylbenzanthracene (DMBA), 3-methylcholanthrene (3-MCA), N-methyl-N'-nitro-N-nitrosoguanidine (MNNG), and 12-O-tetradecanoyl-phorbol-13-acetate (TPA).

[b]Carcinogenicity data taken from IARC, NCI/NTP, or OSHA analyses; R, rat; M, Mouse; O, OSHA candidate carcinogen; U, unevaluated.

[c]Doses given in μg/mL. Doses listed were those giving the maximum observed response (positives) or the maximum tested dose (negatives).

[d]Lowest transf rming dose.

evaluated in the SHE cell assay and about 33 have been applied to the C3H/10T½ assay (see ref. *34*). The nine chemicals listed in Table 2 are those for which data has been published for all three transformation assays and therefore these are the available data from which direct chemical activity comparisons can be made. In a qualitative sense, the results summarized in Table 2 show good agreement among the three assay systems. Thus, "positive" assay results were obtained by all three assay systems for AAAF, Ara-C, B(a)P, CP, DBA, DMBA, 3-MCA, and MNNG (see footnote to Table 2 for abbreviations used). Each of these chemicals is a known or presumptive carcinogen and each has been found to be active in other short-term in vitro tests. None of the three assay systems were responsive to TPA, an in vivo tumor promoter (1) for which consistent in vitro activity in other test systems has not been found. Evidence for activity for TPA has, however, been described under conditions of chronic treatment using Balb/c-3T3 cells (*59*) and observations of in vitro enhancement of transformation by TPA have been published for C3H/10T½ (*46*) and SHE cells (*52*). The potential importance of TPA activity in these assays will be discussed later.

Problem Areas and Developmental Considerations

The data and observations described in the preceding sections are representative of the results available for an assessment of the state of the art of Balb/c-3T3, C3H/10T½, and SHE cell transformation assays. The results show that all three transformation assays exhibit a number of qualities that are of intrinsic interest as well as of practical interest in relation to chemical carcinogen screening. Perhaps the most significant of these qualities is the expression by morphologically transformed cells of secondary phenotypes that are associated with in vivo carcinogenesis. Thus, as shown in Table 1, a significant proportion of morphologically transformed cells isolated from in vitro transformation assays exhibited either the ability to grow in soft agar or were transplantable. These secondary phenotypes were often found to be co-expressed, which supports the idea that in vitro phenomenon of morphological transformation and the in vivo phenomenon of carcinogenesis are related. Additional studies are required for the purpose of systematically studying the relationship between the several morphologies observed and the expression of the secondary phenotypes. The latter is possibly of special importance in view of the work of Ts'o and his colleagues (*2*, *3*), which suggests that SHE cells may acquire malignant properties sequentially over a significant number of population doublings. No evidence bearing on this possibility was reported by the authors cited in Table 1. Furthermore, no systematic studies of the relation of the heterogeneity of the morphological transformed phenotypes observed for SHE cells and any secondary phenotype have been reported.

As was shown in Table 2, each of the assays presently under consideration responded to treatments with a limited set of carcinogens. In other words, within the constraints of the sample size, the Balb/c-3T3, C3H/10T½, and SHE cell transformation assays were found to be sensitive to treatments with the same kinds of chemicals that are of interest in carcinogen screening. This is, of course, a prerequisite to the use of any short-term test in carcinogen screening. However, the significance of the high degree of the activity correlations shown in Table 2 is unclear because the materials tested were, on the whole, archetypical mutagens and carcinogens. Also, very few chemicals generally accepted as being noncarcinogens have been tested in all three systems (TPA may be the only example) and thus little data bearing on the question of assay accuracy has been collected. Clearly, additional comparative data regarding both the sensitivity and the accuracy of these three assay systems needs to be collected before their relative predictive powers can be fairly calculated. Problems in addition to those cited above remain, including those associated with provision for an exogenous metabolic activation system for these assays. In this regard, only a handful of observations have been published (e.g., see refs. 8 and 51) and none of these have been of general usefulness in the context of activation system development because the authors of these studies did not address questions of system optimization (i.e., the effects of the operant variables were not analyzed). Several laboratories, including ours, have been actively investigating the problems associated with the use of both microsomal enzyme and cell-mediated activation systems in cell transformation assays. The experimental emphasis in our laboratory has been toward the development of a cell-mediated activation system for the Balb/c-3T3 cell transformation assay. Using rat liver cells co-cultivated with Balb/c-3T3 1-13, C-14 cells, we have found evidence for activation of nitrosamines and the alkylating procarcinogen, cyclophosphamide. In this context, reports of the use of cell-mediated activation systems in mammalian cell mutagenesis assays have been published (e.g., see refs. 36 and 43) and arguments for the development of cell-mediated rather than microsomal enzyme-mediated exogenous activation systems have been formulated (43).

One final point bearing on the question of the usefulness of the Balb/c-3T3, C3H/10T½, and SHE assays should be made. Currently, the dominant hypothesis on the mechanism of carcinogenesis has somatic cell mutagenesis as its central theme. The process(es) of carcinogenesis is thought to be initiated by a heritable change in target cell DNA as a result of exposure to a mutagen. This mutational event may not, however, always lead directly to *in situ* transformation to malignancy. The progression to malignancy of these altered (mutated) cells may require one or more additional steps and these requirements may be met by exposures to promoting substances such as croton oil or its purified derivatives. These ideas have been codified as the initiation–promotion hypothesis of tumorigenesis and are supported by several important in vivo observations such as those reported by Berenblum et al. (7) and others (1, 12). Since tumor promoters such as TPA are not known to be mutagens their effects are thought to be a result of their epigenetic activities. The importance of this process is that tumor promoters, which may constitute a significant public health concern, are undetected by screening assays measuring point mutations, clastogenicity, or direct DNA damage. Reports of initiation–promotion studies using classic mutagens such as MNNG and well-characterized promoters such as TPA have been published for Balb/c-3T3 (59), C3H/10T½ (46), and SHE (52) cells. These observations have obvious implications for carcinogen screening, but considerable additional work remains to be done before it can be concluded that a cell transformation assay for tumor promoters is feasible.

Summary and Conclusions

The results described in this chapter show that the Balb/c-3T3, C3H/10T½, and SHE cell transformation asssay systems share several important features. Among these are their expression of similar primary as well as secondary transformed phenotypes and their qualitatively similar responses to treatments with a variety of chemical carcinogens. As was previously shown, the morphologically transformed phenotype exhibited by carcinogen-treated Balb/c-3T3, C3H/10T½, and SHE cells was characterized by evidence of cellular disorientation and loss of growth control (see Fig. 1). Accordingly, each of these three transformation assay systems are scored using criteria that are remarkably similar at the level of cellular focal or colonial morphology. The biological relevance of morphological transformation is that cells exhibiting these altered morphologies also exhibit secondary phenotypes that are characteristic of those expressed by cells isolated from *in situ* rodent and human tumors. In other words, as was shown in Table 1, morphologically transformed Balb/c-3T3, C3H/10T½, and SHE cells may co-express the anchorage independence and tumorigenic phenotypes (i.e., they grow in soft agar and are transplantable into appropriate hosts) and these qualities are also expressed by cells cultured from malignant tumor masses. This strongly suggests that in vitro cell transformation of Balb/c-3T3, C3H/10T½, and SHE cells occurs by a mechanism(s) that is closely allied to the cellular events leading to *in situ* carcinogenesis.

The fact that morphologically transformed Balb/c-3T3, C3H/10T½, and SHE cells are malignant and that these phenotypes can be induced in vitro by treatments with chemical carcinogens supports the usage of these cells in research into the mechanism(s) of carcinogenesis as well as for the use of screening of chemicals for carcinogenic potential. However, the use of the these transformation assay systems for screening is additionally dependent upon the accuracy of in vivo rodent carcinogenicity studies in order to assess the predictability of in vitro cell transformation studies. Though the data base is small, the results summarized in Table 2 show that Balb/c-3T3, C3H/10T½, and SHE cells are morphologically transformed by chemical carcinogens, but not by noncarcinogens; i.e., the assays accurately predicted chemical carcinogenic potential. This observation, coupled with the aforementioned data bearing on the issue of biological relevance, supports the contention that these assays, if properly designed, conducted, and evaluated, should be powerful and useful predictors of chemical carcinogenic potential.

References

1. Baird, W. M., and Boutwell, R. K., *Cancer Res.* **31,** 1074 (1971).
2. Barrett, J. C., Crawford, B. D., Grady, L. D., Hester, P. A., Jones, P. A., Benedict, W. F., and Ts'o, P .O. P., *Cancer Res.* **37,** 3815 (1977).
3. Barrett, J. C., and Ts'o, P. O. P., *Proc. Natl. Acad. Sci. USA,* **75,** 3751 (1978).
4. Benedict, W. F., Banerjee, A., Gardner, A., and Jones, P. A., *Cancer Res.* **37,** 2202 (1977).
5. Benedict, W. F., Banerjee, A., and VenKatesan, N., *Cancer Res.* **38,** 2922 (1978).
6. Benedict, W. F., Rucker, N., Faust, J., and Kouri, R. E., *Cancer Res.* **35,** 857 (1975).
7. Berenblum, I., *Cancer Res.* **14,** 471 (1954).
8. Bertram, J. S., *Cancer Res.* **37,** 514 (1977).
9. Bertram, J. S., and Heidelberge, C., *Cancer Res.* **34,** 526 (1974).
10. Berwald, Y., and Sachs, L., *J. Natl. Cancer Inst.* **35,** 641 (1965).
11. Borek, C., Hall, J. E., and Rossi, H. H., *Cancer Res.* **38,** 2997 (1978).

12. Boutwell, R. K., *Critical Rev. Toxicol.* **2,** 419 (1974).
13. Cahn, R. D., Coon, H. G., and Cahn, M. B., Cell culture and cloning techniques, in: *Methods in Developmental Biology,* Wilt, F. H., and Wessels, N. K., eds., Crowell, New York, 1967.
14. Casto, B. C., *J. Virol.* **3,** 513 (1969).
15. Casto, B. C., Janosko, N., and DiPaolo, J. A., *Cancer Res.* **37,** 3508 (1977).
16. Casto, B. C., and DiPaolo, J. A., *Progr. Med. Virol.* **16,** 1 (1973).
17. Colburn, N. H., Koehler, B. A., and Nelson, K. J., *Terato. Carcino. Mutagen,* **1,** 87 (1980).
18. Colburn, N. H., Vorder Bruegge, W. F., Bates, J., and Yuspa, S. H., Epidermal Cell Transformation In Vitro, in *Carcinogenesis,* Vol. 2, *Mechanisms of Tumor Promotion and Cocarcinogenesis,* Slaga, T. J., et al., eds., Raven Press, New York, 1978, pp. 257–271.
19. di Mayorca, G., Greenblatt, M., Trauthen, T., Soller, A., and Giordano, R., *Proc. Natl. Acad. Sci. USA* **70,** 46 (1973).
20. DiPaolo, J. A.: *J. Natl. Cancer Inst.* **64,** 1485 (1980).
21. DiPaolo, J. A., and Donovan, P. J., *Exptl. Cell Res.* **48,** 361 (1967).
22. DiPaolo, J. A., Donovan, P. J., and Nelson, R. L., *J. Natl. Cancer Inst.* **42** 867 (1969).
23. DiPaolo, J. A., Nelson, R. L., and Donovan, P. J., *Science* **165,** 917 (1969).
24. DiPaolo, J. A., Nelson, R. L., and Donovan, P. J., *Cancer Res.* **31,** 1118 (1971).
25. DiPaolo, J. A., Takano, K., and Popescu, N. C., *Cancer Res.* **32,** 2686 (1972).
26. Doniger, J., and DiPaolo, J. A., *Cancer Res.* **40,** 582 (1980).
27. Dunkel, V. C., Pienta, R. J., Sivak, A., and Traul, K. A., *J. Natl. Cancer Inst.* **67,** 1303 (1981).
28. Earle, W. R., and Nettleship, A., *J. Natl. Cancer Inst.* **4,** 213 (1943).
29. Evans, C. H., and DiPaolo, J. A., *Cancer Res.* **35,** 1035 (1975).
30. Freedman, V. H., and Shin, S., *Cell* **3,** 355 (1974).
31. Freeman, A. E., Price, P. J., Igel, H. J., Young, T. C., Maryak, J. M., and Huebner, R. J., *J. Natl. Cancer Inst.* **44,** 65 (1970).
32. Gotlieb-Stematsky, T., Yaniv, A., and Gosith, A., *J. Natl. Cancer Inst.* **36,** 477 (1966).
33. Huberman, E., Donovan, P. J., and DiPaolo, J. A., *J. Natl. Cancer Inst.* **48,** 837 (1972).
34. Heidelberger, C., Freeman, A. E., Pienta, R. J., Sivak, A., Bertram, J. S., Casto, B. C., Dunkel, V. C., Francis, M. W., Kakunaga, T., Little, J. B., and Schechtman, L. M., *Mutat. Res.* in press, 1982.
35. Huberman, E., and Sachs, L., *Proc. Natl. Acad. Sci. USA* **56,** 1123 (1966).
36. Jones, C. A., and Huberman, E., *Cancer Res.* **40,** 406 (1980).
37. Jones, P. A., Benedict, W. F., Baker, M. S., Mondal, S., Rapp, U., and Heidelberg, C., *Cancer Res.* **36,** 101 (1976).

38. Jones, P. A., Long, W. E., Gardner, A., Nye, C. A., Fink, L. M., and Benedict, W. F., *Cancer Res.* **36,** 2863 (1976).
39. Kakunaga, T., *Intl. J. Cancer* **12,** 463 (1973).
40. Kakunaga, T., *Proc. Natl. Acad. Sci. USA* **75,** 1334 (1978).
41. Kouri, R. E., Jurtz, S. A., Price, P. J., and Benedict, W. F., *Cancer Res.* **35,** 2413 (1975).
42. Kuroki, T., and Sato, H., *J. Natl. Cancer Inst.* **41,** 53 (1968).
43. Langenbach, R., Freed, H. J., and Huberman, E., *Proc. Natl. Acad. Sci. USA* **75,** 2864 (1978).
44. Landolph, J. R., and Heidelberger, C., *Proc. Natl. Acad. Sci. USA* **76,** 930 (1979).
45. Milo, G. E., and DiPaolo, J. A., *Nature* **275,** 130 (1978).
46. Mondal, S., Brandow, D. W., and Heidelberger, C., *Cancer Res.* **36,** 2254 (1976).
47. Nesnow, S., and Heidelberger, C., *Cancer Res.* **36,** 1801 (1976).
48. Pienta, R. J., A Transformation Bioassay Employing Cryopreserved Hamster Embryo Cells, in *Advances in Modern Environmental Toxicology,* Vol. 1, *Mammalian Cell Transformation by Chemical Carcinogens,* Mishra, N., Dunkel, V., Mehlman, M., eds., Senate Press, NJ, 1981.
49. Pienta, R. J., Lebherz, W. B., III, and Schuman, R. F., The Use of Cryopreserved Syrian Hamster Embryo in a Transformation Test for Detecting Chemical Carcinogens, in *Short-Term Tests for Chemical Carcinogens,* Stich, H., San, R. H. S., eds., Springer-Verlag, NY, 1981.
50. Pienta, R. J., Poiley, J. A., and Lebherz, W. B., III, *Int. J. Cancer* **19,** 642 (1977).
51. Poiley, J. A., Raineri, R., and Pienta, R. J., *J. Natl. Cancer Inst.* **63,** 519 (1979).
52. Popescu, N. C., Amsbaugh, S. C., and DiPaolo, J. A., *Proc. Natl. Acad. Sci USA* **77,** 7282 (1980).
53. Puck, T. T., Marcus, P. I., and Cieciura, S. J., *J. Exptl. Med.* **103,** 273 (1956).
54. Purchase, I. H., Longstaff, E., Ashby, J., Styles, J. A., Andeson, D., Lefevre, P. A., and Westwood, F. R., *Nature* **264,** 624 (1976).
55. Quarles, J. M., and Tennant, R. W., *Cancer Res.* **35,** 2637 (1975).
56. Reznikoff, C. A., Bertram, J. S., Brankow, D. W., and Heidelberger, C., *Cancer Res.* **33,** 3239 (1973).
57. Rundell, J. O., Guntakatta, M., and Matthews, E. J., Criterion Development for the Application of Balb/c-3T3 Cells to Routine Testing for Chemical Carcinogenic Potential, in *Third Symposium on the Application of Short-Term Bioassays in the Analysis of Complex Environmental Mixtures, Proceedings,* Waters, M. D., et al., eds., Plenum, New York, in press, 1982.
58. Sivak, A., Charest, M. C., Rodenko, L., Silveira, D. M., Simons, I., and Wood, A. M., Balb/C-3T3 Cells as Target Cells for Chemically Induced Neoplastic Transformation, in *Advances in Modern Environmental Toxicol-*

ogy, Vol. I, *Mammalian Cell Transformation by Chemical Carcinogens* Mishra, N., et al., eds., Senate Press, Princeton Junction, NJ, 1980, pp. 133–180.

59. Sivak, A., and Tu, A. S., *Cancer Lett.* **10,** 27 (1980).
60. Styles, J. A., *Br. J. Cancer* **36,** 558 (1977).
61. Sun, N-C., Sun, C. R. Y., Chao, L., Fung, W-P., Tennant, R. W., and Hsie, A. W., *Cancer Res.* **41,** 1669 (1981).
62. Terzaghi, M., and Little, J. B., *Cancer Res.* **36,** 1367 (1976).
63. Traul, K. A., Kachevsky, V., and Wolff, J. S., *Int. J. Cancer* **23,** 193 (1979).

Chapter 5

Lung Tumors In Mice

R. J. M. Fry and H. P. Witschi

Introduction

Despite the fact that researchers have been studying lung tumors of mice since Livingood's observation in 1896 (*1*), the question of the cells of origin and other fundamental facets of these tumors are still being investigated. The biology of these tumors is of interest since the mouse lung tumor assay developed by Shimkin and his coworkers is now being considered for more general use as a method of screening chemicals (*2*). This assay is discussed in detail in this volume (*3*).

The development of the strain A albino mouse by Strong (*4*) provided a good inbred experimental system for the study of lung tumors. The finding by Murphy and Sturm (*5*) that the application of coal tar and distillates to skin produced lung tumors was a stimulus to studies of chemical carcinogenesis. Since that time workers, particularly at the National Cancer Institute (see the reviews in refs. *2* , and *6*), have carried out many studies that not only increased the understanding of the biology of these tumors, but also initiated the development of the use of the mouse lung tumor for the assessment of carcinogenicity of a range of chemicals. A chance finding by Nettleship et al. (*7*) that ethyl carbonate (urethane) produced multiple lung tumors in mice proved important since urethane has provided a suitable reference carcinogenic compound for use in the assay.

Structure of the Lung

The right lung is divided into four lobes: anterior, middle, posterior and a small lobe that is called accessory, median, or cardiac. The left lung is not lobed. As in other mammals the surface of the lung is covered by the visceral pleura. The trachea divides into the left and right bronchi that are completely encircled by irregular cartilaginous plates. These large primary bronchi divide upon entering the lungs. There is no cartilage in the bronchi within the lungs. The trachea is lined by pseudostratified, ciliated, columnar epithelium and goblet cells. In the bronchi the epithelium and terminal bronchioles are lined with cuboidal epithelial cells most of which are Clara cells (Fig. 1). Clara cells are of importance in the metabolism of certain chemical compounds and may show toxic effects after exposure at dose levels that may cause little or no damage to the rest of the epithelium (8). The terminal bronchioles merge into the alveolar ducts

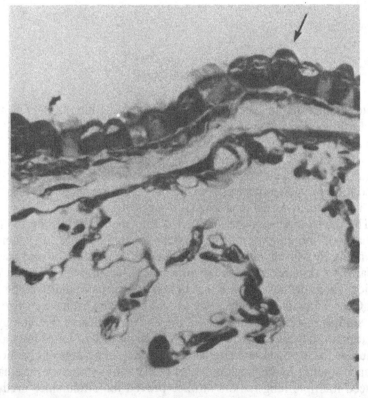

Fig. 1.   Photomicrograph of bronchiolar epithelium showing ciliated-low columnar epithelial cells and Clara cells (arrow). 700 × .

that lead to the alveoli, several of which compose the alveolar sacs. The alveoli consist of flat epithelial cells and a network of capillaries. There are two types of epithelial cells most frequently referred to as type 1 alveolar cells (type A alveolar cells, membraneous pneumocytes). Both the cytoplasm and the cytoplasmic organelles are more evident in type 2 cells than in the type 1 cells. Osmiophilic lamellar structures, which are seen in type 2 cells, are characteristic of the alveologenic lung tumors and are the basis of the proof that these tumors arise from type 2 cells. The ultrastructure of these cells and the tumors thought to arise from them have been described (9, 10). There are also free macrophages, some of which are seen in contact with the alveolar epithelium.

Tumor Classification and Characteristics

Epithelial

Alveologenic carcinoma, adenoma, type 2 cell tumor, type A tumor, type B tumor, bronchiolar–alveolar tumors, and other terms have all been used to describe murine lung tumors. Clearly, the lack of a single term for these tumors underlines the diversity of opinion about the cell of origin and the malignancy of the tumors. Perhaps the degree of frustration with the difficulties in finding an acceptable term that covers the various characteristics of the range of tumors found in various strains is shown by the use of the term ''common pulmonary tumor of the mouse.'' At least this term cannot offend those with firmly held dogmas, although it cannot win awards for brevity.

We have found a higher incidence of tumors in untreated $B6CF_1/An1$ mice in the right lung than in left lung (unpublished data). It is not known whether or not this just reflects a difference in the number of cells that have a potential for tumor formation. Amorales-Mendes (11) reported a non-random distribution of the tumors but within the lobes.

The tumors appear as clearly circumscribed, pearly white nodules that are frequently subpleural. The tumors compress the surrounding pulmonary tissue as they grow, but in the early stages they seldom show any of the aggressive infiltration associated with malignancy. Microscopically, many of the tumors consist of columns of cuboidal cells supported by a small amount of connective tissue without any capsule; apart from capillaries, blood vessels are not a feature. The epithelium is not ciliated and mitotic figures are few and far between. These characteristics and the relatively slow and benign growth have been the basis for the classification of adenoma. Some workers, especially Stewart and coworkers (12), believe that transplantability and the lack of encapsulation fulfill the criteria of malignancy and, therefore, they say that these tumors should be called carcinomas. Other workers prefer to call the tumors adenomas, because they are impressed by the fact that in many strains the tumor cells appear highly differentiated with little evidence of atypia or marked cell proliferation, and that the tumors grow slowly, and when they cause death it is most frequently as a space occupying lesion.

Perhaps of more importance is the question of the cell type of origin. Although it is clear that type 1 cells are the progeny of type 2 cells (13) and thus type 2 cells are considered stem cells, it is not known whether there are one or more stem cells for the alveolar and bronchiolar cell populations. It is the lack of identification of the stem cell(s) that hinders a resolution of the problem of the cell of origin of these lung tumors.

A number of workers consider that the tumors can be divided into two groups described as alveolar (Fig. 2), and bronchiolar (Fig. 3), implying a different cellular origin. However, the initial studies using electron microscopy suggested that the tumors consisted of a single cell type, namely, type 2 alveolar cells. Therefore, there did not appear to be a cellular explanation for the separation of tumors into two types. Recently, Kauffman and her colleagues (14, 15) have suggested that some of the lung tumors arise from Clara cells. Lung tumors induced by transplacental exposure to ethylnitrosourea were classified into bronchiolar or alveolar on the basis of their histological appearance using the light microscope. These two classes could not be distinguished on the basis of their macroscopic appearance, although the alveolar form was more frequently subpleural. Of the 33 tumors examined by electron microscopy, 18 (55%) were found to consist of Clara cells and were classified as bronchiolar tumors by light microscopy. The remaining 15 tumors, which were considered alveolar, consisted of type 2 alveolar cells. Clara cell tumors showed a tubular or papillary pattern. Fluid was often seen in the lumen of the papillary form. The individual neoplastic Clara cells appear columnar or sometimes cuboidal with basal nuclei. Other distinguishing features are dense particles about 30–50 μm in size, elongated mitochondria, and a well-marked smooth endoplasmic reticulum. The free surface of the cells has microvilli and there are complex interdigitations between adjoining cells. In fact, the appearance, including membrane-enclosed crystals, is similar to normal Clara cells except for the presence of a considerable amount of glycogen in the cytoplasm of the cells. The distinction between the Clara cell and type 2 alveolar cell tumors was thought clear-cut, except for a few cases in which the presence of myelin figures, so characteristic of type 2 alveolar cell tumors, introduces questions about the tumor cell type and the homogenicity of cell types within the tumor. Even this apparent heterogeneity might be ex-

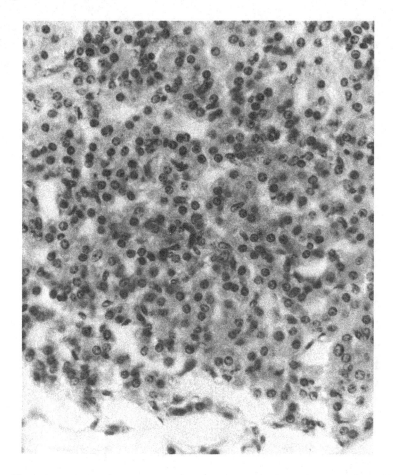

Fig. 2. Photomicrograph of lung tumor in strain A mouse classified as alveolar. 350 × .

plained if the observations of Reznik-Schüller (*16*) in the hamster can be extrapolated to mice. She found lamellar bodies similar to those considered characteristic of type 2 cells, in nonciliated cells of the bronchioles in hamsters treated with nitrosamine. In hamsters exposed to polonium-210, all of the induced tumors were considered to be of Clara cell origin (*17*).

The controversy about the cell of origin of the murine lung epithelial tumors is long standing, with some authorities favoring type 2 cells as the sole origin (*12, 18*), whereas other workers suggest that at least some of the tumors arise from bronchiolar cells (*11, 19–22*).

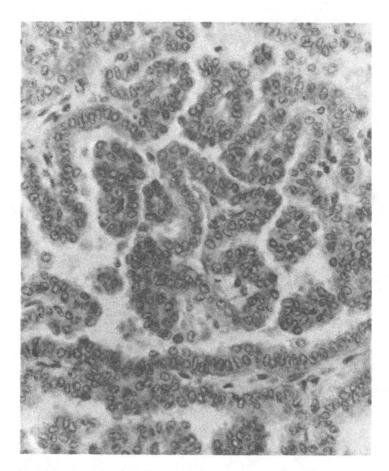

Fig. 3. Photomicrograph of lung tumor in strain A mouse classified as bronchiolar. 350 × .

Shimkin astutely recommended a noncommital term "primary adenomatous pulmonary tumors" (6). The accumulated knowledge and the newer techniques should soon lead to a resolution. If it is established that tumors with different morphology do arise from different cell types, it will be necessary to re-examine strain-, age-, and sex-dependent differences and also dose–response relationships for tumors of different cell origin.

Despite the common use of the term adenoma, both the tumors that occur naturally or after exposure to carcinogens may metastasize and can be transplanted into suitable hosts. It can be seen in Table 1 that lung tumors are more frequently malignant in male $B6CF_1$ mice than in females.

TABLE 1

Malignancy of Lung Tumors in B6CF$_1$/An1 Mice[a]

Sex	No. of mice examined	No. of tumor bearing mice	Incidence, %	Incidental (nonlethal)	Lethal	Incidental with metastases	Lethal with metastases	Incidental/lethal
Female	307	106	34.5	84	18	1	3	4.0
Male	298	180	60.4	96	51	0	33	1.1

[a]Unpublished data.

Metastasis is a late event and spread is characteristically to the mediastinal lymph nodes (23). Metastases are also found in the heart, kidney, liver, and other organs; transpleural spread to the chest wall has also been noted (23, 24). The frequency of metastases is strain-dependent and is increased after exposure to chemical carcinogens (25). A characteristic of both lung metastases and tumor transplants is a remarkably sarcomatous appearance. In the case of metastases the site influences the morphology. Secondaries in the heart are often like fibrosarcomas while metastases in the kidney or liver are similar in form to the primary tumor. None of the discussions about the cell of origin of lung tumors has taken into consideration the sarcomatous form of the secondary and transplanted tumors. There is no information on whether the cell of origin of the lung tumors determines the probability of metastasis.

Squamous Cell Carcinoma

This type of tumor is very rare in untreated mice. In a study of a large number of mice, an incidence of 0.005% of squamous cell carcinomas was reported (23). However, such tumors can be induced. Intratracheal instillation of methylcholanthrene in gelatin has been shown to be an effective method of induction (26).

Vascular Tumors

The natural incidence of the vascular tumors is extremely low but they can be induced by chemical carcinogens (27, 28). The neoplastic nature of these tumors is supported by the results of transplantation studies. The tumors occur as hemorrhagic masses often with cavernous spaces. The blood channels are lined by neoplastic endothelial cells and the tumors are invasive.

Natural Incidence; Age and Strain-Dependency

We can use data for lung tumors in $B6CF_1/An1$ (C57BL/6 × BALB/c) mice to examine a number of aspects of murine pulmonary tumors. In this F_1 hybrid, lung tumors are found at autopsy and may be diagnosed as incidental in mice dying from various causes or in some cases as the cause of death.

Although the natural incidence of lung tumors is high in this hybrid, the life-span is long (mean life span is more than 950 days). This suggests that many of the lung tumors either develop late in life or grow slowly. We have determined the incidence of lung tumors in mice allowed to live out their life span and also the prevalence by serial killing. When the age-specific mortality rates for mice that died from lung tumors are deter-

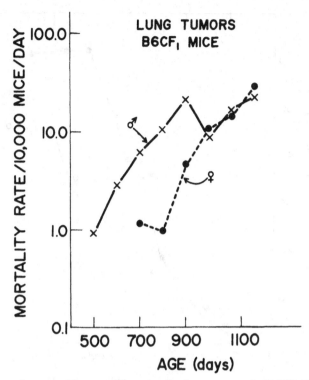

Fig. 4. Age-specific mortality rates for lung tumors in B6CF₁/Anl mice. By permission from *Environment International*, Pergamon Press Ltd.

mined it can be seen that there is a marked sex difference (Fig. 4). Lung tumors that cause death occur at an earlier age in males than in females. About 50% of male mice having a lung tumor at time of death were considered to have died from the tumor, whereas, in about 18% of the female mice the lung tumor found at autopsy was considered lethal.

The prevalence of lung tumors in male and female B6CF₁ mice is shown in Fig. 5. The prevalence was determined from the number of tumor-bearing animals at various ages throughout the life span (29). Tumors can be found quite early in life, suggesting that initiated lung cells were present at birth or shortly afterwards. In males the prevalence rises rapidly in midlife, but plateaus at about 800 days of age. The fact that the curve for prevalence as a function of age reaches a plateau at about 63% indicates that not all of the mice are susceptible to lung tumors. The prevalence of lung tumors in female mice is similar to that in males for the first 400 days, but the subsequent prevalence is lower. It is clear that both the incidence of lung tumors and their contribution to mortality is signifi-

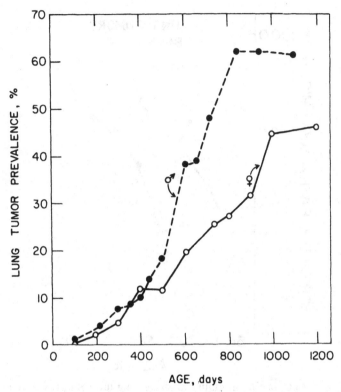

Fig. 5.   The prevalence of lung tumors in B6CF₁/Anl mice serially killed.
By permission from *Environment International*, Pergamon Press Ltd.

cantly less in the female B6CF₁ mice compared to that in the males. It is
not clear whether the tumors appear late in life because they grow more
slowly than those appearing early or because they begin to grow at a later
time. It is possible that the curves for prevalences shown in Fig. 5 reflect
distributions of growth rates and that all the initiated cells were present at
birth. The serial killing data indicate that many of the tumors have been
present for a long time. The long residence time of these tumors is suggested by the finding that the prevalence in animals dying from other
causes is similar to that in animals serially killed (28). This would not be
the case if lung tumors grew rapidly and were very malignant.

     The strain-dependent difference in susceptibility is well-illustrated in
the prevalence data for the parent strains of this F₁ hybrid (Fig. 6). A
dominant inheritance is indicated by the similarity of the prevalence rates
in the more susceptible parent strain, BALB/c, and the F₁ hybrid progeny. The sex-dependent difference is seen in both parent strains. Most
studies report a lower incidence in female mice.

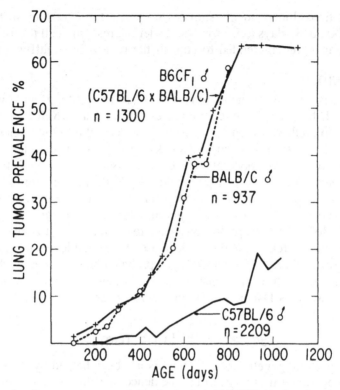

Fig. 6. Lung tumor prevalence in the hybrid B6CF$_1$/Anl male mice, x; o, male BALB/c mice; —, C57BL/6 male mice. The prevalence of lung tumors in C57BL/6 females (not shown) is lower than in male mice (shown).

Cell Proliferation

Normal Lung

The cells throughout the respiratory epithelium are constantly renewed, but at a slow rate. There is not yet as complete a description of cell turnover in the airways and alveoli as there is for many other cell-renewing systems. In the early work, using a metaphase-arrest technique, Bertalanffy and Leblond (30) suggested that there were two principal cell renewal populations in the alveoli. At that time, the cell types were identified as vacuolated and nonvacuolated alveolar cells. Later work established the relationship between the two populations and that type 1 cells were derived from type 2 cells (31, 32). Spencer and Shorter (33) using ^{3}HTdR estimated the turnover time of these alveolar cells to be about 7 and 2–3 weeks, respectively. Evans and Bils (34) concluded that type 2 alveolar cells were a stem cell-type population with a long cell turnover time. Independent estimates suggest a turnover time of type 2 cells to be 20–80 days (35, 36). The reader interested in cell proliferation in the lung is recommended to consult the review by Kauffman (37).

Lung Tumors

After exposure to urethane there is an increase in proliferation; however, there are differences in the reported results. Kauffman (38) found that the response to urethane given in the drinking water fell into three phases. In the first phase, which lasts about 3 weeks, type 2 cells were killed and the labeling indices of the populations were depressed transiently. Between 3 and 6 weeks, the type 2 cell population doubled; the labeling index decreased to almost normal levels independent of tumor formation. Dyson and Heppleston (39, 40) did not identify separate alveolar cell populations, but found that the proliferative rate reached a peak at 2 weeks after the injection of urethane and then decreased to normal levels in another 2 weeks. The difference in the results can probably be explained by the difference in the route of administration. Kauffman (38) used a protracted treatment whereas Dyson and Heppleston (39) used acute single doses.

Genetics of Lung Tumors

The study of the genetics of lung tumors has been helped by the marked strain-dependent differences in the incidence of naturally occurring lung tumors. Also, the effect of chemical carcinogens appears to be easier to detect in strains that show a high natural incidence. The importance of genetic factors in the susceptibility of mice for lung tumors was first shown by Lynch (41), but the most detailed studies have been carried out by Heston (42–45). Heston determined that there were multiple genetic factors influencing susceptibility in two strains, A and C57L, and that they differed at least in four pairs of factors and that about 86% of the susceptibility depended on the inherited factors. It appears that the inheritance of susceptibility to induction of tumors is similar to that of the naturally occurring lung tumors. It has been shown that the primary action of genes controlling the occurrence of lung tumors is in the lung tissues and not some general systemic mechanism (44, 46).

Bloom and Falconer (47) suggested that a single gene ptr determined the difference in susceptibility to lung tumors between C57BL and strain A mice and in a breeding experiment demonstrated that about 75% of the resistance to lung tumors resulted from the action of a single gene. There appears to be a consensus about the predominance of a single gene in the case of C57BL but not for other strains (48).

More recently Mühlbock's group in the Netherlands has studied the relationship of H-2, the major histocompatibility complex in congenic strains of mice on B10-A and C3H backgrounds (49). The results obtained with the congenic strains on the B10-background suggested that the strains could be divided into two groups: One with a low frequency of spontaneous lung tumors carrying the haplotypes H-6, H-2h4, H-2d, H-wi, H-2r, and another group with a significantly higher incidence of lung tumors carrying the haplotypes H-2f, H-2m, H-2h2, H-2a.

When recombinant strains were analyzed, the results indicated that genes in the IB region determined the susceptibility of the naturally occurring lung tumors. The role of other genes was suggested by results for the B10 A strain with the haplotype H-2a, derived from the highly susceptible A strain (H-2a), on the resistant background strain B10 (H-2b), which showed a lung tumor incidence that is intermediate between these two strains.

Factors Influencing Lung Tumors

The Immune System

Attempts to demonstrate antigenicity in murine pulmonary tumors have not been very successful (50). However, there have been a number of investigations of the role of the thymus in the immunological control of lung tumors (51–54) with conflicting results.

Trainin and Linker-Israeli (52, 53) interpreted their extensive studies to indicate that immune surveillance does influence lung tumors. Other studies suggest that cellular immunity does have a small effect on the time of appearance and multiplicity of lung tumors (55, 56). There is no indication that either the natural or induced incidence of lung tumors is higher in athymic nude mice than in normal mice (57, 58). Athymic nude mice do have natural killer cells that may be sufficient to influence the incidence of lung tumors.

A surface protein with a molecular weight of 180,000 has been found on the cells from a naturally occurring alveologenic carcinoma in a BALB/c mouse (59, 60). There was no evidence of cross-reactivity with a range of normal mouse cells or human or rat lung tumor cells. Carcinoma cells from two other mouse strains and from six other BALB/c lung carcinoma cell lines displayed this protein on their surface, whereas natural occurring or induced tumors classified as adenomas were at best weakly positive.

Influence of Viruses

Despite extensive work and many demonstrations of the presence of viral particles in cells of lung tumors, there is no evidence that viruses play a major role in the production of lung tumors.

There have been numerous investigations of the effect of virus infection, in particular, influenza viruses either alone or in combination with chemical carcinogens (*61, 62*) and the subject has been reviewed by Roe and Rowson (*63*). Influenza-infected mice seem to be more susceptible to esposures to some carcinogenic agents, but not all studies have demonstrated a cocarcinogenic effect.

Summary

Studies of murine lung tumors have been as varied in their approach as their contribution to knowledge. Collectively, the past studies have provided a broad base for future experiments. It has been well-established that genetic factors play a predominant role in determining not only the natural incidence in, but the susceptibility of an organism to chemical carcinogens. The evidence that susceptibility to carcinogens is influenced by the natural incidence is of general interest to carcinogenesis. With the new techniques available for studying genes, it seems timely for further studies of lung carcinogenesis at a genetic level.

The tools to answer the question about the cell(s) of origin of the lung tumors are at hand and a final answer should be obtained in the near future.

Acknowledgments

We are grateful to Dr. W. M. Haschek for advice and photomicrographs and to Katherine Allan and Everett Staffeldt for assistance.

Research sponsored by the Office of Health and Environmental Research, U.S. Department of Energy, under contract W-7405-ENG-26 with the Union Carbide Corporation, and under contract W-31-109-ENG-38 with Argonne National Laboratory. By acceptance of this article, the publisher acknowledges the U.S. Government's right to retain a nonexclusive, royalty-free license in and to any copyright covering the article.

References

1. Livingwood, L. E., *Bull. Johns Hopkins Hosp.*, **7**, 177 (1896).
2. Shimkin, M. B., and Stoner, G. D., *Adv. Cancer Res.* **3**, 223 (1975).
3. Smith, L. H., and Witschi, H. P., Lung tumor assay, in this volume.
4. Strong, L. C., *J. Hered.* **27**, 21 (1936).
5. Murphy, J. B., and Sturm, E., *J. Exp. Med.* **42**, 693 (1925).
6. Shimkin, M. B.. *Adv. Cancer Res.* **3**, 223 (1955).
7. Nettleship, A., Henshaw, P. S. and Meyer, H. L., *J. Natl. Cancer Inst.* **4**, 309 (1943).
8. Boyd, M. R., *Nature* **269**, 713 (1977).
9. Svoboda, K. J., *Cancer Res.* **22**, 1197 (1962).
10. Brooks, R. E., *J Natl. Cancer Inst.* **41**, 719 (1968).
11. Amorales-Mendes, J. J., *J. Pathol.* **97**, 415 (1969).
12. Stewart, H. L., Dunn, T. B., Snell, K. C., and Deringer, M. K., Tumors of the Respiratory Tract, in *Pathology of Tumors in Laboratory Animals, Vol. II, Tumors of the Mouse*, Sturosov, V. S., ed., IARC Scientific Publ. No. 23, Geneva, Switzerland, 1977, pp. 251–267.
13. Kapanci, Y., Weibel, E. R., Kaplan, H. P., and Robinson, E. R., *Lab. Invest.* **20**, 101 (1969).
14. Kauffman, S. L., Alexander, L., and Sass, L., *Lab. Invest.* **40**, 708 (1979).
15. Sato, K., and Kauffman, S. L., *Lab. Invest.* **43**, 28 (1980).
16. Reznik-Schuller, M., *Amer. J. Path.* **85**, 549 (1976).
17. Kennedy, A. R., Grandy, R. B., and Little, J. B., *Eur. J. Cancer* **13**, 1325 (1977).
18. Mostofi, F. K., and Larsen, C. D., *J. Natl. Cancer Inst.* **11**, 1187 (1951).
19. Tyzzer, E. E., *J. Med. Res.* **21**, 479 (1909).
20. Slye, M., Holmes, H. F., and Wells, H. G., *J. Med. Res.* **30**, 417 (1914).
21. Magnus, H. H., *J. Path. Bact.* **49**, 21 (1939).
22. Orr, J. W., *Brit. J. Cancer* **1**, 316 (1947).
23. Wells, H. G., Slye, M. and Holmes, M. F., *Cancer Res.* **1**, 259 (1941).
24. Turusov, V. S., Breslow, N. E., and Tomatis, L., *J. Natl. Cancer Inst.* **52**, 225 (1974).
25. Matsuyama, M., Suzuki, H., and Nakamura, T., *Brit. J. Cancer* **23**, 167 (1969).
26. Nettesheim, P., and Hammons, A. S., *J. Natl. Cancer Inst.* **4**, 309 (1971).
27. Andervont, M. B., *J. Natl. Cancer Inst.* **7**, 455 (1950).
28. Toth, B., *J. Natl. Cancer Inst.* **50**, 181 (1973).
29. Fry, R. J. M., Staffeldt, E., and Tyler, S. A., *Environ. Internat.* **1**, 361 (1978).
30. Bertalanffy, F. D., and Leblond, C. P., *Anat. Rec.* **115**, 515 (1953).
31. Evans, M. J., Cabral, L. J., Stephens, R. J., and Freeman, G., *Am. J. Pathol.* **70**, 175 (1973).
32. Adamson, I. Y. R, and Bowden, D. H., *Lab. Invest.* **30**, 35 (1974).

33. Spencer, H., and Shorter, R. G., *Nature* **194**, 880 (1962).
34. Evans, M. J., and Bils, R. F., *Amer. Rev. Resp. Dis.* **100**, 372 (1969).
35. Simnett, J. D., and Heppleston, A. G., *Lab. Invest.* **15**, 1793 (1966).
36. Bowden, D. H., Davies, E., and Wyatt, J. P., *Arch. Path.* **86**, 667 (1968).
37. Kauffman, S. L., *Int. Rev. Exp. Pathol.* **22**, 131 (1980).
38. Kauffman, S. L., *Cell Tissue Kinet,* **9**, 489 (1976).
39. Dyson, P., and Heppleston, A. G., *Brit. J. Cancer* **31**, 405 (1975).
40. Dyson, P., and Heppleston, A. G., *Brit. J. Cancer* **33**, 105 (1976).
41. Lynch, C. J., *J. Exp. Med.* **43**, 339 (1926).
42. Heston, W. E., *J. Natl. Cancer Inst.* **3**, 60 (1942).
43. Heston, W. E., *J. Natl. Cancer Inst.* **3**, 79 (1942).
44. Heston, W. E., and Dunn, T. B., *J. Natl. Cancer Inst.* **11**, 1057 (1951).
45. Heston, W. E., *J. Natl. Cancer Inst.* **15**, 775 (1954).
46. Shapiro, J. R., and Kirschbaum, A., *Cancer Res.* **11**, 644 (1951).
47. Bloom, J. L., and Falconer, D. S., *J. Natl. Cancer Inst.* **33**, 607 (1964).
48. Severi, L., ed., *Lung Tumors in Animals* (Perugia-Quadrennial Conference on Cancer, 3rd, 1965), Perugia, Division of Cancer Research (Perugia Univ) 1965.
49. Faraldo, M. J., Dux, A., Mühlbock, O., and Hart, G., *Immunogenetics* **9**, 383 (1979).
50. Prehn, R. T., *Ann. NY Acad. Sci.* **101**, 107 (1963).
51. Duhig, J. T., *Arch. Pathol.* **9**, 180 (1965).
52. Trainin, N., and Linker-Israeli, M., *Cancer Res.* **29**, 1840 (1969).
53. Trainin, N., and Linker-Israeli, M. *J. Natl. Cancer Inst.* **44**, 893 (1970).
54. Sanford, B. H., Kohn, H. I., Daly, J. J., and Soo, S. F., *J. Immunol.* **110**, 1437 (1973).
55. Colnaghi, M. I., *Europ. J. Cancer* **11**, 633 (1975).
56. Menard, M. I. S., and Dalla Porta, G., *J. Natl. Cancer Inst.* **47**, 1325 (1971).
57. Stutman, O., *Science* **183**, 534 (1974).
58. Holland, J. M., Mitchell, T. J., Gipson, L. C., and Whitaker, M. S., *J. Natl. Cancer Inst.* **61**, 1357 (1978).
59. Kennel, S. J., *Cancer Res.* **39**, 2934 (1979).
60. Kennel, S. J., Lankford, P. K., Foote, L. J., Tsakeres, F. S., Adams, L. M., and Ullrich, R. L., *Cancer Res.* **40**, 2153 (1980).
61. Stein, P. E., and Loosli, C. G., *Cancer Res.* **10**, 383 (1950).
62. Kotin, P., and Wiseley, D. V., *Prog. Exp. Tumor Res.* **3**, 186 (1963).
63. Roe, F. J. C., and Ronson, K. E. K., *Int. Rev. Exp. Pathol.* **6**, 181 (1968).

Chapter 6

Tissue Genotoxic Effects

D. J. Koropatnick and J. J. Berman

Tests using cultured cells (in vitro test) are limited in their predictive value for genotoxic effects in whole animals (in vivo tests), since they do not reproduce the actual conditions of cellular exposure, metabolism, and reaction to toxic compounds that take place in the animal. However, by treating the whole animal with test compounds, allowing reaction to the treatment, and then examining particular tissues for any of a host of genotoxic effects developed for in vitro protocols, one maintains the advantage of rapid and quantitative in vitro testing while gaining the advantage of the relevance of in vivo conditions of exposure. In vivo in combination with in vitro testing permits examination of particular organs and particular cells in organs that are of special interest with regard to particular compounds or classes of compounds. This type of testing is relatively new and limited only by available techniques for preparing cells from different tissues and the ability to measure valid parameters of genotoxic damage in cells under study.

The in vivo tests that are presently in use to assay the primary genotoxic events following carcinogen treatment include:

(a) Tests that assay for single-strand DNA breaks, including the alkaline elution assay (10–12) and alkaline sucrose gradient sedementation assays (13–15).

(b) Tests that assay for adhesion of carcinogen to DNA (the DNA adduct assay (2, 16, 17).

79

(c) Tests that assay for repair of genotoxic lesions, such as the detection of the unscheduled uptake of tritiated (^{3}H-TdR) (*18*).

(d) Mammalian cytogenetic assays, including the detection of chromosome aberrations (*8*), the induction of micronuclei (*19*), and the induction of sister chromatid exchanges (*20*).

(e) Mammalian mutagenesis assays, including specific locus mutations (*21–23*).

(f) The sperm anomaly test (*24*).

(g) Tests for the induction of preneoplastic tissue in vivo (*25*).

These tests can be divided into three groups: those that test the rapid primary genotoxic events following carcinogen administration (*a,b*), those that assay for the immediate or nearly immediate response of the cells to the primary damage (*c,d,f*), and those that assay for mutagenic and precarcinogenic events that occur only after primary initiation events have ended, and an ''eclipse'' period of from several days to months or years has passed, for example.

The alkaline elution assay developed by Kohn (*10*) and Swenberg (*11*) is based on the property of mammalian DNA to elute from membrane filters at a rate proportional to the length of single strands. Different types of DNA damage (single-strand breaks, alkali-labile sites, interstrand crosslinks, DNA–protein crosslinks) induce different elution profiles (single-strand breaks will cause more rapid elution of DNA from the filters than is the case with control DNA). Elution of DNA with induce alkali-labile sites varies in accordance with the type of alkali-labile site induced, allowing some assessment of the nature of the sites. The test system may be used with cultured mammalian cells or with tissue cells prelabeled with ^{3}H-TdR or an appropriate DNA precursor.

DNA fragmentation can also be measured by alkali sucrose gradient sedimentation (*15, 25, 27*). Cells from selected tissues of animals treated with carcinogens or mutagens are excised and squashed to release nuclei. The nuclei are lysed and sedimented through an alkaline sucrose gradient to measure the extent of single-strand DNA breakage. This method assays the induction of anomalies in chromatin as well as breaks in isolated DNA, since density gradient sedimentation properties depend upon the protein associated with chromatin as well as with the DNA itself. ''Relaxation'' of DNA–protein complexes may retard sedimentation on alkaline sucrose gradients in a manner that may be mistakenly assumed to be the result of induction of single-strand breaks. In addition, alkali-labile sites induced in DNA may be converted to single-strand breaks on the gradient. Thus, the type of damage assayed for on alkaline density gradients may not be as specific (i.e., single-strand cleavage) as is sometimes implied, and several types of DNA lesions may produce retardation of DNA sedimentation. Both alkaline sucrose gradients and the alkaline elution assay provide only qualitative data with respect to predicting carcinogenic or mutagenic potential. Although increasing dose produces increasing DNA fragmentation, this does not necessarily mean that a compound that produces 10% DNA fragmentation is a less potent carcinogen than a compound producing 50% DNA fragmentation. Both assays involve events that are associated with both mutagenicity *and* toxicity.

The alkaline sucrose gradient sedimentation and alkaline elution assays share the disadvantage that incorporation of radioactive precursors is necessary to detect DNA. This restricts the tests to analysis of rapidly proliferating tissue where such precursors may be administered and incorporated into DNA days or hours prior to experimentation. Prelabeling may be avoided if DNA and DNA fragments can be detected by reaction of DNA samples with ethidium bromide, a dye that intercalates duplex DNA with a 25-fold enhancement of its fluorescence. Neutralization of the alkaline gradient fractions allows formation of such duplex DNA by intramolecular hydrogen bonding (28). DNA from practically all cells, both dividing and nondividing, may be detected in this way, and expensive and troublesome prelabeling may therefore be avoided.

Both assays may be used to detect repair of lesions in DNA by following the gradual increase in size of DNA from small fragments (shortly after carcinogen administration) to nearly control-sized pieces. In this case, however, prelabeling of cells beforehand is necessary, since detection of DNA by a method that does not distinguish between cells that are present during treatment and those that arise by cell division afterwards may give rise to spurious "repair" that results from the *de novo* scheduled synthesis of DNA rather than repair synthesis.

Tests for DNA repair are based on the uptake of ^{3}H-TdR because of repair replication following carcinogen treatment (29). In this case, an organism may be treated with a carcinogen that induces lesions in DNA recognizable to endogenous cellular repair enzymes. During a selected portion of the repair period (usually 1–2 h immediately following carcinogen treatment), tissues are removed, exposed to ^{3}H-TdR and prepared for sectioning and autoradiography (18, 30). Unscheduled DNA synthesis is readily detectable in nondividing tissues, but particular care must be taken to distinguish DNA replication synthesis from repair synthesis in tissue that contains dividing cells, usually by discounting cells with extreme levels of ^{3}H incorporation (31).

Another test assaying for direct damage to DNA is the analysis of adduct formation to DNA bases. In this case, chemical modification of DNA has the capacity to alter base-pairing by interfering with the template function of DNA. The miscoding that results may lead to mutation, either by base-substitution or by frameshift mutation. In vivo assays of DNA adduct formation involve treatment of test animals with radioactively labeled carcinogen followed by excision of organs from 12 h to 6 months following administration. DNA isolation followed by acid hydrolysis results in deoxyribonucleotides that include those with aryl or alkyl adducts, and these may be separated by column chromatography or high pressure liquid chromatography (2, 17, 32). Care must be taken (at least where high doses of high specific-activity carcinogen are forcefed in vivo) that only aryl or alkyl adducts of DNA are detected rather than the entire amount of label associated with DNA. A large and variable proportion of the radioactivity may be nonspecifically associated with non-alkyl or arylated bases (P. Kleihues, personal communication). In addition, evidence suggests that the events that lead ultimately to tumor formation tend to involve covalent guanine products rather than other pyrimidine-bound products (33). When repair of adduct lesions is to be observed, these other nontumorigenic adducts represent a high and variable background radioactivity in samples. Repair of DNA adducts may be evaluated by removing tissue samples and determining the adduct level at various times following carcinogen administration. The number of adducts of a selected type (generally O^6-alkylguanine) is inversely proportional to the amount of repair that has taken place (2).

All of these assays are suited for the determination of DNA damage and repair of that damage in order to observe species or organ specificity. However, the endpoints have not been causally linked with the induction of tumors. A second series of assays employs observations of chromosome anomalies rather than DNA lesions, in order to use endpoints more closely associated with tumorogenesis (34). These assays include the induction of de novo chromosome aberrations, including translocations, breaks, and exchanges that arise during the metaphase following carcinogen or mutagen treatment (35), the induction of micronuclei in dividing tissue by genotoxic agents (19, 36) and the induction of sister chromatid exchanges (20). Such cytogenetic effects can be observed only in tissues with actively dividing cells. This usually means that the polychromatic erythocytes found in bone marrow are the cells of choice, because of their active division and ease of preparation. However, the use of the limited number of cell types available ignores the problem of organ-specificity of carcinogens so that care must be taken to ensure that proper in vitro testing be done to unmask mutagenic potential. Of the listed tests, sister chromatid exchanges generally occur in detectable levels at chemical concentrations one or two orders of magnitude lower than those found necessary to cause chromosome aberrations (20). This means that induction of sister chromatid exchanges is the most sensitive of the cytogenetic tests, and good correlation of induction of sister chromatid exchanges with carcinogenicity appears to be the case with both strongly mutagenic carcinogens and weak carcinogens such as saccharin (37).

The sperm anomaly test (38) depends upon the observation that the proportion of sperm abnormalities in individual males may be related to the dose and time of exposure to various mutagens, teratogens, and carcinogens. It has been proposed that the measure of the fraction of sperm with head shape abnormalities may constitute a rapid and simple assay for damage induced by such agent on spermatogenic stem cells in vivo. This test may be employed prospectively in animals or retrospectively in humans exposed to suspected biohazards.

The last of the short-term in vivo assays includes those that actually measure mutation or that assess whether cells have taken on preneoplastic characteristics. Of the mammalian mutagenesis assays, specific locus mutations such as the HGPRT assay based on 6-thioguanine resistance of peripheral blood lymphocytes (21) and the use of fluorescent antibodies against sickle hemoglobin to detect sickle-trait red cells in normal nonsickle trait inducers (22) are among those presently available for use.

However, the correlation between mutagenicity and carcinogenicity is by no means complete. There remains the need for short-term in vivo tests to assay for characteristics beyond those in the initial stages of carcinogenesis, but more closely associated with tumor tissue. One technique addressing itself to this need is the detection of resistant preneoplastic liver cells in carcinogen-treated animals (39). This is based on the hypothesis that some initiating dose of a carcinogen may induce an alteration in a rare hepatocyte such that that hepatocyte is no longer subject to inhibition of cell proliferation that is characteristic of most carcinogen-treated cells. A stimulus for proliferation (e.g., partial hepatectomy) may be applied in the presence of a mitosis-inhibiting environment [e.g., dietary administration of the liver carcinogen, 2-acetylaminofluorene (2-AAF)]. Only those rare carcinogen-induced cells resistant to the mitosis inhibition will respond to the partial hepatectomy and undergo rapid cell proliferation. The sites of proliferation are visible nodules of new hepatocytes that are positive for gamma-glutamyl transpeptidase (GGT) activity (40). Elevated levels of GGT activity (an enzyme involved in glutathione metabolism) have been detected in rodent hepatomas (41) and in hepatocytes of early focal lesions induced in rat livers by treatment with potent but unrelated carcinogens (42). This assay requires that at least two rounds of replication take place (to "fix" initiation events and then to stimulate resistant hepatocyte proliferation), and this may usually be induced by the necrogenicity of the administered carcinogen, application of carbon tetrachloride if the administered carcinogen is not necrogenic, or application of a chemical mitogen such as alpha-hexachlorocyclohexane (AHCH) (25). The advantage of this assay is that epigenetic effects of carcinogens are taken into consideration, as well as genotoxic effects. The resistant liver cells positive for GGT that are induced resemble very closely those cells induced by diethylnitrosamine that ultimately become cancer cell foci. It is very likely that the resistant cells seen with all the other carcinogens are also precursors for liver cancer. However, the test takes from 1 to 3 months to perform (as opposed to approximately 1 wk for other more direct genotoxic assays) and the rate of induction of resistant hepatocytes is variable. Although many carcinogens are effective with a single dose, compounds such as ethionine and 4-dimethylaminobenzene and its derivatives require up to a 4-wk exposure before a significant number of foci are induced. When the number of foci induced is small, more animals exposed for longer times must be used to obtain statistically meaningful results. Inherent in this procedure is the assumption that hepatocytes are the appropriate target cells for the compound in question.

The short-term in vivo tests may be thought of as the second level of testing for assessment of human biohazard. In general, short-term in vitro tests provide the valuable service of assaying the theoretical potential for carcinogenicity of a compound. The use of a battery of ultrasensitive microbial, yeast, or cultured cell assays minimizes the prospect of producing a false negative result, but does so at the risk of producing false positives (in terms of the ability of the compound to actually produce tumors in mammalian hosts). The role of in vivo testing should not be to take the place of such in vitro tests, but rather to assess the ability of known genotoxic agents (determined by the use of in vitro tests) to produce similar results in cells when administered under the influence of the multitude of complex and poorly understood processes that occur in vivo. Since the great danger of in vivo testing is the possibility of rendering false negative results (as a result of species specificity, organotropy, or a host of other factors), in vitro assays are necessary to counter this danger. The correlation of in vitro assays for mutagenicity with in vivo assays for mammalian biohazard may then provide information, not only on the environmental danger of compounds, but also on the in vivo events themselves that affect carcinogenicity.

References

1. Heidelberger, C., in *Carcinogenesis—A Comprehensive Survey*, R. I. Freudenthal, P. Jones, eds., p. 1, Raven Press, New York, 1976.
2. Swenberg, J. A., Cooper, H. K., Bucheler, J., and Kleihues, P., *Cancer Res.* **39**, 465 (1979).

3. Ames, B. N., McCann, J., and Yamasaki, E., *Mutation Res.* **31,** 347 (1975).
4. Yahagi, T., Nagao, M., Matsushima, T., Seino, Y., Sawamara, N., Shirai, A., Kawachi, T., and Sugimura, T. *Mutation Res.* **53,** 285 (1978).
5. Brusick, D. J., *Clin. Toxicol.* **10,** 79 (1977).
6. Felton, J. S., and Nebert, D. W., *J. Biol. Chem.* **250,** 6769 (1975).
7. Martz, G., and Straw, J. A., *Drug Metab. Disp.* **5,** 482 (1977).
8. Legator, M. S., and Rinkus, S. J., Mutagenicity Testing Problems in Application, in *Short Term Tests for Chemical Carcinogens,* H. F. Stich, R. H. C. San, eds., New York, Springer-Verlag, 1980.
9. Connor, T. H., Stoeckel, M., Evrard, J., and Legator, M. S., *Cancer Res.* **37,** 629 (1977).
10. Sweenberg, J. A., Utilization of the Alkaline Elution Assay as a Short Term Test for Chemical Carcinogens, in *Short Term Tests for Chemical Carcinogens,* H. F. Stich, R. H. C. San, eds., New York, Springer-Verlag, 1980.
11. Kohn, K. W., and Grimek-Ewig, R. A.: *Cancer Res.* **33,** 1849 (1973).
12. Parodi, S., Taningher, M., Santi, L., Cavanna, M., Sciaba, L., Maura, A., and Brambilla, G., *Mutation Res.* **54,** 39 (1978).
13. Cox, R., Damjanov, K., Abanobi, S. E., and Sarma, D. S. R., *Cancer Res.* **33,** 2114 (1973).
14. Laishes, B. A., Koropatnick, D. J., and Stich, H. F., *Proc. Soc. Exp. Biol. Med.* **149,** 978 (1975).
15. Koropatnick, D. J., and Stich, H. F., *Biochem. Biophys. Res. Comm.* **92,** 292 (1980).
16. Hawks, A., and Magee, P. N., *Brit. J. Cancer* **30,** 440 (1974).
17. Kleihues, P., and Margison, G. P., *J. Nat'l Cancer Inst.* **53,** 1839 (1974).
18. Stich, H. G., Lam, P., Lo, L. W., Koropatnick, D. J., and San, R. H. C., *Can. J. of Genet. Cytol.* **17,** 471 (1975).
19. Heddle, J. A., and Salamone, M. F., The Micronucleus Assay. 1. *In Vivo,* in *Short Term Tests for Chemical Carcinogens,* H. F. Stich, R. H. C. San, eds., New York, Springer-Verlag, 1980.
20. Wolff, S.: The Sister Chromatid Exchange Test, in *Short Term Tests for Chemical Carcinogens,* H. F. Stich, R. H. C. San, eds., New York, Springer-Verlag, 1980.
21. Strauss, G. H., and Albertini, R. J. *Mutation Res.* **61,** 353 (1979).
22. Papayannopoulou, T., McGuire, T. C., Lin, G., Gaszel, E., Nute, P. E., and Stamatoyannopoulos, G.: *Brit. J. Haematol.* **66,** 25 (1976).
23. Mendelsohn, M. L., Short-Term Genetic Tests Extended to the Human, in *Short Term Tests for Chemical Carcinogens,* H. F. Stich, R. H. C. San, eds., New York, Springer-Verlag, 1980.
24. Wyrobek, A. J., Heddle, J. A., and Bruce, W. R., *Can. J. Genet. Cytol.* **17,** 675 (1975).
25. Farber, E., and Tsuda, H., Induction of a Resistant Preneoplastic Liver Cell as a New Principle for the Short-Term Assay in vivo for Carcinogens, in *Short Term Tests for Chemical Carcinogens,* H. F. Stich, R. H. C. San, eds., New York, Springer-Verlag, 1980.

26. Damjanov, I., Cox, R., Sarma, D. S. R., and Farber, E., *Cancer Res.* **33,** 2122 (1973).
27. Abanobi, S. E., Popp, J. A., Chang, S. K., Harrington, G. W., Lotlikar, P. D., Hadjiolov, D., Levitt, M., Rajalakshmi, S., and Sarma, D. S. R., *J. Nat'l Cancer Inst.* **58,** 263 (1977).
28. Morgan, R. A., and Pulleybank, D. E., *Biochem. Biophys. Res. Commun.* **61,** 396 (1974).
29. Rasmussen, R. E., and Painter, R. B., *J. Cell Biol.* **9,** 11 (1966).
30. Stich, H. F., and Kieser, D., *Proc. Soc. Exp. Biol. Med.* **145,** 1339 (1974).
31. Stich, H. F., San, R. H. C., and Freeman, H. J., DNA Repair Synthesis (UDS) as an *In Vitro* and *In Vivo* Bioassay to Detect Precarcinogens, Ultimate Carcinogens, and Organotropic Carcinogens, in *Short Term Tests for Chemical Carcinogens,* H. F. Stich, R. H. C. San, eds., New York, Springer-Verlag, 1980.
32. Nicoll, J. W., Swann, P. F., and Pegg, A. E., *Nature* **254,** 261 (1975).
33. Gerchmann, L. L., and Ludlum, D. B., *Proc. Am. Ass. Cancer Res.* **14,** 13 (1973).
34. Harnden, D. G., and Taylor, A. M. R., *Adv. Human Genet.* **9,** 1 (1979).
35. Barthelmess, A.: Mutagenic Substances in the Human Environment, in *Chemical Mutagenesis in Mammals and Man,* F. Vogel, G. Rohrborn, eds., New York, Springer-Verlag, pp. 69–147, 1970.
36. Schmid, W., *Mutation Res.* **31,** 9 (1975).
37. Wolff, S., and Rodin, B., *Science* **200,** 543 (1978).
38. Bruce, W. R., Furrer, R., and Wyrobek, A. J. *Mutation Res.* **23,** 381 (1974).
39. Solt, D., and Farber, E.: *Proc. Am. Assoc. Cancer Res.* **18,** 52, (1977).
40. Ogawa, H., Medline, A., and Farber, E. *Lab. Invest.* **40,** 22 (1979).
41. Fiala, S., Fiala, A. E., and Dixon, B., *J. Nat'l Cancer Inst.* **48,** 1393 (1972).
42. Laishes, B. A., Katsuhiro, O., Roberts, E., and Farber, E., *J. Nat'l Cancer Inst.* **60,** 1009 (1978).

Section B

Carcinogenesis

Chapter 7

Basic Principles of Chemical Carcinogenesis

J. M. Ward

Classifications of Chemical Carcinogens

Classically, chemicals that have been demonstrated to "cause or induce malignant neoplasms in humans or animals are termed 'carcinogens'." The basis for determining whether a chemical causes or induces malignant neoplasms is a complete evaluation of the carcinogenesis experiment or toxicology experiments involving the chemical, including a detailed histopathology review and statistical analyses. The inherent limitations of the test and evaluation methods should be carefully reviewed prior to the time final conclusions are drawn. More recently, chemicals that are found to cause or induce benign and/or malignant neoplasms have been termed carcinogens. It has been shown that benign neoplasms often progress to malignant neoplasms in humans and animals, and also that what are benign neoplasms to one may well be malignant to another pathologist. Chemical carcinogens that cause benign or malignant tumors in animals thus may cause benign tumors that are life threatening in humans. And chemicals that are known to cause malignant tumors often cause benign tumors as well. No chemical has been shown to cause only benign tumors. For the purposes of this article, however, carcinogens shall be those chemicals that cause benign or malignant tumors in humans or animals (1–9).

TABLE 1
A Classification of Chemical Carcinogens
by Possible Mechanisms of Action[a]

Genotoxic
  Direct-acting
  Bio-activated
  Indirect-acting
    Chronic tissue toxin

Nongenotoxic (possibly epigenetic)
  Solid state
  Hormone
  Immunosuppressor
  Promotor
  Cocarcinogen
  Chronic tissue toxin
    Toxic
    Traumatic
    Inflammatory

---

[a]Modified From Weisburger and Williams
(*10*).

Substances that have been demonstrated to be carcinogenic in humans or animals occur in many chemical classes of both organic and inorganic compounds. Aromatic polynuclear hydrocarbons, halogenated aliphatic and olefinic hydrocarbons, aromatic amines, nitrosamines, pyrrolizidine alkaloids, epoxides, lactones, halo ethers, alkylating agents, metals, and steroids are but a few examples of chemical carcinogens.

The most recent classification for chemical carcinogens proposed (*10*) is based on possible mechanisms of action (Table 1). Until further research identifies the exact mechanisms of carcinogenesis, and develops methods for identifying a chemical's biological activity as falling into one or another of these mechanistic classes, any classification based on these possible mechanisms is necessarily drawn from limited information, and thus may be artificial. Other aspects of this classification are discussed elsewhere in this book.

Metabolism of Chemical Carcinogens

Chemicals are metabolized by cells or tissues and are changed into other chemicals or excreted from the organism unchanged. Direct-acting carcinogens must react with cell membranes and organelles prior to any reaction with DNA presumably to result in cell tranformation. Chemicals that are not direct acting must be metabolized, most frequently by the hepatocytes, to form detoxification products or biologically active metabolites that may cause cell damage or cancer (*6, 7, 11*). The metabolism of a chemical depends on dose, species, sex, route of administration, and other factors. Procarcinogens are metabolized to reactive compounds that are responsible for the events leading to cancer. Some of the possible ultimate carcinogens include epoxides, carbonium ions, and *O*-esters.

Mechanisms of Carcinogenesis

Molecular and Biologic Events Leading to Cancer

The actual molecular events leading to cell transformation are unknown (*12, 13*). However, some related biologic phenomenon have been postulated. Electrophilic chemicals react with nucleophilic atoms in macromolecules to initiate changes in the macromolecules, such as DNA, which may produce alterations at important informational sites that control cell division and biology and differentiation (Fig. 1). These altered

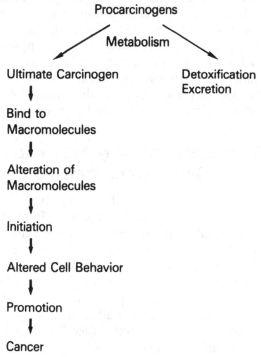

Fig. 1. A simplified genesis of carcinogenic metabolites and cancer.

macromolecules may not be detected morphologically for some time until specific growth or morphologic abnormalities are allowed to be expressed. More recently, changes in the expression of normal cellular genes have been shown to be associated with cancer (*14*). The expression of the altered genotype may depend on extracellular promoters that promote cell growth or allow expression of the abnormal phenotype. Thus, carcinogenesis may go through stages of initiation and promotion. The evidence for these stages has been seen for only a limited number of tissues; however, additional tissues are added each month as more information becomes available. The evidence for promotional stages of carcinogenesis in humans is also accumulating. Thus it is known that cigaret smoking increases the risk of lung cancer in asbestos workers and uranium miners, and chemical promoters of carcinogenesis are found in cigaret smoke. The situation has been most thoroughly studied for rat liver (*15, 16*).

Experimentally, an initiator (complete or incomplete carcinogen) is given once to the animal. Thereafter, the promoter is given for a longer period of time. The promoter must be given after the initiator in order not to interfere with the metabolism and pharmacokinetics of the initiator. The effects of promoters on experimental carcinogenesis is usually measured by an increase in tumor incidence, multiplicity, and malignancy and a decrease in the latency period. The results often show changes suggestive of an increased dose of carcinogen to the animal or an increased growth rate of the tumors. The actual effect of promoters on the carcinogenic process is not known, although promotors may be "carcinogens" by definition in a given experiment and may have specific bioeffects such as enzyme induction or growth promotion in vivo or vitro, or may induce toxic lesions in target sites for promotion.

Chemical Carcinogens That May Act by Epigenetic or Other Mechanisms

The list of chemical carcinogens that have been shown to be nongenotoxic (*17–19*) is growing daily. They come from many chemical classes and "induce" many types of tumors. For these chemicals, the exact mechanisms of carcinogenesis are not known. Some of these nongenotoxic chemicals are found to induce changes in genetic material that may be considered genotoxic for that in vitro system. The definition, however, of a genotoxic carcinogen depends on those who define them. It has been recently suggested that almost all chemicals are genotoxic in at least one in vitro system. Gene unmasking (depression) by several possible mechanisms may help explain cancer development (*12*). Chronic tissue toxins may lead to tissue regeneration with its increased mitotic rate. Increased mitotic rate has been shown to eventuate in increased rate of mutation (20). Tissue damage may also lead to carcinogenesis by other mechanisms. Attack of mitochondrial DNA by carcinogens, rather than or in addition to nuclear DNA, has been suggested in a few recent papers (21).

Use of the mouse liver as a target organ in bioassay tests has been attacked because so many mouse hepatocarcinogens may not be mutagenic (40%) and 20–24% may induce only liver tumors in mice. In a recent survey by the author, 50% of the rat hepatocarcinogens surveyed were not mutagenic as well (Table 2) (19). Further work is needed.

Principles of Dose Response to Carcinogens

Many of the basic principles of the biological response to exogenous substances apply to chemical carcinogens with few exceptions. Thus, many carcinogens act in a predictable way. The uncertainties arise in the shape of the tumor response curve (Fig. 2) and the uncertain bioeffects of low

TABLE 2
Nonmutagenic Rat Liver Carcinogens

Aromatic amines	*Metabolites*
3-Aminotriazole	Griseofulvin
2-Aminoanthraquinone	Luteoskyrin
1-Amino-2-methylanthraquinone	Ethionine
Cupferron	*Amides*
N-Nitroso compounds	Urethane
N-Nitrosodiisopropylamine	Thioacetamide
N-Nitrosomethylethylamine	*Methylenedioxy compounds*
N-Nitrosodiethanolamine	Safrole
Hydrazo compounds	*Cyclic ether*
1,2-Dimethylhydrazine	1,4-Dioxane
Halogenated compounds	*Miscellaneous compounds*
Carbon tetrachloride	Phenobarbital
Kepone	Methapyrilene
Myrex	2,3,7,8-Tetrachlorodibenzo-p-dioxin
	Hexachlorodibenzo-p-dioxins
	Di-(2-ethylhexyl) phthalate

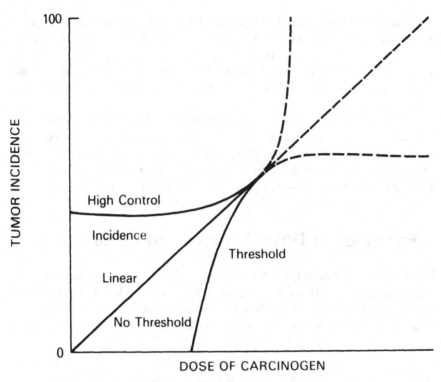

Fig. 2.   Hypothetical responses to different doses of carcinogens. When the induced tumor is morphologically and biologically similar to that of a tumor occurring in a high spontaneous incidence, the interpretation is more difficult than if the induced tumor is rare spontaneously. A threshold would be easier to define if the induced tumor occurred only rarely in controls or if many animals were used.

doses. Further complicating these two parameters are variations in responses between sexes, species, and even different target organs in the same animal. An example of the latter is EDO1 mouse AAF study performed at NCTR (22) where the liver and bladder responded in different ways to the carcinogen.

In general, the greater the dose, the shorter the latent period, the higher the incidence of tumors at any given time, and the greater bilaterally of the tumors and tumors per animal. Even after dosing is stopped, tumor incidence rises with time. Target sites for tumor induction may vary with dose.

An important subject for interspecies comparisons and human risk assessment from animal bioassay concerns the dose dependency of the detoxification, and the metabolism and excretion of the metabolites of carcinogens (*23, 24*). High doses, such as the maximally tolerated doses used in animal bioassays, may result in the production of artificial metabolites and unique tissue responses to these products. Are the results of these studies relevant to humans? The species differences in handling toxic chemicals is sometimes remarkable. Although all human carcinogens have been shown to be carcinogenic in animals (with the recent positive animal experiments for benzene and arsenic), can any given chemical that causes tumors only in one organ of one species be a cancer risk for humans?

Other aspects of carcinogenesis and further details about the subject discussed above are considered elsewhere in this book.

References

1. Shimkin, M., *Contrary to Nature,* Washington, DC, US Government Printing Office, 1977, p. 498.
2. Fraumeni, J. F., ed., *Persons at High Risk of Cancer,* Academic Press, New York, 1975, p. 544.
3. Hiatt, H. H., Watson, J. D., and Winsten, J. A., eds., *Origins of Human Cancer. Book C,* Cold Spring Harbor Laboratory, Cold Spring Harbor, 1977, pp. 1307–1889.
4. Higginson, J., and Muir, C.S., *J. Natl. Cancer Inst.* **63,** 1291 (1979).
5. International Agency for Research on Cancer, An Evaluation of Chemicals and Industrial Processes Associated with Cancer in Humans Based on Human and Animals Data, IARC Monograph vol. 1–20, *Cancer Res.* **40,** 1 (1980).
6. Miller, E.C., and Miller, J.A., *Int. Rev. Biochem.* **1979,** 27.
7. Becker, F.F., ed., *Cancer, A Comprehensive Treatise,* vol. I, Plenum Press, New York, 1975, p. 524.
8. Interagency Regulatory Liaison Group, *J. Natl. Cancer Inst.* **63,** 241 (1979).
9. Occupational Safety and Health Administration, *Fed. Reg.* **45,** 5001 (1980).
10. Weisburger, J.H., Williams, G.M., Chemical Carcinogens, in *Toxicology,* Doull, J., Klaassen, C.D., Amdur, M.O., eds., Macmillan, New York, 1980, pp. 84–138.
11. Searle, C.E., ed., *Chemical Carcinogens,* American Chemical Society, Washington, 1976, p. 788.
12. Hull, L.A., *Med. Hypoth.* **6,** 35 (1980).
13. Rubin, H., *J. Natl. Cancer Inst.* **64,** 995 (1980).
14. Klein, G., *Nature* **294,** 313 (1981).
15. Colburn, N.H., Tumor Promotion and Preneoplastic Progression, in *Chemical Carcinogenesis,* Vol. 5: *Modifiers of Chemical Carcinogenesis,* Slaga, T.J., ed., Raven Press, New York, 1980, pp. 33–56.

16. Pitot, H.C., and Sirica, A.E., *Biochim. Biophys. Acta* **605,** 191 (1980).
17. Bartsch, H., Malaveille, C., Camus, A.M., Martel-Planche, G., Brun, G., Hatefeuille, A., Sabadie, N., Barbin, A., Kuroki, T., Drevon, C., Piccoli, C., and Montesano, R., Bacterial and Mammalian Mutagenicity Tests: Validation and Comparative Studies on 180 Chemicals, in *Molecular and Cellular Aspects of Carcinogen Screening Tests,* Montesano, R., Bartsch, H. Tomatis, L., eds., IARC, Lyon, 1980, pp. 179–241.
18. McCann J., Choi, E., Yamasaki, E., Ames, B.N., *Proc. Natl. Acad. Sci.* **72,** 5135 (1975).
19. Ward, J.M., Griesemer, R.A., and Weisburger, E.K., *Toxicol. Appl. Pharmacol.* **51,** 389 (1979).
20. Berman, J.J., Tong, C., Williams, G.M., *Cancer Lett.* **4,** 277 (1978).
21. Niranjan, B.G., Bhat, N.K., and Avadhani, N.G., *Science* **215,** 73 (1982).
22. Staffa, J.A., and Mehlman, M.A., eds., J. Environ. Pathol. Toxicol. **3,** 1 (1979).
23. Smyth, R.D., and Hottendorf, G.H., *Toxicol. Appl. Pharmacol.* **53,** 179 (1980).
24. Young, J.D., Braun, W.H., and Gehring, P.J., *J. Environ. Pathol. Toxicol.* **2,** 263 (1978).

Chapter 8

Pathology of Toxic, Preneoplastic, and Neoplastic Lesions

J. M. Ward

The morphological sequences of events (histogenesis) in cancer pathogenesis may be similar in all animal species studied. However, specific differences in the histogenesis and morphology of tumors between strains of a given species and between species have been found. The basic definitions of and the nature of the pathology characteristic of the carcinogenic process is the same. In order to study the carcinogenic process definitively, a thorough necropsy is necessary (*1–5*). This chapter will concern all species, with a strong emphasis on rats and mice and their use in chronic bioassays.

Definitions

In order to understand the nature and natural history of cancer, we must first define the terms commonly used in tumor pathology.

A *lesion* is an abnormal gross or histological change in an organ or tissue. It may be naturally occurring without a known cause or it may be experimentally induced. *Hyperplasia* is the increase in the number of cells in a tissue or organ, which number usually returns to normal after the insulting agent is removed. Hyperplasia may be focal, multifocal, or diffuse. *Dysplasia* is an abnormal cytologic change of cells, usually focal, and possibly preneoplastic or precancerous. It is characterized by nuclear and cytoplasmic atypia and loss of the usual cell polarity. *Hypertrophy* is the gross enlargement of an organ or increased size of a cell. A *neoplasm* is a new growth in a tissue that is progressive in nature and generally uncontrolled by the body. *Tumor* is synonymous with neoplasm. Tumors may be benign or malignant. *Benign tumors* are neoplasms of characteristic limited behavior (Table 1), are nodular, always compress adjacent tis-

TABLE 1
Differential Features of Benign and Malignant Tumors

Characteristic	Benign	Malignant
Growth rate	Slow	Fast
Gross appearance	Round, regular	Irregular shape, hemorrhagic, ulcerated, necrotic
Mode of growth	Expansion	Expansion and invasion
Capsule	Yes	No
Mitotic figures	Few	Many
Differentiation	Well differentiated, resembles normal tissue	Poorly differentiated, tends toward anaplasia
Polarity of tissue	Similar to normal	Loss of normal polarity; "piling up" of cells
Cell size	Similar to normal	Larger or smaller than normal
Nucleus	Similar to normal	Hyperchromatic, diffuse chromatin pattern, vesicular, prominent nucleolus, atypical
Cytoplasm	Similar to normal	Basophilic, atypical, sparse or abundant
Stroma of tumor	Prominent	Usually sparse, sometimes prominent
Lymphatics	No invasion	Invasion
Blood vessels	No invasion	Invasion
Metastasis	None	May be present (ultimate proof of malignancy)
Death of animal	Depends on organ, usually rare	Common

sues, and do not invade these tissues or metastasize to other tissues. For example, an *adenoma* is a benign tumor of nonsquamous epithelial tissue and a *papilloma* is a benign tumor of squamous epithelium. "Oma" is a general suffix indicating benign tumor when used after a proper descriptive term. *Malignant tumors* are neoplasms with various degrees of infiltrative and metastatic behavior. They tend towards anaplasia, a state of high cellular undifferentiation. A *carcinoma* is a malignant tumor of epithelial tissue and an *adenocarcinoma* is a malignant tumor of glandular epithelium which forms glandular structures. A squamous cell carcinoma is from squamous epithelium and a transitional cell carcinoma is from transitional epithelium. A *sarcoma* is a malignant tumor derived from mesodermal tissues and cells (fibroblasts, chondroblasts, osteoblasts, etc.). For example, a fibroma is a benign tumor of fibroblasts or fibrocytes while a fibrosarcoma is a malignant tumor of the same cell. *Cancer* is any malignant tumor. The tumor may contain a *stroma* composed of supporting connective tissue and blood vessels. The stromal lymphoid reaction is the presence of lymphocytes, macrophages, and plasma cells within the tumor stroma. This reaction may represent the immune response to tumor antigens. *Invasion* is the process by which tumor cells spread or grow into tissue adjacent to the tumor. *Metastasis* is the presence of tumor cells in tissues that are not part of the tumor. Metastases commonly occur in regional lymph nodes via lymphatic system migration and in distant tissues such as lung and liver via migration through blood vessels. Carcinomas generally metastisize via lymphatics and blood vessels, while sarcomas usually spread via blood vessels. *Tumor regression* is the decrease in the size of a tumor from natural causes (immune response, dietary factors, and so on) or therapy. A *carcinogen* is an agent (chemical, viral, physical, and so on) that causes tumors, either benign or malignant. Carcinogens also usually cause toxic, hyperplastic, and preneoplastic lesions in the same tissues in which they ultimately cause tumors. *Carcinogenesis* is the process of development of a tumor. Table 1 differentiates benign and malignant tumors. Although we have attempted to define the terms and characteristics in general, there may be exceptions to the rules. In rodents, some malignant tumors appear to be malignant when first seen in tissue sections, while others go through stages of progression from focal hyperplasia to benign neoplasia to malignancy (Figs. 1, 2). Adenomas (Fig. 3) may progress to cancer through the appearance of focal atypical cells or malignant cells within the adenoma that represents carcinoma within the adenoma, especially in rodent liver. Evidence has been presented that all benign tumors in rodents are in fact low grade malignant tumors or stages in the development of metastatic cancer *(6)*. These aspects of tumor formation will be discussed later.

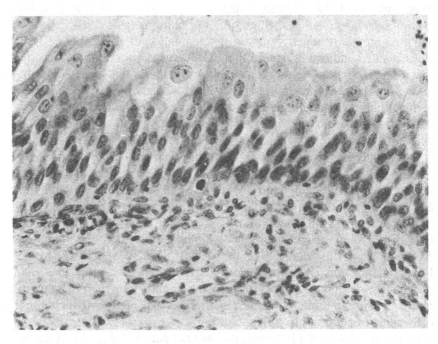

Fig. 1. Diffuse bladder hyperplasia and hypertrophy. The large epithelial cells on the luminal side of the epithelium are hypertrophied.

Pathogenesis of Cancer

The pathogenesis of cancer may be defined and characterized from the molecular level to death of the animal. In pathology, the sequential morphologic changes in the tissue of origin of the cancer is best defined as the histopathogenesis or morphogenesis of cancer from the initiating events. Figure 4 illustrates potential sequences of events based on naturally occurring and induced tumors of rodents. The exact causes of these transitions are not known. They may be associated with continuous carcinogen administration, promoters (especially in the diet), mutational events, epigenetic events, "spontaneous" transformation, immunocompetence of the host, and other unknown factors. Atypia is defined as the presence of cells with characteristic abnormal phenotypes and behavior. Some of these characteristics may be identical to those in cancer and include increased cytoplasmic basophilia, nuclear hyperchromatism, large nucleolus, presence of mitotic figures, abnormal cellular forms, and disorientation of the cells on basement membranes or in their usual order. Atypical

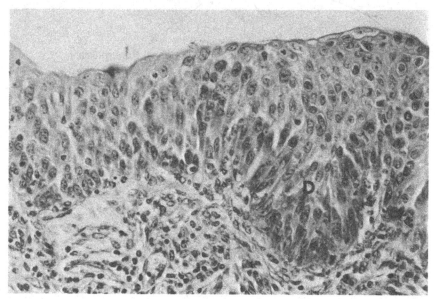

Fig. 2. Urinary bladder of mouse given methylazoxyoctane, a bladder carcinogen. The lesion is diffuse hyperplasia (several cells thick) and a focus of dysplasia (D) or atypia is seen.

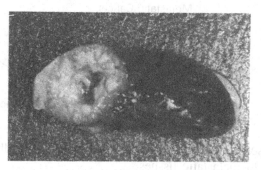

Fig. 3. Renal tubular cell adenoma induced by Aflatoxin B_1 in F344 rat. The tumor is well circumscribed and the center is necrotic.

areas may progress to cancer. Occasionally focal hyperplasias may be composed of cells that are identical to those in benign neoplasms, the primary difference in classification resulting from the nodular and compressing nature of the benign neoplasm. Focal cancer may appear morphologically malignant from its smallest (earliest) origin (5, 6). Primary tumor growth requires vascularization. Metastases require tumor cell

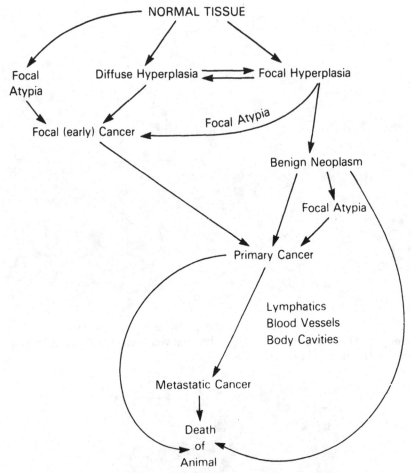

Fig. 4. The histopathogenesis of cancer. The exact sequence depends on the chemical carcinogen, the species, and the tissue involved.

transport in vessels, arrest in the capillary bed of the lung, adherence, and extravasation into metastatic tissues.

Essentially all epithelial tissues may undergo the sequences of events noted in Fig. 4. The rat liver has been the most extensively studied tissue, and the histogenesis of liver cancer in rats is illustrated in Fig. 5. Foci of cellular alteration have been called focal hyperplasias and foci of altered cells. Typically, they contain hepatocytes with gamma-glutamyl transpeptidase or with loss of other enzymes, including ATPase and G-6 Pase. The former is not normally present in hepatocytes. Nodules and carcinomas also have these enzyme profiles. Foci and nodules may regress, especially when carcinogen administration is stopped at specific times after

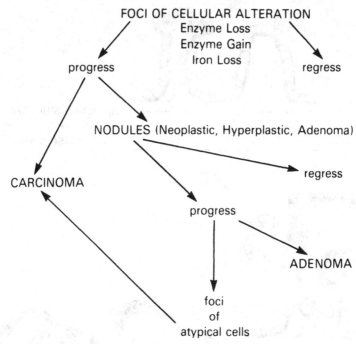

Fig. 5. Genesis of hepatocellular tumors induced by carcinogens in rats.

exposure. Nodules have been termed neoplastic nodules, hyperplastic nodules, and hepatocellular adenomas. They do appear as progressively growing lesions and as neoplasms. If they grow large and do not develop into carcinomas, they would be true adenomas.

The growth of tumors in tubular epithelial organs is more easy to follow than in liver, because of easily identifiable anatomic structures in these tissues. For example, colon tumors arise on the surface of colonic glands. When small, they may be seen as superficial cancer or carcinomas in situ in the epithelium only. As they grow in size, they either grow into the lumen as polypoid adenocarcinomas or into the colon wall as invasive tubular adenocarcinomas. In the wall, they progressively invade the muscularis mucosae, submucosa, tunica muscularis, and serosa. They invade lymphatics and metastasize to regional lymph nodes and/or the peritoneal cavity by extension and seeding (Figs. 6, 7). Stomach tumors act similarly (Figs. 8, 9).

Growth of the tumor, whether benign or malignant, may lead to death of the host in several ways (Figs. 10, 11). Identifying the actual cause of death for individual animals is difficult. Clinical pathology and measurements of specific organ function may be required. The pathologist, however, may make a best judgment about the possible occurrence

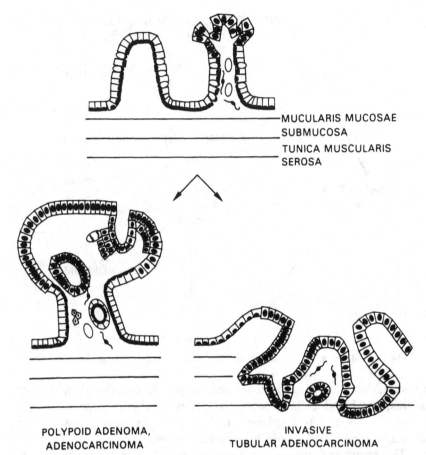

MUCULARIS MUCOSAE
SUBMUCOSA
TUNICA MUSCULARIS
SEROSA

POLYPOID ADENOMA,   INVASIVE
ADENOCARCINOMA   TUBULAR ADENOCARCINOMA

Fig. 6. Morphogenesis of polypoid and invasive tubular adenocarcinomas of the rat colon. Note the polypoid tumors grow into the lumen of the intestine while invasive tubular adenocarcinomas grow through the progressive layers of the gut.

of a tumor-related death. Some contributing causes of death from cancer in rodents include cachexia, interference with the functioning of tissue in which a primary or metastatic tumor is found, infection, accentuated of aging lesions (nephropathy, periarteritis, cardiomyopathy), and other effects (hypercalcemia, uremia). When highly malignant neoplasms are induced by a carcinogen, early mortality eventuates from the devastating effects of metastatic tumors (Fig. 9). Life table methods have been used to evaluate statistically the relationship between dose and mortality. Others have suggested use of detailed methods of evaluation for cause of death including describing at necropsy whether a tumor was (a) definitely incidental, (b) probably incidental, (c) probably fatal, or (d) definitely fatal.

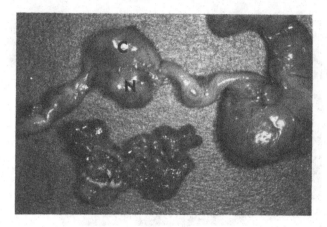

Fig. 7. Rat colon carcinoma (c) metastastic to the regional lymph node (N) and mesentery (M).

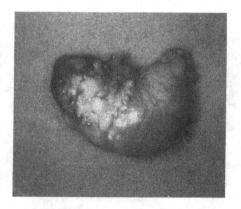

Fig. 8. Squamous cell carcinoma of forestomach invading to serosa in Osborne-Mendel rat given ethylene dibromide.

Tumor Pathology

Natural Tumors in Different Species

Tumors, preneoplastic, and nonneoplastic lesions of rats and mice used in toxicity and carcinogenicity tests are generally similar to those seen in other animals and man. There are, however, differences between species in the nature and incidences of characteristic lesions. The criteria for diagnosis of these lesions have been noted previously in this chapter and elsewhere (7–13). Tumor incidence in major rodent strains have been reported (7, 9, 14–18). The incidence of many naturally occurring tumors is

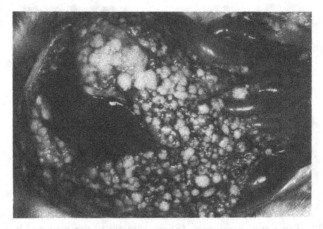

Fig. 9. Peritoneal metastases from gastric squamous cell carcinoma induced by gavage of ethylene dibromide in an Osborne-Mendel rat.

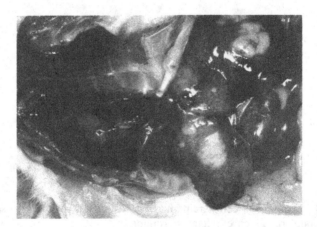

Fig. 10. Multiple hepatocellular carcinomas that metastasized to the lungs causing severe hemothorax in a F344 rat given aflatoxin B_1.

age-dependent (8). Tumor incidence is also variable, depending on statistical and other considerations (19–22).

Chemically Induced Tumors

Sites of rare tumors in control animals are often the site of chemically induced tumors, including those in nasal epithelium, oral cavity, esophagus, stomach, intestine, blood vessels, brain, liver, pancreas, Zymbal's glands, and splenic connective tissue. Thus, in these cases, induced tu-

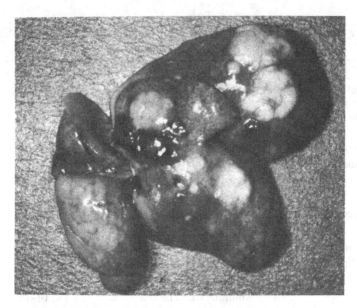

Fig. 11.   Multiple hepatocellular carcinomas in liver of rat fed aflatoxin B_1. The two dark (hemorrhagic) areas are hemangiosarcomas.

mors may have the characteristics of rare tumors. More common tumors, such as leukemias, and those of liver, pituitary, and adrenal glands may be more difficult to distinguish induced tumors from those in controls. It may, however, be frequently difficult to distinguish beteween control and induced tumors in any given case. An attempt should be made to do so in rodent bioassay studies. Characteristic human (hepatic angiosarcoma—vinyl chloride and thoratrast; mesothelioma—asbestos; pulmonary bronchogenic carcinoma—cigarette smoke; vaginal clear cell adenocarcinoma—diethylstilbestrol) and rodent tumors have been induced by specific carcinogens. Carcinogens also induce unique tumors in a given species with a characteristic metastatic rate (Tables 2–5). The metastic rate depends on the chemical, the species, and sometimes, the dose of carcinogen. As noted later, many malignant tumors induced by carcinogens in rodents do not metastasize, an observation made previously for mouse liver tumors in an attempt to discredit their classification as malignant neoplasms.

The induction of tumors by chemicals may be quantified by various methods. The number of grossly visible tumors may be counted at necropsy and quantitated histologically per unit area or volume of tissue. The number of tumors per animal in each group for a specific tissue may be compared for treated and control groups, and statistics may then be used

TABLE 2
Examples of Metastatic Rate of Chemically Induced Carcinomas in Mice
(Other Than Liver)[a]

Chemical	Induced tumor	Metastatic rate (%)[b] (to any tissue),
1,2-Dimethylhydrazine	Colonic adenocarcinoma	0
Azoxymethane	Colonic adenocarcinoma	0
1,2-Dibromo-3-chloro- propane	Forestomach squamous cell carcinoma	34–50
1,2-Dibromoethane	Forestomach squamous cell carcinoma	40–50
1,2-Dibromo-3-chloro- propane	Nasal carcinoma	10–30
p-Cresidine	Urinary bladder carcinoma	10–20
o-Anisidine	Urinary bladder carcinoma	0
1,2-Dichloroethane	Mammary carcinoma	0–22
Sulfallate	Mammary carcinoma	14–18
Reserpine	Mammary carcinoma	14

[a]From the NCI Carcinogenesis Technical Reports.
[b](Number of rats with metastatic tumor/number of rats with primary tumor) × 100.

to determine the significance of differences in the mean number of tumors. The size or weight of tumors may be measured and compared in treated and control groups. We have used an image analyzer computer to compare the morphology of liver tumors in both control mice and mice exposed to a pesticide. Significant differences in tumor cell morphology were detected. The quantitation of the findings from pathological studies lends more credence to pathology as a science and allows the results to be analyzed in a more meaningful manner.

A Classification of Toxic Nonneoplastic Lesions Induced by Chemicals

In order to understand the effects of chemical carcinogens on their target sites and the histopathogenesis of cancer in these sites, one must consider the types of toxic lesions induced in tissues by chemical carcinogens. The most common sites of toxicity of chemicals in rodents are liver and lung, perhaps because of the metabolism and excretion of xenobiotics by these organs. Classification of toxic nonneoplastic lesions for liver and other tissues are given in Tables 6 and 7.

TABLE 3

Examples of Metastatic Rate of Chemically Induced Carcinomas in Rats
(Other Than Those of the Liver)[a]

Chemical	Induced tumor	Metastatic rate (to any tissue), (%)[b]
Methyl (acetoxymethyl) nitrosamine	Intestinal adenocarcinoma	0–14
1,2-Dimethylhydrazine	Colonic polypoid adenocarcinoma	0
	Colonic tubular adenocarcinoma	0–5
	Colonic mucinous adenocarcinoma	50
N-Methyl-N-nitrosourea	Colonic cystadenocarcinoma	0
N-Methyl-N-nitrosourea	Urinary bladder carcinoma	0
N-Butyl-N-(4-hydroxy-butyl) nitrosamine	Urinary bladder carcinoma	0
4-Amino-2-nitrophenol	Urinary bladder carcinoma	0–9
4-Chloro-o-phenylenediamine	Urinary bladder carcinoma	0–14
m-Cresidine	Urinary bladder carcinoma	0
p-Cresidine	Urinary bladder carcinoma	0–3
o-anisidine	Urinary bladder carcinoma	0
N-Methyl-N-benzylnitrosamine	Esophagael carcinoma	0
1,2-Dibromoethane	Forstomach squamous cell carcinoma	30–70
N-Methyl-N'-nitro-N-nitrosoguanidine	Glandular stomach adenocarcinoma	0
Lead acetate	Renal carcinoma	10–40
Tris(2,3-dibromopropyl) phosphate	Renal carcinoma	0
2,4-Diaminoanisole sulfate	Thyroid follicular cell carcinoma	0
4,4'-Methylene-N,N-dimethyl-benzamine	Thryoid follicular cell carcinoma	0–2
Ethylene thiourea	Thyroid follicular cell carcinoma	0–12
1,2-Dibromo-3-chloropropane	Nasal carcinoma	0–3
1,2-Dichloroethane	Mammary carcinoma	11
Sulfallate	Mammary carcinoma	0–22
1,2-Dibromo-3-chloropropane	Mammary carcinoma	10–16

[a]Data predominantly from the NCI Carcinogenesis Technical Report Series.
[b](Number of rats with metastatic tumor/number of rats with primary tumor) × 100.

TABLE 4

Metastatic Rate of Induced Hepatocellular Tumors in F344 Rats at 2 yr[a]

Chemical or group	Neoplastic nodule	Hepatocellular carcinoma	Metastatic rate to lung, %[b]
Tumors in controls	+		0
p-Nitrosodiphenylamine	+		0
1,4-Dioxane	+		0
Cupferron		+	0
1-Amino-2-methylanthraquinone		+	0
Selenium sulfide		+	0
Myrex		+	0
p-Cresidine	+	+	0–33
3-Amino-9-ethylcarbazone		+	0
2-Amino-anthraquinone		+	0
Hydrazobenzene		+	15–20
Michler's ketone		+	15–55
N-Nitrosodiethanolamine		+	10–90

[a]Data from the NCI Carcinogenesis Technical Report Series.
[b]Percent of primary hepatic tumors noted that metastasized to the lung.

Rodent liver responds to toxins in a similar fashion to the livers of other species (Table 6). Other unique lesions, however, are seen only in rodents. Rat and mouse differ somewhat from each other. *Necrosis* is the usual acute response to high doses of toxins. The pattern of necrosis in the liver lobule depends on the type of chemical and the dose administered. It has been noted that water-soluble chemicals tend to cause periportal lesions and lipid-soluble chemicals generally cause centrilobular lesions. Although these facts may be true, many exceptions exist. A commonly overlooked pattern is midzonal necrosis. The exact causes of the pattern of necroses are not known, but may be related to carcinogen metabolism, solubility, conjugation, excretion, and mechanism of toxicity. *Degenerative* hepatocyte lesions frequently lead to necrosis. If the animal survives the insult, these lesions may persist or regress, especially if the toxin is no longer administered to the animal. These lesions represent specific morphologic alterations in the cell as a result of metabolism or detoxification of the toxin. For example, proliferation of agranular endoplasmic reticulum, a common result of induction of drug-metabolizing enzymes, appears as hyaline areas within the cell. Interference with lipid metabolism by hepatocytes leads to marked vacuolization of hepatocytes. Cholestasis is the increased amounts of bile in hepatocytes, in Kupffer's cells, or in

TABLE 5

Metastatic Rates of Hepatocellular Adenomas and Carcinomas to the Lung in B6C3F1 Mice[a]

Chemical or group	Metastatic rate to lung, %[b]
Controls 96 weeks of age (all liver tumors)	0–10
Controls 110 weeks of age	
Hepatocullular carcinomas	20–40
Hepatocellular adenomas	0–2
Toxophene	0
Hexachloroethane	0
Tetrachlorvinphos	0–4
2,3,7,8-Tetrachlorodibenzo-*p*-dioxin	0–6
2,6-Dichloro-*p*-phenylenediamine	0
Selenium disulfide	0
2-Nitro-*p*-phenylenediamine (adenomas only)	0
Eugenol	18
2-Aminoanthraquinone	0
Tris(2,3-dibromopropyl)phosphate	0–8
Hexachlorodibenzo-*p*-dioxins	33
Nitrofen	10–25
Di(2-ethylhexyl)phthalate	16–38
Di(2-ethylhexyl)adipate	25–45

[a]Data from the NCI Carcinogenesis Technical Report Series.
[b](Number of mice with lung metastases/number of primary hepatocellular carcinoma) × 100, unless adenoma noted.

bile canaliculi. Intranuclear inclusions may occur from the modification of nuclear membrane activity and appear as pseudo-inclusions with the nuclear membrane surrounding the cytoplasmic contents. True nuclear inclusions are rare in rodents, but may occur. Nuclear chromatin may be modified in appearance from normal, depending on cellular activity. Active nuclei may be larger than normal, have a large prominent nucleolus, and display a dispersed chromatin pattern. Inactive nuclei or those in atrophied hepatocytes may be small in size and have a clumped chromatin pattern. Cytomegaly may occur as a result of the inhibition of cell division or decreased cell turnover (Figs. 12, 13). This lesion is common in the hepatocytes of some strains of aging mice, but rare in others. Multinucleated hepatocytes on the other hand may be seen in many rats and mice in normal livers. Binucleate forms are most common, but multinucleate forms are seen only after toxic insult, especially by chlorinated pesticides

TABLE 6
A Classification of Toxic Hepatic Lesions of Rodents

Necrosis
  Focal (multifocal)
  Centrilobular (periacinar)
  Midzonal
  Periportal
  Massive

Degenerative Hepatocyte Lesions
  Atrophy
  Glycogen
  Glycogen depletion
  Hydropic change
  Hyaline
  Lipidosis (fatty metamorphosis)
    Macroglobular, microglobular,
      granular
  Cholestasis
  Inclusions
    Intranuclear (true, pseudo-
      invaginations of
      nuclear membrane)
    Intracytoplasmic
  Nuclear chromatin change
  Cytomegaly
  Karyomegaly
  Multinucleated hepatocytes
  Storage Diseases

Kupffer's Cell Lesions
  Hypertrophy
  Hyperplasia
  Granulomas
  Amyloid
  Pigments
    Endogenous
      Bile (cholestasis)

      Hemosiderin
      Lipofuscin
    Exogenous (injected or
      ingested materials)
  Storage diseases

Biliary Lesions
  Hyperplasia of bile ducts
  Hyperplasia of cholangioles (oval
    cell hyperplasia)
  Cholangiofibrosis

Cirrhosis (degeneration, fibrosis,
  regeneration)
  Postnecrotic
  Biliary
  Pericellular

Vascular Lesions
  Peliosis
  Endothelial hyperplasia

Regeneration
  Hepatocyte
    Diffuse (mitotic figures)
    Focal
    Nodular
  Kupffer's Cell
  Biliary
    Oval cell
    Bile duct

Fibrosis
  Biliary
  Parenchymal
  Postnecrotic
  Pericellular

in mice. Storage of cellular materials such as lipid and glycogen occurs in hepatocytes of mice with genetic storage diseases similar to those in humans.

Kupffer's cells are phagocytic cells of the liver. Thus, they ingest endogenous and exogenous materials including blood pigments and in-

TABLE 7
Types of Tissue Responses to
Toxins

1. Cell Degeneration
   a. Reversible
2. Cell Death (Necrosis)
   a. Nonreversible
3. Regeneration
   a. Hyperplasia
   b. Mitotic figures
4. Chronic Tissue Damage
   a. Fibrosis
   b. Inflammation
   c. Immunopathology
5. Preneoplasia and Neoplasia

gested or injected substances. Biliary lesions involve the gall bladder (mice), extrahepatic and intrahepatic bile ducts, and cholangioles (formed by oval cells). The latter cannot be seen in normal liver. Ligation of the

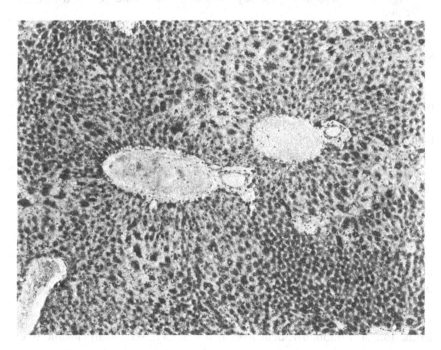

Fig. 12.   Centrilobular cytomegaly in liver of mouse given aldrin.

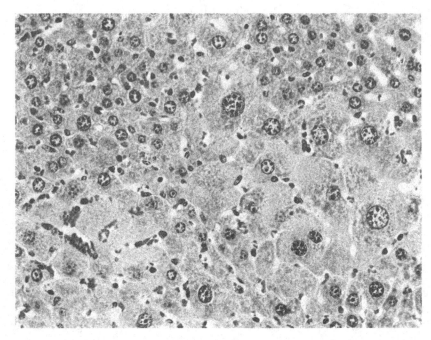

Fig. 13. Hepatic cytomegaly in mouse liver induced by α-benzene hexachloride.

common bile duct in rats stimulates the oval cells to divide and oval cell hyperplasia is visible in tissue sections. Specific toxins, primarily carcinogens, induce this lesion (Fig. 14). Cholangiofibrosis is a unique hepatic lesion of rats. It is characterized by atypical hyperplastic bile duct hyperplasia in fibrotic tissue (Fig. 15).

Cirrhosis in rodents differs from that in humans. Cirrhosis is defined as a chronic fibrosis of the liver with nodular regeneration induced primarily by chronic toxic hepatic insult. Degenerative and necrotizing hepatocyte lesions lead to fibrosis. The origin of fibrotic connective tissue in the liver may be from fibroblasts in portal areas or hepatocytes. It has been recently shown that hepatocytes can synthesize collagen and its precursors. In rodents, cirrhosis is most commonly of the biliary or pericellular type (Figs. 16–20). Biliary cirrhosis originates from portal areas or extensions of biliary tissue into hepatic lobules. Pericellular cirrhosis is a unique rodent lesion characterized by the presence of individual or bundles of reticulin fibers around individual hepatocytes. Fewer collagen fibers may be seen. Postnecrotic cirrhosis is rare in rodents and is a response to severe chronic necrotizing damage (Figs. 21, 22). The formation of a nodular rodent liver is not always seen with chronic liver

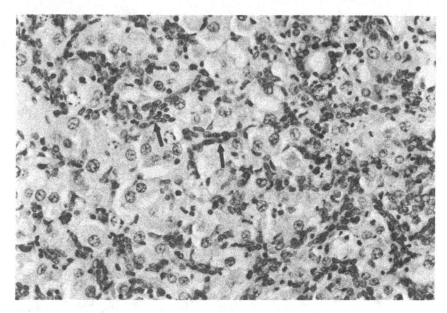

Fig. 14. Oval cell (cholangiolar) hyperplasia in F344 rat receiving direct benzidine-based dye for 90 days. Oval cells form cholangioles in the liver in some areas (arrows).

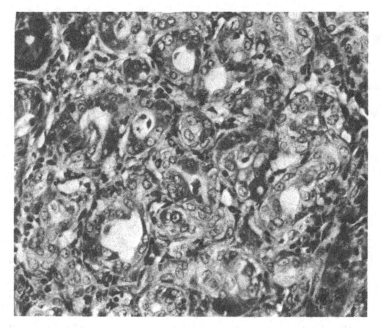

Fig. 15. Cholangiofibrosis in rat liver induced by methapyrilene.

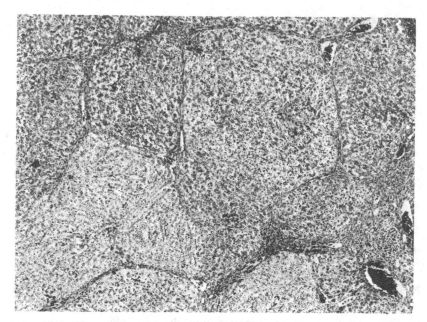

Fig. 16.   Biliary cirrhosis in liver of F344 rat given benzidine-based direct dye for 90 days.

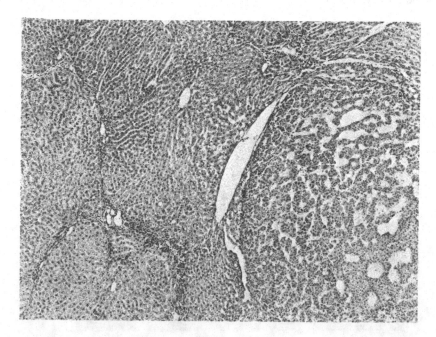

Fig. 17.   Trabecular hepatocellular carcinoma (on right) in cirrhotic (biliary) liver of rat given acetylaminofluorene.

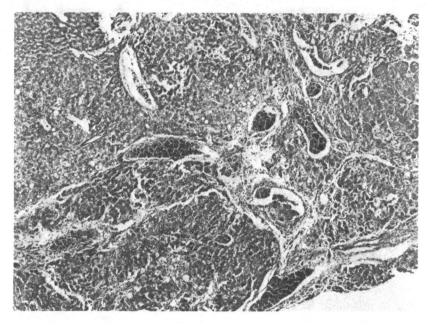

Fig. 18.   Advanced cirrhosis in liver of mouse given carbon tetrachloride. The entire liver is disorganized and it is difficult to ascertain normal architecture.

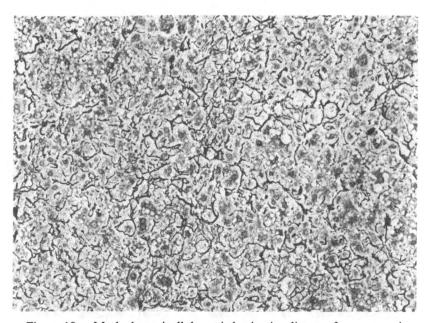

Fig. 19.   Marked pericellular cirrhosis in liver of mouse given tetrachlorvinphos. Note large numbers of reticulin fibers surrounding individual hepatocytes. Reticulin stain.

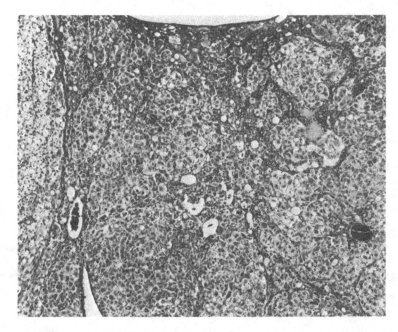

Fig. 20. Hepatic pericellular cirrhosis in rat given hexachlorodibenzo-*p*-dioxin. Portion of neoplastic nodule on left.

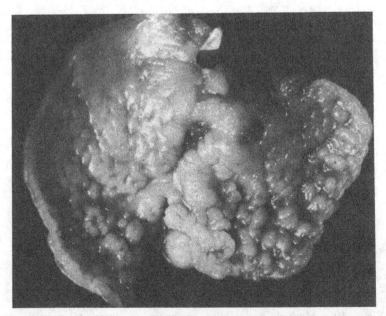

Fig. 21. Postnecrotic cirrhosis in a rat 90 days after continuous feeding of diallyl phthalate. Nodules are remnants of normal liver.

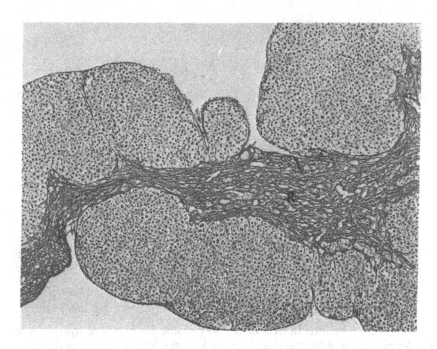

Fig. 22. Postnecrotic cirrhosis induced by diallyl phthalate in F344 rat liver after 90 days. Reticulin stain shows collapsed reticulin network and remaining areas of regenerating liver (apparent nodules).

damage. In mice, nodular cirrhotic livers are unusual unless tumors appear. When nodular rodent livers are seen, the nodularity is usually not the result of nodular regeneration, but rather to the accentuation of liver lobules or of surviving liver lobules that may be in various phases of regeneration. True nodular hyperplasia is difficult to define. Lobules or areas that show regeneration by the presence of active nuclei and mitotic figures often appear nodular only because of biliary fibrosis in the surrounding areas.

Regeneration is the process in which tissues repopulate their cells. In rodent liver, partial hepatectomy leads to true regeneration. The only evidence of regeneration in these livers is the presence of many mitotic figures. In fact, with toxic subchronic–chronic liver damage in rats and mice, degenerative and necrotizing hepatocyte lesions are seen without the formation of nodules (Fig. 23). Commonly associated with degenerative and necrotizing lesions in these livers, mitotic figures are seen to be evidence of regeneration (Figs. 24, 25). Nodules are first seen as early as 20–30 weeks in rats and 30–50 weeks in mice after initial carcinogen exposure. These nodules are the earliest evidence of neoplasia and have

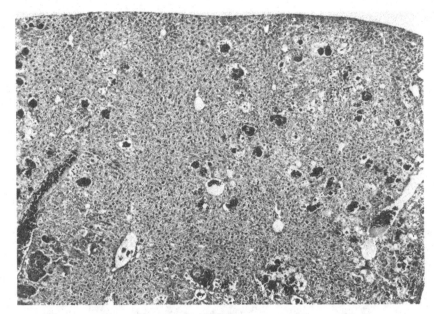

Fig. 23.   Peliosis in liver of B6C3F1 mouse fed butylated hydrotoluene for 2 years. Note dilated sinusoids throughout the lobules and no nodules.

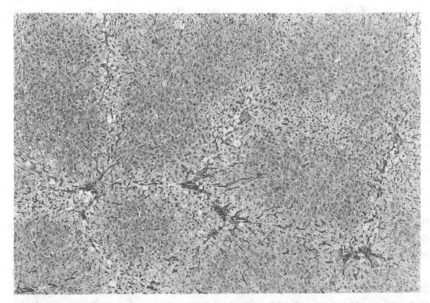

Fig. 24.   Rat liver with mild lipidosis after 90 days of dosing with bromodichloromethane. Note lack of nodule formation. Dark areas are erythrocytes in sinusoids.

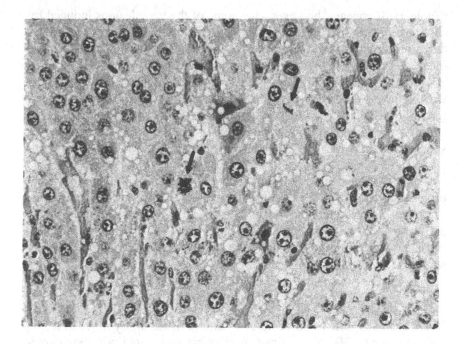

Fig. 25. High magnification of Fig. 24 showing lipid droplets in hepatocytes and mitotic figures (arrows) in hepatocytes, indicating regeneration procedes in this manner and not by nodular hyperplasia.

been termed neoplastic nodules in rats and hepatocellular adenomas in mice. These lesions may progress to carcinomas.

Toxic renal lesions are similar to those of liver. They are classified by anatomic location, morphologic type, and cause (toxic or vascular). In rodents, the location of the lesions may be dependent on the chemical and dose. The typical sequence of events is degeneration, necrosis, and regeneration. If the toxin is removed, regeneration may be complete, but may require several months to reach normal histology. Continuous exposure to the toxin eventuates in marked chronic renal damage. The chronic renal lesion may resemble the nephropathy of aging rats or may be characterized by unique lesions such as lead inclusions or adriamycin-induced vacuolization of glomerular epithelial cells.

Unique Toxic Lesions Induced by Carcinogens

It has been proposed that some unique toxic lesions are induced primarily by carcinogens (23). Chemicals, including chemical carcinogens, when given in lethal doses induce tissue damage, much of which is nonspecific

(Table 7). It appears, however, that some of the toxic lesions induced by carcinogens are specific for carcinogens (22). Although specific procedures or a certain few chemicals may also induce these unique lesions, over 95% of the chemicals that have induced these lesions are carcinogens for the same tissue. If this hypothesis holds up under closer scrutiny, we will have a relatively quick rodent bioassay. Thus, if a chemical tested for carcinogenicity in a bioassay induces these unique lesions, the chemical may be presumed to be a carcinogen from the results of an acute or subchronic bioassay. These lesions may be produced in hours, days, or weeks after chemical administration.

Some of these unique lesions may be preneoplastic, e.g., they may progress to cancer. These include the majority of hyperplasias and foci. They are usually reversible, however, especially after cessation of chemical exposure. Other lesions are toxic, such as oval cell hyperplasia, cirrhosis, and cytomegaly. The latter are responses to tissue damage and are sometimes reversible (Figs. 26, 27).

Toxicity and Carcinogenesis

It has been suggested that acute and chronic tissue injury may, in itself, lead to cancer (24). Rare human tumors are associated with bone frac-

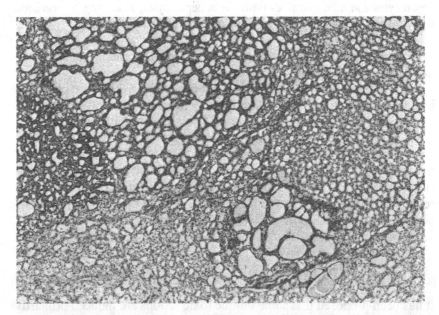

Fig. 26.   Diffuse and focal thyroid hyperplasia (goiter) induced in a rat by ethylene thiourea.

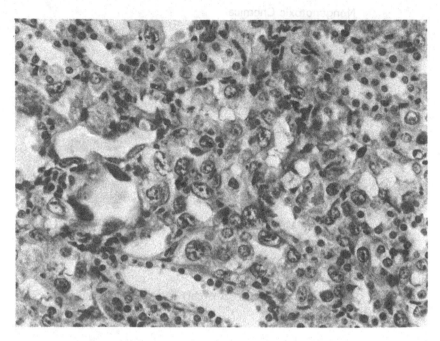

Fig. 27.   Giant nuclei (karyomegaly) in renal tubules of F344 rat 7 days after initial dose of Tris-(2,3-dibromopropyl) phosphate. At this stage it is difficult to distinguish between regenerative cytomegaly and a toxic cytomegaly.

tures, wounds, and so on. Horn core carcinoma in Indian cattle has been associated with irritation caused by halters. Solid state carcinogenesis in rodents may be associated with chronic tissue irritation. Yet direct evidence for the role of tissue damage *per se* leading to cancer is unconvincing and unproven. Genotoxic chemicals may cause mutations that lead to cancer. Nongenotoxic chemicals may cause cancer by as yet unknown mechanisms. A suggestion has been made that nongenotoxic chemicals may cause cancer via chronic tissue damage and its subsequent effects (Fig. 28). Abnormal mitotic figures can occasionally be found in rodent livers damaged by carcinogens, but prior to tumor formation (Fig. 29) (*25*). Some differences between genotoxic and nongenotoxic carcinogens are listed in Table 8. The classification of a chemical as a nongenotoxic carcinogen, or one that acts by an epigenetic mechanism, may depend, in part, on limited or incomplete information. The information is limited by the types of present day in vitro tests. Thus, nongenotoxic carcinogens are only those that have not yet been demonstrated to be genotoxic.

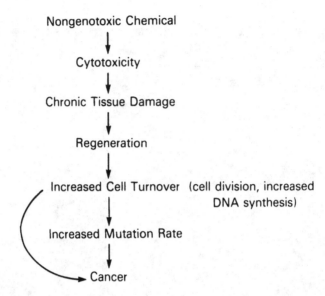

Nongenotoxic Chemical

↓

Cytotoxicity

↓

Chronic Tissue Damage

↓

Regeneration

↓

Increased Cell Turnover (cell division, increased
                                            DNA synthesis)

↓

Increased Mutation Rate

↓

Cancer

Fig. 28.   Hypothetical sequence of events if toxicity leads to cancer.

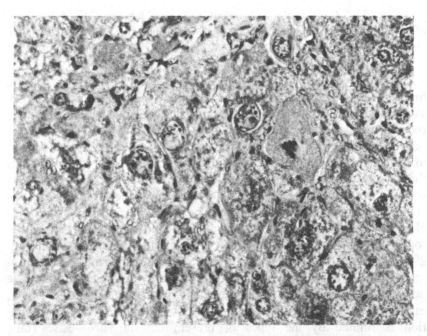

Fig. 29.   Abnormal mitotic figure in severely damaged liver (cytomegaly, oval cells) of mouse given *N*-nitrosodiethanolamine for 6 months.

TABLE 8

Differentiation of Genotoxic and Nongenotoxic Mechanisms of Carcinogenesis

Characteristic	Genotoxic carcinogen	Nongenotoxic carcinogen
Alkylates DNA in target tissue	Yes	No
DNA synthesis in target tissue	Not increased	Increased
Tissue damage at carcinogenic MTD[a]	No	Yes
Tumors not induced at doses below those causing chronic tissue damage	No	Yes
Morphology and biology of induced tumors compared with tumors in controls	Usually different	Similar or different

[a]Maximally tolerated dose.

In general, carcinogens that are genotoxic may be given at maximally tolerated doses (MTD) that do not produce either chronic toxic lesions or severe chronic tissue damage in tissues at the site of the carcinogenic process. This phenomenon depends in part, however, on the dose of the carcinogen. Most genotoxic carcinogens may be given at doses that cause chronic lesions and subsequent cancer, which then occurs at a dose-related earlier time than when lower MTD doses may be given. On the other hand, several nongenotoxic carcinogens have been shown to significantly increase tumor incidence only at MTD that cause chronic tissue damage (Table 8). As the dose is lowered, the amount of tissue damage is reduced and fewer tumors appear. This phenomenon is also true for genotoxic carcinogens. The maximum carcinogenic response, however, appears to be more dependent on tissue damage for nongenotoxic chemicals, especially for chlorinated pesticides and mouse liver (Tables 9, 10). Recently, six aromatic chemicals (Figs. 30–32) were shown to cause sarcomas of the spleen. They also cause methemoglobinema, hemosiderosis in the spleen, and splenic fibrosis. Without nonneoplastic splenic lesions, no tumors are seen. Since several nongenotoxic chemicals "induce" tumors at MTD or 1/2 MTD doses that do not cause chronic tissue damage (Table 10), other mechanisms of carcinogenesis may be postulated for these chemicals. For example, chlordane, 1,4-dioxane, chloroform, and tetrachloroethylene induce liver

TABLE 9

Carcinogens Inducing Liver Tumors in B6C3F1 Mice at Maximally Tolerated
Doses That Also Induce Chronic Hepatotoxic Lesions[a]

Compound	Type of Lesion
Genotoxic Chemicals	
Tetrachloroethylene	Cytomegaly
Trichloroethylene (males)	Cytomegaly, oval cell hyperplasia
Toxophene (males)	Cytomegaly
Chemicals Not Demonstrated to Be Genotoxic	
Aldrin	Cytomegaly
Dieldrin	Cytomegaly
Chlordane	Cytomegaly
Tetrachlorvinphos	Cirrhosis, granulomas
Chloroform	Cytomegaly, oval cell hyperplasia
Kepone	Cytomegaly
1,4-Dioxane	Cytomegaly
Chloramben (males)	Multinucleated hepatocytes
2,3,7,8-Tetrachlorodibenzo-*p*-dioxin	Cirrhosis
Hexachlorodibenzo-*p*-dioxin	Cirrhosis

[a]From the NCI Carcinogenesis Technical Report Series.

TABLE 10

Carcinogens "Inducing" Liver Tumors in B6C3F1 Mice at Maximally Tolerated
Doses without Chronic Hepatotoxic Lesions[a]

Genotoxic Chemicals	Chemicals Not Demonstrated to Be Genotoxic
2,4-Toluenediamine sulfate	Chloramben (females)
5-Nitroacenaphthene	2-Aminoanthraquinone
2-Nitro-*p*-phenylenediamine	1-Amino-2-methylanthraquinone
Sulfallate	*o*-Toluidine
Tris (2,3-dibromopropyl) phosphate	Di-(2-ethylhexyl)phthalate
Toxophene (females)	Di-(2-ethylhexyl)adipate
Trichloroethylene (females)	Eugenol
	Hexachloroethane
	Selenium disulfide

[a]From the NCI Carcinogenesis Technical Report Series, available from the National
Technical Information Service, US Department of Labor, 5285 Port Royal Road,
Springfield, VA 22161.

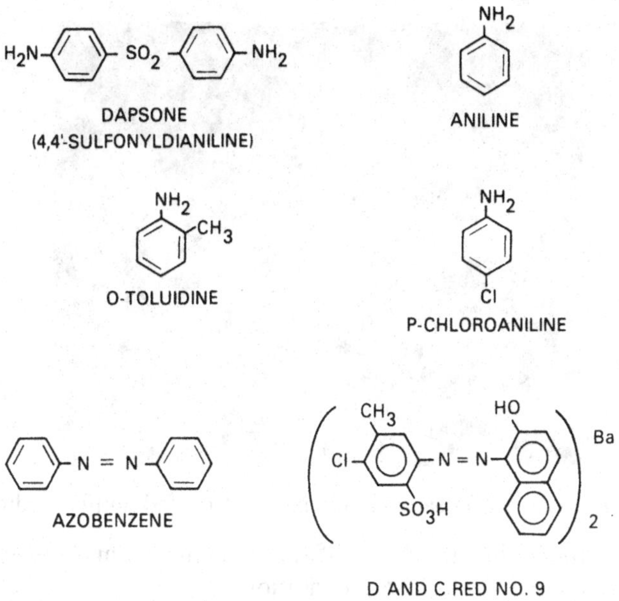

DAPSONE
(4,4'-SULFONYLDIANILINE)

ANILINE

O-TOLUIDINE

P-CHLOROANILINE

AZOBENZENE

D AND C RED NO. 9

Fig. 30. Structures of chemicals inducing splenic sarcomas and fibrosis and methemoglobinemia.

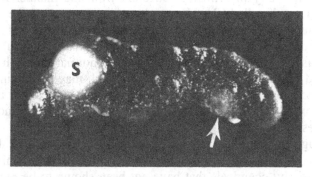

Fig. 31. Small (early) splenic sarcoma(s) and area of parenchymal fibrosis (arrow) in rat given aniline hydrochloride.

tumors in B6C3F1 mice at the MTD and 1/2 MTD and also chronic hepatic damage at the MTD but not at 1/2 the MTD. Promoters might not cause chronic tissue damage, but would promote tumors that morphologically and biologically resemble those in controls. On the other hand, some chemicals cause chronic hepatic damage in rodents without "inducing" liver tumors. For example, butylated hydroxytoluene induces hepatic cytomegaly in mice, and methotrexate administration leads

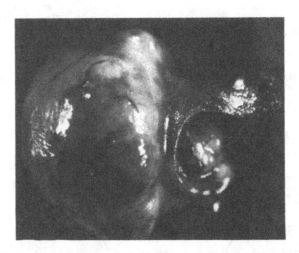

Fig. 32.   Large fibrosarcoma in spleen of rat fed aniline hydrochloride.

to hepatic cirrhosis in rats. None of these chemicals are hepatocarcinogens or carcinogens under other conditions.

Associated with chronic tissue damage caused by nongenotoxic chemicals is the use of possible inappropriate doses in rodent bioassays. The high doses used in these chronic studies may be metabolized and handled by the body in a manner different from the manner in which lower doses are handled. The lower dosage responses of the animals would of course more appropriately mimic human exposure and metabolism. High doses also may not be detoxified normally as would lower doses because of glutathione depletion. Thus abnormal metabolites may be produced by these high doses, some of which may be carcinogenic. The pharmacokinetics and tissue distribution of metabolites may also differ from normal, as might their effect on initiation and promotion of carcinogenesis.

Although the chronic tissue damage theory has some appeal, much information is lacking at present to explain the mechanisms of carcinogenesis by chemicals that have not been shown to be genotoxic. The definition of genotoxicity has yet to be finalized. Our classification is dependent on the test systems used. Perhaps most chemicals are genotoxic in at least one in vitro system, a suggestion recently made. If so, the classification into genotoxic and nongenotoxic is irrelevant. Hypothetically, the chronic tissue injury carcinogenesis theories may be limited, based on a lack of information, on the existence of unknown mechanisms of carcinogenesis by genotoxic and nongenotoxic chemicals, on the dose-response phenomenon and the limitations of present in vitro methods of testing for carcinogenicity.

Acknowledgments

The author is grateful for the editorial assistance of Fran Harris and photomicrography by Larry Ostby and Jack Romine. Some of the data presented in this chapter is derived from the NCI Carcinogenesis Technical Report Series on the carcinogenesis bioassays of more than 200 chemicals performed under contract to the National Cancer Institute and National Toxicology Program. The reports on individual chemicals are available from the National Technical Information Service, Springfield, Virginia. The data is derived from the Carcinogenesis Bioassay Data System. The pathology diagnoses in the CBDS is put into the system by pathologists at contract laboratories and their participation is acknowledged. Many of the diagnoses have been reviewed by NCI and NTP pathologists and verified.

References

1. Ward, J. M., Goodman, D. G., Griesemer, R. A., Hardisty, J. F., Schueler, R. L., Squire, R. A., and Strandberg, J. D., *J. Environ. Pathol.* **2**, 371 (1978).
2. Frith, C. H., *J. Environ. Pathol. Toxicol.* **3**, 231 (1979).
3. Kulwich, B. A., Hardisty, J. F., Gilmore, C. E., and Ward, J. M., *J. Environ. Pathol. Toxicol.* **3**, 281 (1979).
4. Frith, C. H., Boothe, A. D., Greenman, D. L., and Farmer, J. H., *J. Environ. Pathol. Toxicol.* **3**, 139 (1979).
5. Stewart, H. L., Dunn, T.B., Sneli, K. C., and Deringer, M. K., Tumors of the Respiratory Tract, in *Pathology of Tumours in Laboratory* Animals, vol. II. *Tumors of the Mouse,* Turusov, V. K., ed., IARC, Lyon, 1979, pp. 251–287.
6. Stewart, H. L., Comparative Aspects of Certain Cancers, in *Cancer—A Comprehensive Treatise,* Becker, F. F., ed., Plenum Press, New York, 320 (1975).
7. Altman, N. H., and Goodman, D. G., Neoplastic Disease of the Laboratory Rat, in *Biology of the Laboratory Rat,* Baker, H. J., Lindsey, J. R., and Weisbroth, S., eds., Academic Press, New York, 334–376, 1979.
8. Burek, J. D., *Pathology of Aging Rats,* CRC Press, West Palm Beach, 1978, p. 230.
9. Squire, R. A., Goodman, D. G., Valerio, M. G., Frederickson, T. N., Strandberg, J. D., Levitt, M. H., Lingeman, C. H., Harshbarger, J. C., and Dawe, C. J., Tumors, in *Pathology of Laboratory Animals,* vol. II. Benirsche, K., Garner, F. M., and Jones, T. C., eds., Springer-Verlag, New York, 1978, pp. 1051–1283.
10. Turusov, V. A., ed., *Pathology of Tumours in Laboratory Animals,* vol. *I. Tumours of the Rat,* part 1, IARC, Lyon, 1973, p. 214.

11. Turusov, V. S., ed., *Pathology of Tumours in Laboratory Animals*, vol. *1. Tumours of the Rat*, part 2, IARC, Lyon, 1976, p. 319.
12. Turusov, V. S., ed., *Pathology of Tumours of the Mouse*, IARC, Lyon, 1979, p. 669.
13. Ward, J. M., Sagartz, J., and Casey, H., *Pathology of the Aging F344 Rat*, Armed Forces Institute of Pathology, Washington, DC, 1980, p. 41.
14. Coleman, G. L., Barthold, S. W., Osbaldiston, G. W., Foster, S. J., and Jonas, A. M., *J. Gerontol.* **32,** 258 (1977).
15. Goodman, D.G., Ward, J. M., Squire, R. A., Chu, K. C., and Linhart, M. S., *Toxicol. Appl. Pharmacol.* **48,** 237 (1979).
16. Goodman, D. G., Ward, J. M., Squire, R. A., Paxton, M. B., Reichardt, W. D., Chu, K. C., and Linhart, M. S., *Toxicol. Appl. Pharmacol.* **55,** 433 (1980).
17. Sheldon, W. G., and Greenman, D., *J. Environ. Pathol. Toxicol.* **3,** 155 (1979).
18. Ward, J. M., Goodman, D. G., Squire, R. A., Chu, K. C., and Linhart, M. S., *J. Natl. Cancer Inst.* **63,** 849 (1979).
19. Gart, J. J., Chu, K. C., and Tarone, R. E., *J. Natl. Cancer Inst.* **62,** 957 (1979).
20. Tarone, R. E., Chu, K. C., and Ward, J. M., *J. Natl. Cancer Inst.* **66,** 1175 (1981).
21. Ward, J. M., *Prog. Exp. Tumor Res.* **26,** 241 (1982).
22. Ward, J. M., and Reznik, G., *Prog. Exp. Tumor Res.* **26,** 266 (1982).
23. Ward, J. M., *Med. Hypotheses* **6,** 421 (1980).
24. Reitz, R. H., Watanabe, P. G., McKenna, M. J., Quast, J. F., and Gehring, P. J. *Toxicol. Appl. Pharmacol.* **52,** 357 (1980).
25. Schrankel, K. R., Hsia, S., and Pounds, J. G., *Res. Comm. Chem. Pathol. Pharmacol.* **28,** 527 (1980).

Chapter 9

Carcinogen Bioassay Design

J. F. Douglas

Bioassay is the measurement or estimation of animal response to a chemical ingredient. "Bioassay," often used instead of the term "carcinogenic bioassay," is time-consuming, expensive, and insensitive. Yet, to date, it is still the only acceptable procedure for assessing carcinogenic potential. Almost all known human carcinogens have also been demonstrated to be animal carcinogens. Although carcinogen bioassay is still an evolving procedure and will improve as the state of the art matures, the long-term solution to this evaluation of carcinogenic potential is to find faster, simpler, and more reliable indices of carcinogenesis. Exploration of substitutes for bioassay has generated considerable effort, a discussion of which forms the basis for the first portion of this book.

It has long been recognized that cancer can be subdivided into a variety of diseases and conditions, all resulting in an uncontrolled growth of tissues. Gene mutation of the DNA has been a unifying endpoint in neoplasia, although other factors may play a significant role in cancer origin. Included in these other factors are turning on of transforming genes, chromosome translocation and, in some cases, viruses. DNA change, which can occur decades prior to clinical manifestation in humans, is small enough so that the cell is undamaged, yet permanent, so that it is transmitted genetically to daughter cells. At some point in time, for reasons as yet poorly understood, the cells proliferate abnormally and produce a tumor. This process has been described as the initiator-promoter concept.

131

The response of experimental animals to a carcinogenic stimulus, although highly complex and dependent upon numerous factors, both endogenous and exogenous, is just one more toxicological endpoint. As such, it follows the classical dose dependence described by Paracelsus and elaborated for cancer by Druckery (1). The response curve to a carcinogen can be one of several patterns, as shown in Figs. 1 (2) and 2 (3). Moreover, the question of a threshold effect (Fig. 2C) versus a linear effect (Fig. 2A or 2B) has never been resolved. This has recently become more of an issue following the findings of the Federal Government's massive "megamouse" study (ED_{01} carcinogen bioassay of 2-acetylaminofluorene [2-AAF]) (4). In this experiment with the known carcinogen 2-AAF, the development of bladder and liver neoplasms was evaluated. The bladder neoplasms had a rapid onset, could be catalogued as following the threshold concept, and developed the high incidence of tumors only with continued application of the carcinogen. The liver neoplasms on the other hand had a slow onset, gave a linear response, and their ultimate incidence was not affected by the withdrawal of the 2-AAF.

Table 1 lists some of the inherent conditions known to affect tumor development. Although there is general qualitative agreement among species and strain in their reaction to administration of a specific chemical, sufficient exceptions exist to exercise care in selection of the experimental animal.

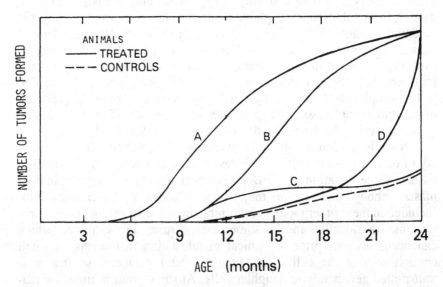

Fig. 1. Theoretical relationship of tumors formed with age of animals.

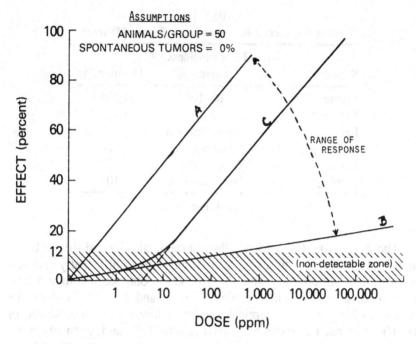

Fig. 2. Possible dose–response curves to carcinogens.

TABLE 1
Physiological Factors Affecting Tumor Development

Species	DNA repair mechanisms
Strain	Mutational state
Age	Hormonal (stress)
Immunologic factors	State of health (infection)

The first of these factors is illustrated in Table 2, where differences were found among six species to the skin painting of benzo(a)pyrene (5). Notable is the finding that some rodents—mouse and rabbit—gave positive responses, whereas others—the rat and guinea pig—were unaffected by this chemical.

TABLE 2
Species Difference in Response to Benzo(a)Pyrene[a]

Species	Tumor incidence (range), %	Duration, yr
Mouse	60–100	0.2–0.6
Rabbit	2–15	0.7–4
Rat	None detected	2
Guinea pig	None detected	2
Fowl	None detected	2
Monkey	None detected	10

[a]Painted (0.1–0.5%) 2 or 3 times weekly.

There is substantial evidence that inbred strains have different backgrounds of spontaneous tumors, and also can respond differently to divergent chemical structures. Table 3 illustrates spontaneous tumor differences in mice (6, 7), while Tables 4 (8, 9) and 5 (10, 11) show the variability of response to chemically induced tumors in various strains of rats. The response range can vary from zero to 100% and, even where the animals give a positive response in the same target organ, the quantitative differences can be significant. The target site may also be a property of animal strain.

Less well-documented but of critical importance are the effects of infective agents, immunologic factors, as well as the inherent capacity of the animal body to repair the deleterious actions of exogenous agents. Al-

TABLE 3
Effect of Mouse Strain on Carcinogenic
Response to Urethan

Strain	Pulmonary tumors	
	Spontaneous, %	With urethan treatment, %
A	17	100
Balb/c	3	100
C3H	None detected	76
FA	None detected	0
DBA	None detected	16

TABLE 4

Mammary Cancer in Rat Strains Induced by Oral
Administration of 7,12-Dimethylbenz(a)anthracene

Strain	Test dose, mg	% With mammary tumors
August	30	90
Wistar	45	100
Chester Beatty	45	92
Marshall	30	0
Sprague-Dawley	20	100
Long Evans	20	16

though stress has been implicated as one of the contributing factors to incidence of cancer in humans, it has not been well-illustrated in the laboratory animals. Della Porta and Terracini (12) have shown that the age at
which a single administration of a known carcinogen is given to female
rats can affect neoplasm production (Table 6).

The tumor development process can be modulated by environmental
parameters, some of which are shown in Table 7.

Items that minimize the probability of infection (Table 8, No. 1) (3)
such as animal derivations including source, animal production, use of
defined flora, and laboratory procedures can all be critical. Although
strong evidence does not exist regarding specific interaction between infection and chemically induced cancer, animal health status does affect
longevity and study reproducibility. Chemical pollutants (Table 8, No. 2)
can affect bioassay results. These contaminants can exert their effect
through a variety of known cancer-producing mechanisms, including di-

TABLE 5

Effect of Rat Strain in Cancer Induction by 2-AAF

Strain	Mammary tumors, %	Liver tumors, %
Osborne-Mendel	62	0
Marshall	0	80
Sprague-Dawley	64	4.5
Copenhagen	0	20

TABLE 6
Starting Age and Effect of a Single Administration
of N-Nitrosodimethylamine in Famale Rats

	Dose, mg/kg	Tumor incidence, %	
		Renal	Liver
> 1 d	21–25	40	44
12–15 wk		8	0
—	Untreated	4	0

rect carcinogenesis, cocarcinogens, promoters, or initiators. It is almost impossible at the present time to completely exclude small amounts of known carcinogens from animal feed in the form of pesticide residues, and most public water systems in the US contain at least micro amounts of unwanted chemicals. Effective animal management is necessary to maximize the usefulness of bioassay data and eliminate testing problems (Table 8, No. 3). Autolysis/cannibalism, for example, can significantly affect the analysis of results if good laboratory practices are not strictly adhered to. Not only must moribund animals be sacrificed promptly, but they also must be autopsied before deterioration sets in.

Diet and nutrition have been shown to alter carcinogenic response. Two examples are shown in Tables 9 (13) and 10 (14), where oxidized corn oil and caloric content significantly modify tumor incidence. Although strong experimental evidence does not exist for these particular experiments, one can speculate that oxidation of corn oil produces peroxides that may interact with DNA. Data are accumulating that minimal caloric intake is consistent with strong immune competence. Excess calories can adversely affect this biological function.

Protein intake has also been shown to be an essential factor in carcinogenic responses. Care should also be exercised to avoid dietary constituents that act as promoters. An example of the latter is the effect of the amino acid L-tryptophan on N-nitrosodiethylamine carcinogenesis (Table 11) (15).

TABLE 7
Environmental Factors Affecting Tumor Development

Animal husbandry practices
Nutritional state and diet
Route of administration
Dosage regimen

TABLE 8
Management, Supply, and Husbandry Factors
That Can Influence Carcinogenesis Tests

1. Infectious diseases
   Viral
   Bacterial
   Parasitic

2. Chemical pollutants in
   Feed
   Water
   Bedding
   Air

3. Operations management
   Cannibalism
   Autolysis
   Vermin infestation
   Cross-contamination

The rationale behind a carcinogen bioassay affects its design, this, in turn, can affect the nature of the bioassay result. Since data evaluation rests largely on the statistical analysis of tumor pathology, it would be imperative to have as sensitive an endpoint as possible. Unfortunately, the cost limitations of lifetime studies with extensive histopathology input place restrictions on the number of animals, or groups of animals, which in turn may affect study sensitivity. Table 12 (16) lists the underlying probability of tumor occurrence needed to attain a statistical significant result ($p = 0.05$) compared to the probability of spontaneous tumors in the control group. An insensitive design resulting from inadequate animal

TABLE 9
Effect of Oxidized Corn Oil on 2-AAF Carcinogenesis in Rats

AAF, %	Oxidized oil, %	Sex	Tumor incidence, %		
			Liver	Ear duct	Mammary gland
0.05	—	M	0	0	0
0.05	—	F	0	0	13
0.05	2.5	M	96	21	70
0.05	2.5	F	89	21	94
0.00	—	M	0	0	0
0.00	—	F	0	0	0

TABLE 10
Effect of Caloric Content in Diet on Mouse
Skin Tumors[a]

Diet during application[b]	Subsequent diet[b]	Tumor incidence, %
High	High	69
High	Low	34
Low	High	55
Low	Low	24

[a]0.05 mg benzo(a)pyrene applied twice weekly.
[b]Caloric content.

group sizes, refractory species/strain, or low dose levels can give a false negative result.

If the test rationale was the risk to a particular level of chemical, it might be impractical to develop the appropriate sensitivity, since that would entail hundreds of test animals per group. If a smaller group size were employed *a priori,* the test might be negative for carcinogenicity when in fact there is a definable risk. The alternative approach to administering a high dose of compound to animals—maximum tolerated does (MTD)—has its limitations: namely, possible alteration of normal metabolic pathways, immunological depression, and the difficulty of extrapolating from large doses in animals to smaller exposure levels in humans. The MTD philosophy is well suited to a screening study in which the test rationale is a simple yes–no answer to the question of carcinogenicity potential. Perhaps the best approach, where possible, would be an initial screening procedure at the MTD, with appropriate toxicologic safeguards to ensure that the dose was not causing some abnormal biological or metabolic effects, followed by a study with smaller doses in which a large animal group could be used. If the latter design was focused only on the target tissue in a relatively sensitive animal, it would be economically feasible.

TABLE 11
Effect of L-Tryptophan in N-Nitrosodiethylamine Carcinogenesis

L-Tryptophan, %	N-Nitrosodiethylamine, mg/d	Tumor incidence, %
1	0.00	0
0	0.79	17
1	0.77	62

TABLE 12

Underlying Probability of Tumor Occurrence in Chemically Treated
Animals Needed to Obtain Significance [a]

Control (spontaneous)	No. of animals per group[b]				
Probability of tumor, %	10	25	50	75	100
0	55.2%	29.5%	15.4%	10.4%	7.9%
2	71.6%	33.2%	20.8%	15.5%	13.3%
5	68.7%	39.7%	27.0%	21.6%	18.8%
10	76.2%	49.1%	35.7%	29.8%	26.6%
20	86.7%	62.2%	49.0%	43.3%	39.7%
30	94.3%	72.6%	61.1%	54.5%	51.2%

[a]Detected with 90% probability by a one-sided Fisher's Exact Test carried out at
the 0.05 level.
[b]Control and treated groups of same size

The dosage regimen, which should be consistent with the test rationale, can markedly alter the test outcome. With some carcinogens, a single administration is sufficient to induce neoplastic responses, whereas at the other extreme, continuous dosing for a lifetime is necessary to produce significant tumor results. The ED_{01} study at the National Center for Toxicological Research (4), which will be discussed in detail later, provides interesting examples of the effects of both duration of treatment and dosage levels.

A carcinogen bioassay may be subdivided into a number of discrete elements as follows:

> Experimental design
> Selection of suitable facility (only if using an outside contractor)
> Prechronic studies
> Chronic study including interim sacrifices
> Histopathology
> Collection of data and analysis
> Report writing and publication

Overlying many of these steps are also safety and health requirements in the handling of a potential carcinogen by the personnel or Laboratory Investigators and an appropriate quality assurance—good laboratory practices function in many of the study phases.

After the study objective has been delineated, selection of the chemical form and purity can pose a problem. Do you test a pure chemical or the form to which the public is exposed, such as a technical grade material? The salt or the nonsalt form? If there are a number of commercial producers with different manufacturing processes and an outside agency is conducting the test, from which is the material chosen? What level of impurities is acceptable? Should certain specific impurities be excluded?

Selection of species and strain is another critical element in bioassay design. Ideally, one would prefer an animal sensitive to carcinogens and with a low or negative spontaneous tumor rate. In practice, rodents have been almost exclusively used as the test animal of choice because of their relatively short life, response to chemicals, ease of handling, modest cost, and the existence of an adequate background on their aging disease state. Dogs, monkeys, and so on, have not proven practical in extended studies because of their longer age span, high maintenance costs, and the difficulty of using groups large enough for statistical accuracy. Of the rodent species used extensively, only a few strains have been utilized to a considerable degree. For rats, the Fischer 344, Osborne-Mendel, and Sprague-Dawley strains are cited most often in the literatures. Currently, the F344 rat, which is used almost exclusively by the NTP Carcinogenesis Testing Program, is employed most frequently. It is small, has good longevity, is docile, can be readily produced, and its background tumor levels have been documented in thousands of animals. Similarly the hybrid mouse B6C3F1, a cross of the C3H/Hen male and the C57BL/6N female, is the current strain of choice by the National Toxicology Program (NTP). Table 13 provides the percent of spontaneous tumors found in untreated animals used in the NTP studies (17).

The number of doses chosen and the dose ranges are a function of test rationale and sensitivity desired. Where information is known or suspected for a particular chemical, Tables 12 and 13 can be helpful in selecting group size. In addition to the number of animals desired at test termination, provision should be made for sentinel animals (quality assurance) and for projected interim sacrifices.

The route of administration, which can include oral (dosed feed, dosed water, and gavage), skin paint, inhalation, implantation, or injection (intraperitoneal, subcutaneous, and intravenous) is usually selected on the basis of reason for testing, chemical stability, and target site.

Study length can vary, although generally a fixed 2-yr duration or lifetime is chosen. If the latter is selected, provision should be made for sacrifice when a minimal number of animals in a group (species and sex) have survived. Multigeneration or *in utero* studies are sometimes conducted when this type of program would yield the desired information.

There are a number of approaches to histopathology sampling. The two principally utilized are examination of all tissues from all animals or initial observation of all tissues from the high dose and control groups only, followed by analyses of the critical target sites in every animal. Another interesting approach is a random statistical selection of tissues followed by examination of all tissues with tumors in the original group observed (18, 19). This procedure should be less costly, preserve a critical bioassay element (pathology time), yet yield accurate results. Recently, Dr. E. E. McConnell at NTP has advocated the use of a smaller number of tissues for histopathology with an initial evaluation only from the highest test group and control based on gross necropsy observations and an analysis of positive tumor findings in several hundred NTP bioassays (20). Dependent upon these results, additional organs are then examined.

It should be remembered that carcinogenicity is a special endpoint in a toxicology study, and therefore the experimental design should take this into account. Often, additional toxicology parameters are also part of the overall design. The latter can include other procedures as clinical chemistry, cytology, hematology, behavioral studies, immunotoxicology, metabolic patterns, and so on. These ancillary designs are useful not only in defining the toxicology of the chemical under tests, but also are frequently useful in clarifying the mechanisms of action.

To properly select the levels of chemical administered in a chronic study, it is necessary to perform a series of dose-ranging studies. The toxicity of the test chemical on the particular strain employed can vary as illustrated in an NTP rat strain sensitivity study now underway using five different rat strains. In this experiment, it was found that toxicity to different strains varied widely to the chemical being used, trichloroethylene. Even with a careful estimation of MTD for chronic studies, an occasional study is aborted because of excessive lethality. The current prechronic studies include an acute one-dose, followed by a 2 wk repeated dose study, and a subchronic study of 90–180 d duration. The data obtained from the previous experiment is the basis for establishing the successive study doses. A valuable addition in planning the prechronic evaluation is to include other appropriate parameters so that a thorough toxicological profile can be obtained for the chemical being examined.

If there is no substantial information on the chemical toxicity, then the first procedure employed is an acute toxicity test. The acute toxicity is generally run with five animals per group in a two species study with both sexes of each species used. A minimum of three (3) dose levels, and preferably five (5) dose levels, are used with a concentration difference between each level being a factor of two. The route generally utilized is gavage administration. Treatment is for one day, followed by a 2-wk observation period. At sacrifice or death, no histopathology is performed, although the tissues should be saved for possible examination based on subsequent findings.

TABLE 13

Percent Spontaneous Primary Tumors in Untreated Species Used at NCI for Carcinogen Bioassays

Species: Strain:	Mouse, B6CF1		Rat, Fischer 344		Rat, Osborne-Mendel		Rat, Sprague-Dawley		Rat, Charles River CD	
Sex:	Male	Female	Male	Female	Male	Female	Male	Female	Male	Female
Number necropsied:[a]	3543	3617	2960	2924	270	270	440	205	184	184
Organ/tissue										
Brain	<.1%	.1%	.8%	.6%	—	—	.7%	.5%	2.7%	1.6%
Skin	3.1	1.7	7.8	3.2	8.9	5.9	3.2	3.4	7.1	3.3
Mammary gland	—	1.3	1.5	20.9	3.7	28.5	1.4	39.0	.5	45.1
Circulatory system[b]	2.9	2.4	.7	.4	4.1	2.6	—	—	2.2	45.1
Lung/bronchi/trachea	13.7	5.2	3.0	1.9	1.5	.7	—	—	1.6	1.6
Liver	24.6	4.7	2.2	1.9	1.1	1.9	.2	.5	.5	2.2
Pancreas	<.1	<.1	.2	—	—	—	—	—	—	—
Stomach	.4	.4	.3	.2	—	.4	—	—	—	.5
Intestines[c]	.5	.2	.6	.3	.4	.4	.2	—	—	.5

Kidney	.3	>.1	.5	.2	3.3	2.6	—		1.6	—
Urinary bladder	<.1	<.1	.1	.3	.4	—	.2		.5	—
Preputial gland[d]	—	—	2.4	1.8	1.6	1.2	—	—	—	NA
Testes[e]	.4	NA	82.3	NA	.7	NA	2.0	NA	3.9	.5
Ovary	NA	.9	NA	.4	NA	1.5	NA	NA	NA	3.8
Uterus	NA	1.6	NA	17.0	NA	3.7	NA	4.4	NA	3.8
Pituitary	.3	3.6	14.7	34.9	7.4	20.0	5.9	40.0	33.2	57.6
Adrenal	1.4	.6	12.4	5.2	10.4	10.0	.7	2.9	7.6	4.3
Thyroid	1.0	1.7	8.2	6.8	9.6	11.1	.9	2.0	3.8	—
Pancreatic islets	.4	.2	3.9	.8	3.0	1.9	.5	.5	2.7	—
Body cavities	.4	.3	2.6	.4	1.9	.4	.5	1.9	2.2	—
Leukemia/lymphoma	10.3	20.6	19.9	13.4	3.3	1.8	4.8	0.5	3.3	3.3

[a] Studies terminated at 21–25 months for mice and 23–25 months for rats.
[b] Hemangioma and hemangiosarcoma.
[c] Duodenum, jejunum, ileum, cecum, and colon.
[d] Clitoral gland in females.
[e] Seminal vesicle and testis.

The second phase, the repeated dose study, is run to set the doses for the subchronic evaluation and consists of groups including controls of five animals each. Generally, two species and sexes are tested. There are usually five dose levels, differing by a factor of two with the highest concentration equal to or less than the LD_{10} calculated from the acute toxicity experiment. These doses are LD_{10}, ½ LD_{10}, ¼ LD_{10}, and so on. The animals are treated daily for 14 d by the route planned for the chronic study, observed 1 d, and sacrificed. Weights are taken weekly and a gross necropsy performed, but generally there is no histopathological examination unless a particular finding so indicates.

The last of the prechronic studies is the subchronic. It is usually run for 90 d, but can be extended for 180 d or longer, depending upon the nature of the chemical, its toxicological profile, and the manner in which the body stores the chemical. Care should be exercised with lipophilic materials that are stored in the fat, since short time periods often do not represent their true toxicity. After the fat depots are saturated, excessive chemical becomes available for biological activity, and this must be fully recognized in an experimental design of a chronic nature. Conversely, subchronic study periods of less than 90 d, such as 6 wk, frequently give unreliable results in terms of estimating 2-yr levels for a maximum tolerated dose. A 90-d minimum for the subchronic has several other advantages, including sufficient time to develop appropriate toxicological observations and occasionally indications of the carcinogenic target site.

Usually the subchronic study consists of groups of 10 animals of each sex and species at each dose level including the controls. Five dose levels are generally employed, with the highest being the dose level in the repeated dose study that showed no clinical signs of toxicity, had no significant pathological changes, or appreciable weight gain depression. Other doses decrease by fractions of the largest dose, usually by a factor of two: ½, ¼, ⅛, and 1/16. The route of administration is that planned for the chronic carcinogenicity experiment. In addition to clinical observations, animals are weighed weekly and sacrificed 1 d after their last treatment. A careful gross necropsy is performed, and a histopathological examination is conducted on the controls and the highest dose of each sex and species that had a survival rate of at least 60%. Target organs are examined histopathologically for all animals of that sex and species until a no-effect dose level is reached.

The long-term or chronic study is the critical procedure for evaluating the carcinogenic potential of a chemical or other substance. The study objective can markedly affect the experimental design, particularly group size, dosage levels, number of doses, route, and pathology sampling.

Group size is a compromise of the resources available, power of the test, target site-spontaneous tumor rate, and previous experimental evidence of tumorogenesis of the test compound. Although the first two items have been discussed earlier, it is worth reemphasizing the carcinogenicity evaluations may not give sensitive endpoints and are highly dependent on statistical analysis of the data. A weak carcinogen can be insidious and, if acting on a specific organ with a moderate spontaneous tumor rate, difficult to detect. For example, a material inducing 10% tumor formation at a site with close to a 0% spontaneous rate would go undetected (statistically insignificant) in the commonly used group size of 50 animals. This, translated into the US population of over 200,000,000 people, indicates how critical it is to identify correctly any chemical with carcinogenic potential. Generally, the group size employed is fifty (50) for each sex and species, which provides a statistical inflection point below which sensitivity is significantly impaired and above which there is minimal gain for the considerable extra expense. Additional animals are often included as health sentinels and for histopathology workup where required. With a chemical for which considerable background is available, it is sometimes possible to limit the study by sex and species and focus on a single tissue. In the situation with a weak-acting carcinogen, it is feasible to increase the group size substantially to a hundred or more animals.

Studies are generally conducted in two rodent species, the rat and the mouse, with the hamster used occasionally.

Control groups of equivalent size to the test chemical group are employed. Selection of the number of control groups can be an important aspect of the experimental design. A matched control group, treated exactly like the test chemical group except for the compound administration, is a must.

Besides the vehicle control, an untreated group (if the route is gavage, injection, and so on) can be employed, particularly when the test laboratory and the species are not well-documented with respect to background tumor development. If several studies are conducted simultaneously, each should have its own control group to avoid the problems that can readily occur with the joint arrangement of common control groups. At present, positive controls are seldom used, but should be considered in specific circumstances.

The age of the animal at initiation of chemical treatment can be critical. Generally, 6 wk has been chosen as the earliest practical time. This permits weaning at 3–4 wk, shipment, and 2 wk of quarantine. Earlier starts have been criticized on the basis of immature metabolic systems. Multigeneration studies can have a number of unusual design features including preconception, *in utero* (transplacental), and immediate onset of chemical treatment at birth.

Route of administration is determined by the best rationale, exposure situation, or the screening test philosophy that delivering the maximum amount of agent to the target site is critical in evaluating the carcinogenic potential of a compound. The methods of treatment generally utilized are dosed feed, dosed water, skin paint, gavage, and inhalation. Usually the first two types of administration are carried out 7 d/wk, whereas the others are principally given 5 d/wk. Also used, although rarely, are intraperitoneal or other parenteral routes.

Perhaps the most controversial aspect of a carcinogenicity study is the selection of the number of doses and their levels. A yes–no study or screen employs the maximum tolerated dose (MTD), i.e., the dose level that does not produce toxicologic signs or histopathologic lesions other than neoplastic that could be considered life-threatening during the course of a chronic study. A weight gain within 10% of the controls is also considered for determination of the MTD. In this procedure a second does usually ⅓ or ½ the MTD is also administered. The MTD concept has been criticized from essentially two viewpoints: namely, (1) that it may significantly alter or overwhelm the metabolic and other patterns (i.e., DNA repair and immune responses), and (2) that the concentration has no relevance to human exposure or risk to the chemical being investigated. The former point has merit in some situations, but it certainly should not be applied in a blanket fashion without extensive comparative metabolic data, particularly considering variation in human metabolic patterns. For risk assessment purposes, the MTD has limited application; however, for a screening rationale it is undoubtedly the best approach to the problem at the present time. Unfortunately, when a chemical has been shown to be an animal carcinogen, the public presssure often dictates that the Governmental regulatory agencies act promptly rather than spend the 3–5 yr needed for a well-designed dose–response and relevant metabolism study that would be more applicable to a risk assessment judgment. In fact, one law—the Delaney Clause (21)—mandates that any material found carcinogenic at any dose level cannot be used as a food additive.

A dose–response carcinogenicity evaluation is designed similarly to any other toxicology study. The number of animals per group is determined by the anticipated tumor percentage at each dose level. This often leads to an unbalanced design that is critical for statistical significance at the lower levels of administered chemical.

Test duration to be effective must be at least 2 yr in length. An earlier sacrifice period does not permit sufficient time for tumor development at most organ sites. If the target tissue is known early evidence of malignancy has been indicated, the experiment can be designed on this basis. There is a body of thought, particularly at the IARC, that the experiment should proceed on a lifetime basis to generate full development of tumors. The main objections to this school of thought are the high background of spontaneous lesions generated in the aging animal and the unresolved discussion of when to terminate the study as deaths occur in various groups. Generally, the additional stress to the animals receiving the test chemical produces earlier deaths than the control group. To have statistical equality, all studies should have a predetermined point of sacrifice of all animals when one group reaches a specific survival level, i.e., 10%, or 20%, and so on.

It is important in all toxicological evaluations to observe the animals frequently for clinical signs and health status. Most laboratories within the NTP Master Agreement have two daily checks, once in the morning and again in the late afternoon. Any moribund or dead animals should be removed and necropsied as soon as possible. It is essential to determine the cause of death or disease to maintain study integrity. As the experiment progresses, the animals should be palpated more frequently. Animal health should also be followed by measuring weight, weekly for the first three months and monthly thereafter.

At termination, the animals are necropsied, the tissues preserved, and histological slides prepared. The gross necropsy procedure is probably the one step in the experimental operation that is most underrated. A well-qualified pathologist, experienced in rodent tumors, should be responsible to carefully supervise this aspect of a carcinogenicity evaluation. All gross observations should be recorded and slides prepared from the appropriate tissue part. Sampling, like many scientific endeavors, is a critical experimental aspect dependent upon experience, art, and science.

With a material of unknown effect, a wide spectrum of tissues is selected for complete histopathologic examination. Table 14 lists the tissues examined microscopically in the NTP Carcinogenesis Testing Program.

In designing a chronic bioassay and in the subsequent interpretation of the data, a variety of fundamental factors relating to the interaction of the chemical and the mammalian organism should be considered.

The National Toxicology Program is considering modifying the pathology protocol. Currently being discussed are (1) the addition of an interim sacrifice of all groups (10 animals/dose/sex/species) at 15 months to better characterize the toxicology lesions. All tissues (Table 14) would be examined histopathologically in these animals; (2) animals that die or are sacrificed before 21 months would have the full microscopic evaluation of

TABLE 14
Complete Histopathologic Examination Will Be Performed on
These Tissues

Gross lesions	*Tissue masses or suspect tumors*
Skin	*and regional lymph nodes*
Mandibular lymph node	Ileum
Mammary glands	Colon
Salivary glands	Cecum
Thigh muscle	Rectum
Sciatic nerve	Mesenteric lymph node
Sternebrae, vertebrae	Liver
or femur including marrow	Gall bladder (mice)
Costochondral junction, rib	Pancreas
Thymus	Spleen
Oral cavity, larynx and	Kidneys
pharynx	Adrenals
Trachea	Urinary bladder
Lungs and bronchi	Seminal vesicles
Heart and aorta	Prostate
Thyroid	Testes, epididymis, vaginal tunics
Parathyroids	of the testis and scrotal sac
Esophagus	Ovaries
Stomach	Uterus
Duodenum	Nasal cavity and nasal turbinates
Dejunum	Brain
Tongue	Pituitary
	Spinal cord
	Eyes
	Preputial or clitoral glands
	Zymbal's glands (auditory sebaceous)
	glands)

all tissues (Table 14); (3) for 24 months sacrific and animals that die after 21 months, after a thorough gross necropsy, only the high dose and control animals would have histopathology. The latter would be limited to selected tissues—16 for females and 18 for males; and (4) target organs detected either at gross necropsy or histopathology would then be examined in all other animals.

The pharmacokinetics of the compound can be important in understanding the study, and they should be relevant to the experimental conditions. Thus, a simple one-dose administration is insufficient. Rather, the various rates that develop under dose load, multiple administration, and long-term dosage need to be evaluated. Any pharmacological–toxicological action should be explored for mechanism. Is the administered chemical a procarcinogen, a direct-acting carcinogen, or does it act through an intermediary such as hormones? Is the administrative regimen altering the metabolic pattern toward or away from a carcinogenic effect? Is an MTD leading to metabolic products not normally present at lower levels of administration?

To appropriately evaluate and analyze the experiment, a variety of data in addition to histopathology must be considered. This includes experimental design, food consumption, clinical signs, survival information, weight patterns, chemical analysis, and other literature information. Survival information includes time of animal death and its nature, i.e., natural, serial sacrifice, or terminal sacrifice. Survival is usually graphically represented by standard means (plot of the probability of surviving versus time in study) or with Kaplan-Meier (plot of the probability of surviving from natural death versus time on study). These curves are then compared by either the Breslow test or the Cox-Tarone test.

In evaluating the significance of the tumors found histopathologically, incidence data is critical: that is, the number of animals with a specific tumor divided by the number of that target site examined. The incidence data is analyzed statistically either unadjusted or by time-adjusted methods. At NTP, the former is accomplished with a series of procedures including the Fisher Exact test (Bonferoni criteria), Cochran-Armitage, and binomial probability. The latter uses the Breslow, the Cox-Tarone, and the cumulative incidence tests.

Although evaluation and interpretation of bioassay results will be discussed in detail in a later chapter, a brief review of the results analysis will be helpful in designing and conducting appropriate studies. Griesemer and Cueto (20) have developed a decision tree that permits variable classification of the experimental evidence for carcinogenicity (Fig. 3). Step one is the adequate design and conduct of the study. An overview of these essential elements, which consist of the desired factors cited elsewhere, are presented in Table 15.

The increased incidence of malignant tumors (step two) is dependent on suitable statistics and evaluation by a multidiscipline team. These include combination of tumors, rare tumors, age adjustment at specific type and site, and appropriate use of various control groups. Equivocal results can arise from several sources, but usually develop when the chemical-treated group varies statistically between the matched controls and the historical controls.

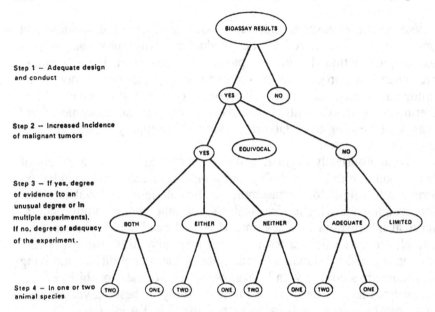

Fig. 3.   Decision steps in evaluating degrees of experimental evidence for carcinogenicity.

The extent of the evidence (step three) can be utilized as an index to the severity of carcinogenicity produced by a particular chemical when sufficient experimentation has been performed. An unusual degree of evidence can be derived from high tumor incidence at a specific site, unusual tumor types, several tumor sites, early onset of tumor, both sexes in-

TABLE 15
Adequacy of Bioassay Design and Conduct

1. Appropriate route of administration
2. Proper test species and strain
3. Contamination in test agent (chemical)
4. Identification of test chemical
5. Adequate group size
6. Long-term administration of chemical
7. Adequate survival
8. Suitable matched controls
9. Adequate pathology review
10. Potential for body retention—body burden
11. Metabolic overload

volved, or corroboration of other literature studies. No evidence of carcinogenicity can be classified into an adequate study and limited information. The latter is derived from an inadequate dose and/or other mitigating factors.

Based on their decision tree, Griesemer and Cueto have divided the weight of carcinogenicity evidence into nine categories, ranging from very strong evidence in two species to no evidence in two animals species. This will be discussed in greater detail in the following chapter.

Care should be exercised in simply classifying a chemical as positive (carcinogen) or negative (noncarcinogen) resulting from one or more animal bioassays. Not only are there degrees of activity by dose and time but also by site of action. Examples are polycyclic hydrocarbons that induce cancer where applied to the skin, and compounds that produce tumors in specific internal organ sites after ingesting. Direct application of the chemical to the target tissue can increase potency. For example, DMBA administered as tracheal implants of 10 μg/d produces tumors in 4 months.

Chemicals that produce early cancer after 3–4 months of administration, such as benzidine-based dyes, ethylene dibromide, dibromochloropropane, or aflatoxin, which produces cancer at feed levels of 1 ppb, are potent carcinogens compared to captan, which was barely carcinogenic to mice at 16,000 ppm in the feed for 80 wk.

Many chemicals require continuous administration to induce neoplasia, as with 2-AAF for mice bladders, whereas other very potent materials, such as diethylnitrosamine, can produce tumors in offspring in 90–120 d when given once to pregnant animals.

Understanding of possible results is fundamental in the designing and conducting of a bioassay. Results of one recent study are given as illustrations of possible endpoints. This is the huge experiment employing over 20,000 mice to evaluate in detail the carcinogenic potential of 2-AAF. The critical data are the nature and extent of neoplasms developed in the bladder and liver. Figure 4 depicts the bladder tumor response with respect to dose at various sacrifice times. A threshold effect can readily be visualized for each sacrifice time.

A similar plot of the liver neoplasm data (Fig. 5) shows a linear dose–response relationship, with the conclusion that the liver cancer formation follows the "one hit theory" dose dependency; that is, a single molecule of a compound interacts chemically with DNA to produce an irreversible genetic change.

If 2-AAF administration is discontinued after 12 months and the animals maintained for 24 months prior to sacrifice, there is again a sharp

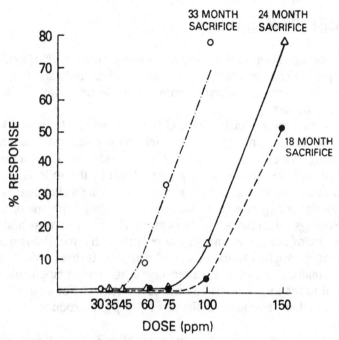

Fig. 4. The prevalence of bladder neoplasms in sacrificed mice with respect to dose.

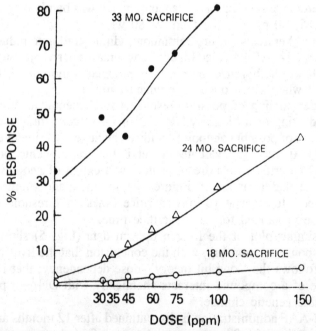

Fig. 5. The prevalence of liver neoplasms in sacrificed mice with respect to dose.

152

difference between the two different sites regarding tumor progression. The bladder neoplasm incidence is sharply reduced relative to the 24-month dosage, while the incidence of liver tumors, on the other hand, is only mildly affected by cessation of chemical treatment and there is no significant effect in cancer growth from the additional administering of 2-AAF (Figs. 6, 7).

There is as yet an untested theory emerging that could account for the sharp differential pattern between the liver and bladder tumor formation. The latter neoplasm could originate by an epigenetic mechanism— tissue injury that must occur repeatedly until tumors are formed, thereby requiring massive doses to (1) overcome DNA repair processes, and (2) constantly injure tissue and require regeneration. Withdrawal of the injury stimulus would shut down the regeneration process and very few cancers would form. The mechanism for the liver neoplasm could be genetic, i.e., interaction with DNA at an early stage, producing a linear dose relationship, and cessation of chemical stimulation would have a minor effect on final cancer incidence.

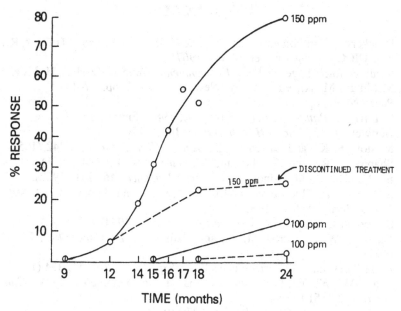

Fig. 6.   The prevalence of bladder neoplasms in mice fed 2-AAF for 12 months and sacrificed at 24 months.

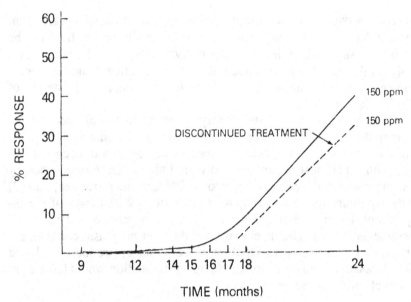

Fig. 7. The prevalence of liver neoplasms in mice fed 2-AAF for 12 months and sacrificed at 24 months.

References

1. Druckery, H., in *Potential Carcinogenic Hazards from Drugs*, Truhaut, R., ed., UICC Monograph Ser. 7, 60 (1967).
2. Modified form. Page, N. P., in *Environmental Cancer*, Kraybill, H. F., and Mehlman, M. A., eds., Wiley, New York, 1977, pp. 87–171.
3. Page, N. P., op. cit.
4. *J. Environ. Pathol. Toxicol.* 3 (No. 3), 1980, Entire issue.
5. Hartwell, J. L., *Public Health Service* 149, 1951.
6. Mostofi, F. K., and Larsen, C. D., *Am. J. Clin. Pathol.* **21**, 342 (1951).
7. Shapiro, J. R., and Kirschbaum, A., *Cancer Res.* **11**, 644 (1951).
8. Boyl and, E., and Sydnor, K. L., *Brit. J. Cancer* **16**, 731 (1962).
9. Sydnor, K. L., Butenandt, O., Brillantes, F. P., and Huggins, C., *J. Natl. Cancer Inst.* **29**, 805 (1962).
10. Symeonidis, A., *J. Natl. Cancer Inst.* **15**, 539 (1954).
11. Dunning, W. F., Curtis, M. R., and Madsen, M. E., *Cancer Res.* **7**, 134 (1947).
12. Della Porta, G., and Terracini, B., *Prog Exp. Tumor Res.* **11**, 334 (1969).
13. Sugal, M., Witting, L. A., Tsuchiyama, H., and Kummerow, F. A., *Cancer Res.* **22**, 510 (1962).
14. Tannenbaum, A., *Cancer Res.* **4**, 673 (1944).
15. Kawachi, T., Hirata, Y., and Sugimura, T., *GANN* **59**, 523 (1968).

16. Haseman, J., personal communication.
17. Chu, K. C., Cueto, C., and Ward, J. M., *J. Toxicol. Environ. Health* **8**, 251 (1981).
18. Fears, T., and Douglas, J. F., *J. Environ. Pathol. Toxicol.* **1**, 125 (1977).
19. Fears, T., and Douglas, J. F., *J. Environ. Pathol. Toxicol.* **1**, 211 (1978).
20. Griesemer, R. A., and Cueto, C., in *Molecular and Cellular Aspects of Carcinogen Screening Tests,* Montesano, R., Bartsch, H., and Tomatis, L., eds, IARC Scientific Publications No. 27, International Agency for Research on Cancer, Lyon, 1980, pp. 259–281.

Chapter 10

Evaluation and Interpretation of Carcinogenesis Bioassay Results

Cipriano Cueto, Jr.

General Considerations

Although various approaches to carcinogenesis testing have been proposed [e. g., Weisburger and Williams (1)] involving short-term in vitro tests and limited or short-term in vivo tests using a tumorigenic endpoint, chronic carcinogenesis bioassay in animals is still the method most commonly used to detect the potential carcinogenicity of chemicals to humans. These bioassay methods have various levels of sophistication, sensitivity, and predictability. The tests are usually performed in mice and rats because of their relatively short lifespan, their known historical control-tumor incidence, their cost, and their availability relative to other species. The results of these tests are used for species and dose extrapolation and as a measure, or more properly an indication, of the potential risk to humans of the compound tested, as well as a means of evaluating the relative carcinogenic activity of chemicals within a specific biological testing system.

It must be recognized that the objective of most carcinogenesis bioassays is to determine whether a chemical, when administered by any route to animals at doses and experimental conditions that maximize the sensitivity of the test, induces or promotes a cellular transformation that leads to the development of a tumor. Such an objective is considered to be

157

the first and most basic step in determining the qualitative capability of a chemical to produce a carcinogenic effect on a specific host. Although this type of testing and the data it generates may be used to predict the ability of the chemical to produce a carcinogenic response in humans, in general it would be going well beyond the scope of the data to predict the actual qualitative site and the quantitative nature of the response in different species, including humans. Thus carcinogenesis bioassays are considered not to be well-designed to generate quantitative "safety data" as are the more classsical toxicological tests involving other endpoints than those of tumor induction.

Within the last three years, the National Cancer Institute and later the National Toxicology Program have published in the Carcinogenesis Technical Report Series the results of the bioassays of over 200 compounds. These studies have generated certain basic approaches to the evaluation and interpretation of carcinogenesis bioassay results (2). It is clear that the evidence for carcinogenicity, or the lack of this effect, differs considerably from one bioassay to another. The evidence for different chemicals may range from overwhelmingly positive to negative or be of a borderline nature and difficult to interpret. The purpose of this presentation is to emphasize some of the basic characteristics and problems with carcinogenesis bioassays in terms of the evaluation and interpretation of results obtained in testing a few selected chemicals. Detailed information about each bioassay in the National Cancer Institute studies can be obtained from the original reports* for each specific chemical.

Overview of Bioassay as Conducted

As a first step in the process of evaluation of the results of a bioassay, the overall experimental design is considered in terms of the limited and specific objectives stated in the above section. For this purpose, it is considered that as a basic requirement each of the major elements of the bioassay specified below should be evaluated as to the degree or extent of their adequacy. It is recognized that many other experimental design factors or elements having a possible impact on bioassays have been considered in the technical literature, and the reader is referred, as a source for these, to pertinent chapters in this treatise and to the International Agency for Research on Cancer, Monographs Supplement 2 (IARC, 1980). The

*Reports from the Carcinogenesis Technical Report Series are available from the National Technical Information Service, US Department of Labor, 5285 Port Royal Road, Springfield, Virginia 22161.

statement of major basic factors is not to imply that other factors may not be important, but only to indicate that the overview evaluation must be accomodated or facilitated by setting some guidelines about what basic elements are indicative of the adequacy of the study. These may be modified as the reviewer's training, experience, or objective dictates.

Suggested major basic elements of bioassay experimental design:

1. Identification of the test material and its relative purity and stability.
2. Periodic documentation of the dose or concentration that the animals received throughout the study.
3. Use of an appropriate route of administration to facilitate the stated objective.
4. Use of an adequate number of animals at risk per group throughout the test.
5. Use of an appropriate randomization of animals, i.e., to cages and dose groups.
6. Administration of the test compound to both sexes of two appropriate species of rodents.
7. Administration of doses at levels approximating a maximum permissible dose based on documented 90-d subchronic results and at least one close, but lower, fraction of this dose.
8. Administration of the test compound for the major part of the animals' normal lifespan.
9. Use of appropriate control animals.
10. The taking of appropriate and detailed observations, involving mortality, weight gain, food consumption, clinical signs, and pathology.
11. Statement of the specific type of statistical analysis to be used.

The sum total of the degree to which each of the above factors is considered either deficient or adequate in a particular study determines the reliability of the results. Each factor can affect the reliability in a different way (qualitatively) or to a different extent (quantitatively). The effect also depends on the characteristics of the results. For example, in the case of a test considered adequate in terms of all the above-indicated major basic factors, except for the number of animals used or surviving, a negative finding would force one to consider the results as questionably reliable based on this inadequate number of animals. On the other hand, a significant positive finding under the same set of conditions would be considered reliable, notwithstanding the reduced sensitivity that results from that low number of animals or poor survival. This should not be misinterpreted as a bias; it should be recognized that the closer the response in dosed animals is to that of the controls (approaching a negative finding) the more "hard data" is needed to consider the response reliable in either a negative or positive direction. An extreme case of an unreliable and unacceptable statistically positive pathological finding at a specific target organ is typified by testicular interstitial-cell tumors in Fischer 344 rats. The incidence of these tumors in undosed control groups of F344 rats at any laboratory ranges between 50 and 100%. Any positive response to a test chemical at this target-site, including a dose-related response, is considered unreliable (unlikely to be a reproducible result). This is true notwithstanding the fact that comparison of the incidence of these tumors in dosed animals with that found in concurrent controls may result in a statistically significant finding. Other possible target-sites representing this extreme situation in the particular species or strain of test animals used in the bioassay should be identified for purposes of proper evaluation.

In a typical chronic bioassay for carcinogenicity, the analytically defined test chemical is adminstered on a daily basis in feed or 5 d/wk for gavage, dermal, or inhalation studies for a period of 18–24 months to both sexes of specifically defined mice and rats. The test compound is usually administered by the route most comparable to that of human exposure or by a route considered to facilitate administration and achieve maximum systemic exposure of the test animal. At least 50 animals of each sex are used per group. Since the animals of each species are usually grouped five to a cage by sex and treatment, they are individually randomized using a table of random numbers into cages, and the cages are then similarly randomized into treatment groups. A minimum of two dose levels is used, and an undosed or vehicle dosed group of animals of each sex serve as controls. The highest dose used is that predicted, on the basis of a 90-d subchronic study, to be the Maximum "Tolerated" Dose (MTD). If only two doses are used, the second dose is generally half of the MTD, since much lower doses could reduce the sensitivity of the test to such an extent that negative results or results approaching a negative finding could be considered unreliable.

The MTD is *defined* as the maximum dose of the test chemical that, when administered under specified conditions during the carcinogenesis bioassay, is predicted not to significantly alter the animals' *survival* compared to controls, except from effects involving carcinogenicity. The MTD is *estimated* from the results of a 90-day subchronic study of the test chemical administered under the same specified conditions as those that will be used in the chronic phase of the bioassay. This estimation is made based on the highest dose considered by a team of experts (consisting of at least a toxicologist, a pathologist and a statistician) to meet the following criteria, *as applied to the subchronic data:*

1. No mortality.
2. Weight gain decrement of approximately 10%.
3. No other sign or clinical finding of life-threatening overt toxicity.
4. No progressive or life-threatening pathological lesion.

These criteria are not intended to be applicable to the findings of the carcinogenesis bioassay; they are intended to be a basis upon which to estimate the maximum test dose that will permit maximum survival of the test animals and facilitate optimum bioassay sensitivity. If later in the chronic phase of the test, the dose that produces a carcinogenic effect also produces an overt toxic effect, the test material is nevertheless considered carcinogenic to the test animals under the conditions of the bioassay; however, further research is warranted, using experimental designs suitable for the new objective of clarifying, if the overall *chronic toxic effects* predisposed the test animal to the carcinogenic response.

Under these considerations, the MTD should be viewed not as a tolerated or nontoxic dose in the bioassay, but rather as a maximum test dose intended to permit optimum test sensitivity, the results of which may warrant further toxicological studies. It seems to follow that the MTD notation then should be considered as more correctly representing a Maximum Test Dose.

During a typical carcinogenesis bioassay, observations of mortality, moribundity, signs and clinical findings of toxicity, palpable masses, body weight, and food consumption are made throughout the study at predetermined frequencies for each of the observations. The duration of the dosing period is typically 18–24 months for mice and 24 months for rats. Animals dying during the chronic phase of the study are necropsied. Moribund animals and animals surviving until the end of the study are killed and necropsied. Twenty-five to 30 different topographical tissues and any masses detected during gross observation are taken from each animal for microscopic examination.

Once the adequacy of the experimental design has been assessed, the second step of the overall evaluation of a carcinogenesis bioassay is that of determining the extent to which the study has been appropriately conducted.

The complexity of conducting a bioassay is discussed in detail in another chapter of this treatise and has been reviewed [Arcos et al. (3); Berenblum (4); Canadian Department of Health and Welfare (5); Golberg (6); Sontag et al. (7); Page (8); IARC (9); Chu et al. (2)], officially published as proposed guidelines [EPA (10, 11); IRLG (12)], and aspects concerning Good Laboratory Practice published as official regulations [FDA (13)]. It is recognized that both experimental design and conduct of the test can vary extensively between laboratories. Perhaps one of the basic reasons for this variation is the lack of recognition that any carcinogenesis bioassay is actually a hypothetical test for an effect of a chemical whose ultimate mechanisms of cancer induction and promotion are not sufficiently understood. The test, because of its hypothetical nature is always considered deficient in one way or another. Although there are pros and cons to these considerations, the test is generally handled as a limited research problem in chemical carcinogenesis and considered primarily to be a relatively standardized diagnostic screening test for qualitative assessment of the possible biological effect of a chemical on a specifically defined biological system. To this end, certain well-established principles or concepts must be recognized and used as basic requirements in the design and conduct of chronic toxicological tests in which cancer is considered as a possible endpoint. This is essential if the results of the test are to be reproducible and valid.

In summary, it must be considered that as part of this initial evaluation of the overall adequacy of a bioassay, statements of experimental design, including materials and methods, the conduct of the test, and eventually the evaluation of the results, must be reviewed with respect to their nature, appropriateness, and the extent to which they consistently meet well-recognized principles. The adequacy of the test, and therefore the reliability of the results, is considered to be proportional to the extent or degree of adherence to these principles.

Nature and Evaluation of Results

The carcinogenesis bioassay, although limited in its scope to testing chemicals for the possible qualitative induction or promotion of a carcinogenesis process in experimental animals, is a complex test providing results that are often very difficult to evaluate. In many areas the evaluation is fraught with controversy. it is quite clear that any one scientist's knowledge of the analysis and evaluation of bioassay results has severe limitations. Expertise or intuition in one field may not be transferable to another field. A multidisciplinary approach must be used not only in designing and conducting the test, but also in evaluating its results. The evaluation should be a joint, interactive, formal team effort of scientists having recognized expertise in at least the following disciplines: chemistry, toxicology, pathology, and statistics.

Having first assessed the degree of adequacy of the design and conduct of the bioassay, the evaluative team formally states the extent of acceptability of these parameters and their possible limitations. Attention is then given to assessing the results in terms of the nature and the extent of the evidence or lack of evidence for the induction or promotion of a carcinogenic process by the test chemical.

Prior to analysis and evaluation of any data generated by the bioassay, the data itself must have attained a final form of validation and presentation. Since the main endpoint of the test involves histo-pathological lesions, uniformity and accuracy of diagnosis and nomenclature must be achieved. All information considered relevant to interpretation of the bioassay findings is collated and tabulated for analysis. Statistical analyses are performed, particularly on the probability of survival and the incidence of neoplasms.

Survival

The chronic administration of the test chemical may decrease the survival of dosed animals compared to controls. This constitutes evidence that the chemical was tested at or near the maximum test dose level possible under the conditions of the bioassay. It is considered essential to the carcinogenesis bioassay that the high dose administered produce some limited sign of toxicity, such as a limited decrease survival of animals. Alternatively, evidence of an MTD must be clearly established based on the 90-d subchronic test. This is particularly true, as stated earlier, for those tests resulting in negative findings. In such cases, a survival rate greater than 35/50 (70%) at the end of the chronic dosing period is usually considered the minimum requirement for maintaining the optimum sensitivity of the test.

The bioassay of the insecticide endosulfan (NCI, *17*) presented negative findings associated with high mortality in both sexes of rats but only in male and not in female mice. Such findings lead to consideration of the possibility that no evidence for carcinogenicity was obtained and that the results are limited because of the reduced sensitivity of the test. The bioassay of 1,2-dibromoethane (NCI, *19*), 1,2-dichloroethane (NCI, *16*), and 1,2-dibromo-3-chloropropane (NCI, *15*) in turn presented statistically significant, highly positive findings in both sexes of rats and mice associated with overt toxicity and high mortality in both sexes of both species. Such findings lead to the conclusion that there is evidence, to an unusually strong degree and in multiple tests, for the carcinogenicity of these compounds in two species of rodents. However, under the conditions of the bioassay, the effects of overt toxicity on the results of such tests need further clarification and may thus require further toxicological studies.

Growth, Feed Consumption, and Morbidity

The dose of the test chemical administered may also adversely affect the growth, feed consumption, and clinical health status of tested animals. As stated earlier, these adverse effects may be taken as evidence that the chemical was administered at or near the maximum possible test dose under the conditions of the bioassay. However, such adverse effects if extensive may compromise the reliability of the results. The extent of the compromise must be evaluated for each set of data. The following are a few examples of how these factors (similar to survival) tend to modulate the evaluation and interpretation of bioassay findings.

Decreased growth or body weight gain of dosed animals compared to controls may lower the rate of tumor formation and thus reduce the total tumor incidence or the number of tumors found at specific anatomical sites in dosed animals. Such effects could result in a false negative finding or in a decreased overall positive response. This decreased overall response could then be attributed to a decreased baseline (spontaneous) incidence of tumors and/or a decreased carcinogenic response to the test chemical. Decreased body weight gain in test animals may result from either test compound toxicity or decreased feed consumption. The decreased food intake, in turn, may also result from either the toxicity of the test chemical or the animals' refractiveness to the dosed diet. Furthermore, it is generally recognized, although the data is somewhat limited, that rats and mice receiving certain test materials by gavage or in drinking water also tend to reduce their intake of standard undosed basal diet. Feed consumption in many instances is not considered reliable data owing to the extensive variation involved in this measurement, particularly with animals that tend to scatter feed and deposit urine and feces in certain types of feeders. The possible causes of decreased feed consumption, toxicity, and/or refractiveness to the feed cannot be dissociated; however, normal or increased feed consumption associated with a decreased weight gain in dosed animals compared to controls is evidence that the animals' weight-gain decrement results from toxicity and not from "starvation".

Mean body weight data associated with poor survival may present "soft" rather than "hard" data. It must be considered that, since the size of a group diminishes because of mortality, the mean body weight may be subject to wide variation as a result of possible weight bias in either dead or surviving animals. The meaningfulness of the data may then be questioned.

All clinical signs relating to survival, growth, morbidity, feed consumption, appearance, behavior, clinical chemistry, and palpable masses should be reviewed, quantitated to the extent possible, and analyzed for any dose-related effects. It should be emphasized again that if the doses that produce a carcinogenic effect also produce an overt toxic effect, the test material is considered carcinogenic to the test animals under the conditions of the bioassay; however, further research should be required to clarify whether the overall chronic toxic effects play a significant role in initiating or promoting the carcinogenic reponse.

Pathology Findings

A carcinogenic response is considered evident when a test chemical administered to groups of animals in an adequately designed and conducted bioassay results in a statistically significant, time-adjusted increase in the incidence of one or more types of malignant neoplasms, or of a combination of benign and malignant neoplasms, in at least one group of dosed animals as compared to controls maintained under identical conditions but not dosed with the test compound. The carcinogenic response is regarded with greater confidence if statistically significant results are obtained in more than one dosed group, sex, or species. This confidence is further enhanced if a dose–tumor response relationship is evident.

Since the criteria for carcinogenicity are based on the extent and accuracy with which the organs and tissues of dosed and control animals can be microscopically examined for lesions, the findings of the primary pathologist must be reviewed and verified by at least two groups of referee pathologists to ensure that proper nomenclature has been used, and that the interpretation and classification of lesions is correct. The quality, accuracy, and extent of pathological examination and documentation are therefore basic requirements for the validity of animal bioassays (2, 7, 12, 13, 21).

Once the pathology diagnoses are verified and their validity accepted, a summary table of neoplastic (and nonneoplastic) lesions in each group of controls and dosed animals of each sex and species is prepared for review and to facilitate statistical evaluation. For this purpose, the professional judgment of the pathologist must be relied upon for the appropriate grouping of tumors. It is considered unacceptable in a long-term bioassay to combine all tumors into one category and analyze the incidence of total tumor-bearing animals in dosed versus control groups. This defeats the purpose of the bioassay since, under the long-term conditions of the test, the majority of animals will develop one type of malignant tumor or another. It is also considered inappropriate to subdivide tumors by anatomical site or morphologically into so many individual groups as to reduce the power of the test to detect an effect. However, it must also be considered inappropriate to combine unrelated tumors in a way that maximizes the power of the test, while disregarding whether such groupings are biologically correct.

It is generally accepted that the incidence of tumor observed at different target sites can be evaluated separately, as if each target site tumor type developed independently from each other. There are exceptions to this, such as in the cases of leukemia and specific tumor types originating in blood vessels of nerves at different sites. These in general are combined for analysis. The judgment of an experienced pathologist must be relied upon in determining whether tumor formation at *different anatomical sites* in histogenically related tissue *or* tumors of different histological types (adenocarcinoma and undifferentiated carcinoma) arising at the *same anatomical site* should be analyzed as combined and/or separate tumors. In the first instance, tumors of the same general histological type that arise at different sites in the same tissue type are usually grouped together for analysis. In the second instance and in all cases where judgment about groupings may be difficult, it is generally considered that the tumor types should be evaluated separately and combined.

The combination of benign and malignant neoplasms in the bioassay is disapproved by some pathologists, who correctly point to the critical scientific difference between a benign and a malignant tumor. Others point out that this distinction is not meaningful in a bioassay and consider further that the statistically significant increase of specific benign tumors alone in dosed animals as compared to controls may be a sensitive indicator of the induction of a carcinogenic process. Regardless of both of these considerations, there are strong arguments (9, 12, 22) based on scientific findings that such benign tumors should be part of the total carcinogenesis evaluation. It is considered likely that many malignant tumors in animals do not metastasize. The differential diagnosis of a tumor's benign or malignant nature is thus largely based on the tumor's histological characteristics. Expert pathologists may disagree about the diagnosis of those tumors that are considered borderline between the two categories. The recognition that the pathologist in some cases may not be able to clearly distinguish between such tumors is often considered as a basis for combining them for purposes of statistical analysis. It has been recognized for many years (22) and recently restated (9, 12,) that the scientific community in general is unaware of a chemical that (when properly evaluated in any species in a carcinogenesis bioassay) induces only benign tumors and no malignant tumors. It is further recognized that very few, if any, benign tumor types are now known that in time, and under appropriate enhancing conditions, do not undergo transition to a malignant neoplasm. Squire and Levitt (23) reviewed the literature describing the pathogenesis of rat liver tumors. Thus chemicals that significantly increase benign tumors are looked upon with as much concern about their potential human hazard as those that induce malignant tumors in an animal carcinogenesis bioassay. For purposes of objective evaluation, these two tumor types, when found in the same type of histogenic tissue and usually at the same anatomical site, are analyzed statistically as both separate and combined tumor categories. If the occurrences of malignant tumors alone or the combination of malignant and benign tumors are statistically significant in dosed animals compared to controls, the test material is considered carcinogenic to the specific test animals under the conditions of the bioassay. If only the benign tumors are statistically significant, the test material is considered a suspect carcinogen to the specific test animals under the conditions of bioassay (2).

Statistical Analysis

Generally, in a carcinogenesis bioassay, statistical analyses are directed at detecting significant survival and tumor differences between dosed groups and controls, as well as any possible dose–response relationship of these parameters. Other observations, such as growth, feed consumption, morbidity, clinical chemistry, and organ weight–body weight ratios, should be quantitated and analyzed to the extent deemed possible by the responsible toxicologist and statistician. Although most of these latter observations have considerable variation, they nevertheless may contribute importantly to the overall evaluation.

In most bioassays (National Cancer Institute/National Toxicology Program) the probability of survival is estimated by the product-limit procedure of Kaplan and Meier (24) and are usually presented in the form of graphs. Analyses for a possible dose-related trend is conducted using the method of Cox (25) for testing two groups for equality and the extension of this method by Tarone (26).

The incidence of neoplastic lesions usually are presented and analyzed as the ratio of the number of animals with such lesions at a specific anatomical site to the number of animals in which that site was examined microscopically. However, the denominator may consist of the total number of animals necropsied when gross examination is used as a basis to determine tissue sampling or when lesions such as lymphomas appear at multiple sites. The traditional Fisher's exact test (27) for pairwise comparison, the Cochran-Armitage linear trend test for dose–response relationship (28, 29), as well as life table methods and time-adjusted analyses, are commonly used. The problem of error rates involved in the statistical analyses of tumor incidence is discussed by Fears et al. (30) and by Chu et al. (2). Difficulties in the interpretation of statistically significant findings for specific "spontaneous" tumors that have a high and variable incidence in a given strain and sex of test animals are discussed by Tarone et al. (31).

Two other methods that adjust for intercurrent mortality are now part of the National Cancer Institute/National Toxicology Program approach to the statistical analysis of bioassay tumor data. The first method assumes that all tumors of the specific type or category being studied either directly or indirectly cause the death of those animals that die before the planned terminal kill. The proportion of animals with these tumors in the dosed and control groups are compared each time an animal dies with the specific tumor. The total number of animals at risk in each group is used as the denominator of these proportions.

The second method of analysis assumes that all tumors of a specific type or category being considered are "incidental" and did not cause the death of animals dying before planned terminal kill. The proportions of animals with these tumors in dosed and control groups are compared at specified time intervals. The number of animals actually necropsied in each group during the indicated time interval is used as the denominator of these proportions.

Details of the two methods have been reported by Peto et al. (9). For those studies in which the test compound produces little effect on survival compared to controls, the results of the different analyses of tumor incidences indicated in this discussion will generally be similar.

The Evidence

The testing of any chemical for carcinogenticity is seriously dependent upon the consistent appearance and the incidence of so-called "spontaneous" (baseline) tumors in the control group of test animals. Evaluation by a team composed of a pathologist, a toxicologist and a statistician is necessary to judge the meaningfulness of an apparent increase of tumors in dosed animals at a site at which control groups have a variable or high baseline tumor incidence. This is also true in the evaluation of a low incidence of rare tumors appearing in dosed animals. In the latter case, tumors thought to be historically rare (that is, they are known to occur with an incidence of less than 1% in a given species, strain, and sex) are considered suspicious with respect to possible carcinogenic (depending on the magnitude) response if they are induced only in dosed animals at levels that are not necessarily statistically significant. The induction of statistically significant rare tumors in dosed animals in a properly conducted bioassay should be considered as strong evidence of carcinogenicity in the test animals and as an indicator of a possible increased carcinogenic risk to humans.

For those tumor lesions appearing in control animals at relatively high incidence, the historical control tumor data is of utmost importance in facilitating the meaningfulness of the bioassay evidence. Since the lesions considered are said to be "spontaneous" primary tumors, i. e., tumors of unknown causes, their appearance and thereby their incidence is subject to variations dependent on the nature of the unknown causes. The variability around the mean incidence of baseline tumors usually is unknown for a particular bioassay. Yet, in most cases, it is this baseline incidence of a specific tumor type with its usually unknown variability that is used as the reference point for determining whether a chemical is carcinogenic in a given biological test system. An indication of the possible variability involved is usually obtained only from historical data in a particular species, strain, and sex of a particular age and under specific conditions in a particular laboratory. Each of these factors has been shown to modulate the incidence of tumors. It is such closely controlled historical data that facilitates the evaluation of the typical or atypical nature of the tumor incidence obtained with concurrent controls.

It must be recognized that the higher the incidence of a baseline tumor, the greater will be the variability. As an example, the mean incidence of hepatocellular carcinoma in male B6C3F1 mice from several untreated control groups in a given laboratory may be 15% and vary between 10 and 20%. In another laboratory, this same tumor in the same strain of mice from the same animal supplier and being fed the same type of feed from the same source, may have a mean incidence of 30% and vary between 15 and 45%. Thus, the endpoint lesion in the B6C3F1 mouse may be adequately evaluated at one laboratory and perhaps not at another because of increased incidence and variation. On the other hand, this same hepatocellular carcinomas in various untreated control groups of female B6C3F1 mice has a mean incidence of 2.5%, which varies between 0 and 5%. Furthermore, this range of incidence is consistent from laboratory to laboratory. Thus, hepatocellular carcinomas appear to be a more reliable (less variable) endpoint lesion in female than in male B6C3F1 mice.

An extreme case of baseline tumor variation is evident in the male Fischer 344 rats, which have a mean incidence of about 76% interstitial cell testicular tumors. The incidence of these tumors in groups of animals in any laboratory varies between 50 and 100%. If one considers a testicular tumor incidence of 25/50 in control animals and an incidence of 50/50 in a test chemical dosed group, a statistical analysis would indicate an effect in the dosed animals at a level of $p < 0.01$ compared to the controls. Yet, it must be considered that an incidence of 100% testicular tumors could have occurred in the control group based on typical historical data. This particular lesion endpoint in the Fischer 344 must be considered unreliable and inadequate for evaluating the possible carcinogenicity of a test compound.

The incidences of baseline pituitary tumors in female F344 and Osborne-Mendel rats of the order of 20–30%, respectively, do not indicate as extensive a problem as does the higher and more variable incidence of testicular tumors in F344 rats. Nevertheless, the variability of the control pituitary tumor incidence in females of each of the two strains of rats presents some difficulties to the adequate evaluation of possible "induced" tumors at this site.

It is clear that both judgment and statistical analysis are required to determine whether the tumor incidence in concurrent control groups differ from that expected for historical groups; this in turn is basic in the evaluation of the possibility of a tumor response to a test chemical.

Quantitative tumor data resulting from the National Cancer Institute/ National Toxicology Program bioassay of a few selected chemicals are presented in Fig. 1 through 5 as examples of the possible spectrum of rodent tumor response.

In the case of nitrofen (NCI, *14*) (Fig. 1), a chlorinated nitrophenoxy benzene compound used as a herbicide, both male and female B6C3F1 mice gave a classical dose–response profile, with a high incidence of hepatocellular carcinomas and a historically typical control tumor incidence. In control male B6C3F1 mice, the incidence of this tumor at 21–24 months of age ranges approximately from 10 to 30% depending upon the test laboratory. On the other hand, female mice of the same strain, from the same animal source, of the same age, and under the same experimental conditions as males, develop hepatocellular carcinomas with an incidence range of 0–5% that does not appear to vary with the test laboratory. The lower incidence of these tumors in female mice and its associated low variability makes the female a more reliable test model than the male for this particular type of tumor. Nevertheless, in this instance, the magnitude of the male mice liver tumor response to nitrofen tend to overcome the limitations of the baseline variability.

The female Osborne-Mendel rat responded to nitrofen (Fig. 2) with a statistically significant dose-related incidence of rare (less than 1%) pancreatic carcinomas. The study was repeated using F344 rats and the B6C3F1 mice. The hepatocellular carcinoma response in the mice was confirmed; however, the pancreatic tumors seen in the Osborne-Mendel females were not induced in either sex of the F344 rats.

The findings with nitrofen indicate the reproducibility of the bioassay results under the same experimental conditions and illustrates the possible sex- and species-oriented response to a chemical. It also of-

Nitrofen

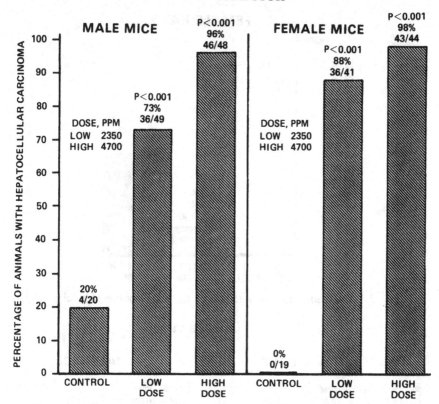

Fig. 1.   Carcinogenesis of nitrofen in B6C3F1 mice.

fers an extreme example, in the case of the female Osborne-Mendel rat, why the combination of data for specific tumor types from both sexes for purposes of analysis is only meaningful if the response of the two sexes separately is not statistically different.

The bioassay of chloramben (32), an amino chlorinated benzoic acid herbicide, presents relatively limited evidence of carcinogenicity. Under the conditions of the test, the chronic administration of the compound in feed caused no significant increased tumor incidence in Osborne-Mendel rats. In mice (Fig. 3), the compound caused an increase in liver tumor incidence in both sexes compared to controls. However, the evidence in males was considered limited because of the variability of this particular endpoint in control male B6C3F1 mice and because of the relatively low magnitude of the response.

In female mice, the response also was of a low magnitude, but the reliability of the baseline incidence of hepatocellular carcinomas in

Nitrofen

FEMALE RATS

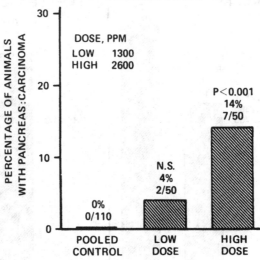

Fig. 2. Carcinogenesis of nitrofen in female Osborne-Mendel rats.

Chloramben

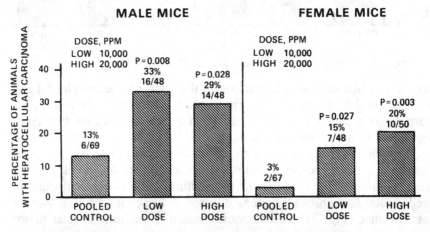

Fig. 3. Carcinogenesis of chloramben in B6C3F1 mice.

B6C3F1 female mice and the significant response, including a dose-related trend, led to the conclusion that chloramben was carcinogenic to the female mice. In male mice the reults were considered equivocal. Thus the overall bioassay of chloramben present segments of the full spectrum of carcinogenic responses, i.e., negative, equivocal, and positive.

The bioassay of 1,2-dibromoethane (NCI, *19*) presents relatively strong evidence of carcinogenicity . Under the conditions of the test, the chronic adminstration by gavage of the test material in corn oil caused a significant increase of tumor incidence in both sexes of Osborne-Mendel rats and B6C3F1 mice. Since the findings were similar in both species, only the results for rats are presented in Fig. 4. Animals died with forestomach tumors as early as 12 weeks for rats and 24 weeks for mice. Survival rates were poor, but most animals died with these characteristically rare tumors for rodents. Other systemic tumors away from the stomach were not detected. The response of the high dose was less than that of the low dose and appears to be explained on the basis of dose-related early mortality.

This bioassay result may indicate the advantage of selecting doses that give a relatively quick maximum response, but it is clear that the doses prevented the distinction between tumors that develop at the site of application and those that might develop at other systemic sites from lower doses. The doses in this case may indeed have prevented a wide spectrum of tumor responses by reducing the survival of the animals.

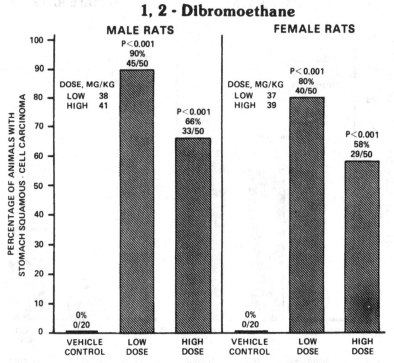

Fig. 4. Carcinogenesis of 1,2-dibromoethane in Osborne-Mendel rats.

An example of such a case is the bioassay of tris(2,3-dibrom-opropyl) phosphate (NCI, *18*), a compound used as a flame retardant. The test was conducted by administering the compound in feed to F344 rats and B6C3F1 mice at doses that permitted relatively good survival of animals for 103 weeks. The compound produced the following wide spectrum of statistically significant tumors in mice:

- Stomach (female and male): Squamous-cell papilloma and carcinoma
- Lung (male and female): Adenoma and carcinoma
- Kidney (male only): Tubular-cell adenoma and adenocarcinoma
- Liver (female only): Hepatocellular adenoma and carcinoma

In F344 rats (Fig. 5), the compound produced a statistically significant increased incidence and dose-related trend of kidney tubular-cell adenocarcinomas alone and in combination with tubular-cell adenomas at the same site. Although not completely the case with this compound, it is, however, considered a supportive example of the fact that a statistical

Tris (2, 3 - dibromopropyl) phosphate

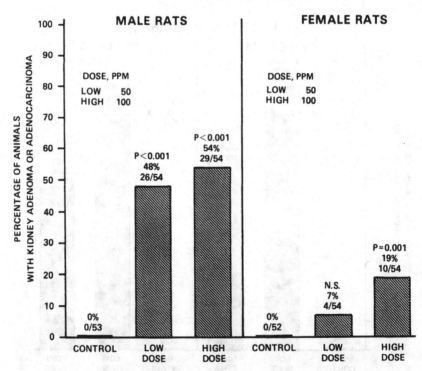

Fig. 5. Carcinogenesis of tris(2,3-dibromopropyl) phosphate in F344 rats.

increase in the incidence of various tumor types in two sexes of two species constitutes a maximum carcinogenic response.

Strength of the Evidence

The degree or strength of the evidence for carcinogenicity in a specific bioassay must be carefully assessed and its limitations recognized. An approach to such an assessment has been reported by the International Agency for Research on Cancer (9, 20). In this approach the evidence in a bioassay that a chemical *produces tumors* in animals is classified as "sufficient" or as "limited." According to this concept, "sufficient evidence" of carcinogenicity is provided by those bioassays that demonstrate a statistically significant increased incidence of tumors: (1) in more than one species or strain, (2) in more than one experiment, preferably using different routes of administration or different dose levels, or (3) with a tumor response of an unusual degree in incidence, site, type, or early onset. "Limited evidence" is considered to be data that suggests a carcinogenic effect, but that is limited, to various degrees, by its qualitative or quantitative scope. In some cases, these limitations may be so restrictive that the findings can then be considered inadequate.

In a recent report (33) a few modifications of the IARC approach were made and the concept was extended to the evaluation of bioassays presenting no evidence of carcinogenicity. The analysis of bioassay data, both biologically and statistically, should permit the grouping of the results into three general categories: (1) those presenting evidence of a statistically significant increased incidence of tumors, (2) those in which there is no such evidence, and (3) those in which the evidence is equivocal.

The criteria used for positive findings required a statistically significant, time-adjusted or life-table computed increase incidence of a specific tumor or acceptable tumor combination at a common site, in dosed animal groups compared to concurrent control groups. A dose-related response enhanced the positive nature of the data. The concurrent control group baseline incidences of specific tumors or tumor combination were required to be within the range expected from historical control data obtained from the same strain of animals. If this latter criteron was not met, evidence of increased tumor incidence was considered equivocal.

In the proposed classification scheme of Griesemer and Cueto, *positive evidence* of carcinogenicity for a single species in a given bioassay is subgrouped into (1) those with multiple positive fingings in terms of route (usually only one is used in a given bioassay), dose, and sex, and (2) those with an unusual degree of tumor response in terms of incidence, histological type, multiplicity of body sites, and early onset. *Strong evidence* of carcinogenicity is defined, for the purpose at hand, as evidence meeting one or both of the above stated criteria. *Sufficient evidence* of carcinogenicity is defined for the purpose at hand, as statistically significant evidence, meeting both of the criteria stated above but to a lesser extent, i.e., not necessarily multiple and not to an unusual exaggerated degree.

Equivocal evidence is defined as data that suggest a carcinogenic effect, but that are limited in various ways and degrees so that no clear conclusion can be drawn.

Evidence for the lack of carcinogenicity was subdivided into three categories of increasing support for the lack of a neoplastic response. The evidence in this case was dependent on the extent or degree to which the bioassay was adequately designed or conducted and to which the test chemical, nevertheless, produced no carcinogenic response in both sexes of one or two species of animals. Such bioassays were considered limited in the case of decreased survival or the lack of evidence that the maximum test dose used was sufficiently high to permit optimum test sensitivity.

For the purpose of facilitating the development of a classification scheme with sufficient categories to accommodate the various levels of degrees of evidence usually generated by carcinogenesis bioassays, the following categories of evidence have been proposed:

1. Very strong evidence with multiple positive findings in terms of route, dose, or sex, and/or unusual degree of tumor response in terms of incidence, type, number of anatomical sites, or early onset in two species.

2. Very strong evidence for carcinogenicity as in Category 1, but in one species and sufficient evidence for carcinogenicity to a lesser degree than Category 1 in a second species.

3. Very strong evidence for carcinogenicity as in Category 1, but in one species and no evidence for carcinogenicity in a second species.

4. Sufficient evidence for carcinogenicity to a lesser degree than Category 1 in two species.

5. Sufficient evidence for carcinogenicity as in Category 4, but in one species and no evidence for carcinogenicity in a second species.

6. Equivocal evidence for carcinogenicity suggesting a possible effect but not permitting a clear conclusion.

7. No evidence for carcinogenicity in a limited bioassay.

8. No evidence for carcinogenicity in one species in an adequate bioassay.

9. No evidence for carcinogenicity in two species in an adequate bioassy.

Perspectives on the Findings

The strength or degree of the evidence for or the lack of carcinogenicity must not be taken to indicate categories of chemical carcinogenic properties. The categories reflect the extent of the evidence and the evidence may change with further test or studies under different conditions. It must be recognized that evidence of carcinogenicity is the result of an interaction between a specific biological system under a specific set of conditions. As the system and conditions change, the qualitative and quantitative responses will also change. It is considered that the overall qualitative nature of the response in a given species is more consistent or reproducible than the quantitative response. However, not only the quantitative effect, but also the qualitative carcinogenic effect itself may be modified in the test animal by both endogenous and exogenous factors (4).

Considerable emphasis has been placed on the possible induction or promotion of cancer through physiological overloading factors precipitated by maximum test doses. Thus overt toxic manifestations owning to high doses is often viewed as an indication of the development of a condition that may lead, through unspecified mechanisms, to cancer. In this approach, emphasis is placed on the overloading of detoxifying mechanisms and the altered metabolism and pharmokinetics of the high doses. Perhaps further emphasis is needed on possibly altered immunological competence and DNA repair mechanisms caused by the chronic administration of the test chemical. It is recognized that a better perspective of the carcinogenicity of a test chemical may be gained from evaluation of the results of other bioassays, mutagenicity testing, and structure-related activities. In addition to this, it is suggested that those chemicals of considerable health and economic benefit that are found first to be mutagenic in short-term bacterial tests should be subjected to an extensive toxicological evaluation *simultaneously* to their evaluation in a long-term carcinogenesis bioassay in order to develop better technical perspectives in the interpretation of the findings in a timely manner.

Predictive Value of the Findings

The qualitative predictive value of an appropriately designed and adequately conducted carcinogenesis bioassay is indicated in the review of the IARC (20) in which 27 chemicals (including some groups of chemicals) generally accepted to cause or probably cause cancer in humans, have been shown, all but two (arsenic and benzene) to cause cancer in at least one animal species. The qualitative predictiveness of the bioassay appears to be substantially established with but limited exceptions. The quantitative aspects are more tenuous.

The ED_{01} study conducted at the National Center for Toxicological Research (*34*) and the subsequently published independent evaluation (*35*) of the reported findings has provided valuable information on the need for further studies on cancer risk assessment procedures. The importance of time-to-response data modeling and the development of new methods for analysis of complex, extensive, and large-scale chronic studies is clearly indicated by this particular study. However, large-scale time-to-response studies are not likely to be performed often and therefore, the question remains about the fitness or specificity of a mathematical model derived from data obtained with one chemical when it is applied to data obtained with another chemical.

It must be considered that mathematical models for carcinogenicity have been set forth for the extrapolation of high dose findings in animals to much lower dose levels. However, the problem is not the mathematics involved, but the biological nature of the carcinogenic process. At low levels of exposure, generally consistent with that of occupational and general public exposure, the endogenous and general environmental factors in the test animal can mask, augment, or inhibit the carcinogenic response to a chemical to the extent that any dose–time response relationship previously established at higher doses is no longer quantitatively meaningful. It must be taken into account that although a chemical carcinogen by itself at low levels of exposure may not produce tumors in a given population, it nevertheless can act as an "initiator" and in the presence of a suitable "promoter" produce cancer. Thus, the significance of a time–dose response curve at low levels of exposure in the establishment of a "standard" or an "acceptable risk" level for a specific environmental chemical carcinogen is rather obscure. Since carcinogens at low dosage can act as "initiators," interacting with "promoters" to produce tumors, the prevalence of tumors induced by environmental chemicals cannot be predicted on the base of a dose–time response curve of the carcinogen alone. This is without considering the differences in species sensitivity that further complicate the interpretation.

Human risk assessment involving animal data is of necessity based on biological evidence having potentially large experimental errors that do not permit precise quantitative statement of risk. The "state of the art" suggests that strong or sufficient evidence of carcinogenicity in animal bioassays should be taken as a pragmatic indication of increased human risk whose quantitation at this time can not be determined.

The problem has been addressed in a recent paper by Squire (*36*), who, recognizing that no rigid system for classification or regulation of animal carcinogens could accommodate all the chemical and biological variables involved in the ill-defined carcinogenic process, pointed out that the weight of "the most relevant toxicological evidence derived from animals and genotoxicity studies" should be used to *rank* carcinogens. The emphasis was placed on test animal data as the most relevant to human risk evaluation since the limited knowledge of carcinogenesis mechanisms itself limits the quantitative assessment of in vitro data in terms of in vivo potential effects. "The weight of scientific evidence should be considered in an appropriate (ranking) system of carcinogen classification." This approach acknowledges and permits the classification of different carcingenic potentials of various chemicals within the spectrum of scientifc evidence available and minimizes tenuous classifications or risk assessments based on limited knowledge of chemical and biological uncertainties.

References

1. Weisburger, J. H., and Williams, G. M., *Science* **214**, 401 (1981).
2. Chu, K. C., Cueto, C., and Ward, J. M., *J. Toxicol. Environ. Hlth.* **8**, 251 (1981).
3. Arcos, J. C., Argus, M. F., and Wolf, G., *Chemical Introduction of Cancer,* vol. 1, New York, Academic Press, 1968.
4. Berenblum, I. (ed.), *Carcinogenicity Testing* (UICC Technical Report Series, Vol. 2), Geneva International Union Against Cancer, 1969.
5. Canadian Health and Welfare, *The Testing of Chemicals for Carcinogenicity, Mutagenicity and Teratogenicity,* Ottawa, Ministry of Health and Welfare, 1973.
6. Golberg, L. (ed.), *Carcinogenesis Testing of Chemicals,* Cleveland, CRC Press, 1973.
7. Sontag, J. M., Page, N. P., and Saffioti, U., Guidelines for Carcinogen Bioassay in Small Rodents, Bethesda, DHEW Publication No. (NIH) 76-801, 1976.
8. Page, N. P., Concepts of a Bioassay Program in Environmental Carcinogenesis, in Kraybill, H., and Mehlman, M. C. (eds.); *Environmental Cancer,* New York, Wiley, 1977, pp. 87–171.
9. International Agency for Research on Cancer: Monographs on the Long-Term and Short-Term Screening Assays for Carcinogens: A Critical Appraisal, Geneva World Health Organization, 1980. Supplement 2.
10. Environmental Protection Agency: Proposed Guidelines for Registering Pesticides in the US.: Hazards Evaluation, *Federal Register* **43** (163), 37336 (1978).
11. Environmental Protection Agency: Proposed Good Laboratory Practice Guidelines for Toxicology Testing, *Federal Register* **45** (77), 26373 (1980).

12. Interagency Regulatory Liaison Group: Scientific bases for identification of potential carcinogens and estimation of risks, *Federal Register* **44** (131), 39858 (1979).

13. Food and Drug Administration, Non-clinical Laboratory Studies: Good Laboratory Practice Regulations, *Federal Register* **43** (248), 59886 (1978).

14. National Cancer Institute: Bioassy of Nitrofen for Possible Carcinogenicity, Technical Report Series No. 26, Bethesda, DHEW Publication No. (NIH) 78–826, 1978.

15. National Cancer Institute, Bioassay of Dibromochloropropane for Possible Carcinogenicity, Technical Report Series No. 28, Bethesda, DHEW Publication No. (NIH) 78–828, 1978.

16. National Cancer Institute, Bioassay of 1,2-Dichloroethane for Possible Carcinogenicity, Technical Report Series No. 55, Bethesda, DHEW Publication No. (NIH) 78–1361, 1978.

17. National Cancer Institute, Bioassay of Endosulfan for Possible Carcinogenicity, Technical Report Series No. 62, Bethesda, DHEW Publication No. (NIH) 78–1312, 1978.

18. National Cancer Institute, Bioassay of Tris (2,3-dibrompropyl) Phosphate for Possible Carcinogenicity, Technical Report Series No. 86, Bethesda, DHEW Publication No. (NIH) 78–1326, 1978.

19. National Cancer Institute, Bioassay of 1,2-Dibromoethane for Possible Carcinogenicity. Technical Report Series No. 86, Bethesda, DHEW Publication No. 78–1336, 1978.

20. International Agency for Reseach on Cancer: Monographs on Industrial Processes Associated with Cancer in Humans, Geneva, World Health Organization, 1979, Supplement 1.

21. Ward, J. M., Goodman, D. G., Griesemer, R. A., Hardisty, J. F., Schueler, J. D., Squire, R. A., and Strandberg, J. D., *J. Environ. Pathol. Toxicol.* **2, 371** (1978).

22. US Department of Health, Education and Welfare: Report of the Secretary's Commission on Pesticides and Their Relationship to Environmental Health, Washington, DC, US Government Printing Office, 1969.

23. Squire, R. A., and Levitt, M., *Cancer Res.* **35,** 3214 (1975).

24. Kaplan, E. L., and Meier, P., *J. Amer. Stat. Assoc.* **53,** 457 (1958).

25. Cox, D. R., *J. R. Stat. Soc.* **B34,** 187 (1972).

26. Tarone, R. E., *Biometriks* **62,** 679 (1975).

27. Cox, D. R., *Analysis of Binary Data, London, Methuen, 1970.*

28. Armitage, P., *Statistical Methods in Medical Research, New York, Wiley, 1971, pp. 362–365.*

29. Thomas, D. G., Breslow, N., and Gart, J. J., *Comput. Biomed. Res.* **10, (1977).**

30. Fears, T. R., Tarone, R. E., and Chu, K. C., *Cancer Res.* **37,** 1941 (1977).

31. Tarone, R. E., Chu, K. C., and Ward, J. M., *J. Natl. Cancer Inst.* **66,** 1175 (1981).

32. National Cancer Institute: Bioassay of Chloramben for Possible Carcinogenicity, Technical Report Series No. 25, Bethesda, DHEW Publications No. (NIH) 77–825, 1977.

33. Griesemer, R. A., and Cueto, C.: Toward a Classification Scheme for Degrees of Experimental Evidence for Carcinogenicity of Chemicals for Animals, in Montesano, R., Bartsch, H., and Tomatis, L. (eds)., *Molecular and Cellular Aspects of Carcinogen Screening Tests,* Lyon (IARC Scientific Publication No. 27), 1980.
34. Staffa, J. A., and Mehlman, M. A. (eds.), *Innovations in Cancer Risk Assessment* (ED_{01} *Study*), Pathotex Publishers, Park Forest South, Illinois, 1979, pp. 1–246.
35. SOT, Society of Toxicology ED_{01} Task Force Symposium, *Fund. appl. Toxicol.* **1,** 26 (1981).
36. Squire, R. A., *Science* **214,** 877 (1981).

Part II

Practical Carcinogenesis and Mutagenesis Assay Methodology

Section A

Gene Mutation Assays

Chapter 11

Bacterial Reverse and Forward Mutation Assays

S. R. Haworth

Theory and Background

The *Salmonella*/mammalian-microsome mutagenicity assay developed by Ames et al. (*1,2*) has proven to be a valuable tool for the rapid detection of potential genetic activity in a wide variety of chemical classes. For general mutagenicity screening purposes, five tester strains are routinely used: TA1535, TA1537, TA1538, TA98, and TA100. These strains possess mutations of the histidine operon, making them dependent upon the presence of histidine in the medium of growth. Mutagenesis is detected as the reversion of these strains to histidine prototrophy on selective medium.

Strain TA1535 possesses a missense mutation, $hisG_{46}$ (*2*). This mutation is a base pair substitution that alters one codon of the mRNA transcribed from the gene coding for the first enzyme of the histidine biosynthetic pathway. The mutation can be reverted by direct back-mutation of *his*G by mutagens that cause base pair substitutions, such as alkylating agents, 2-aminopurines, and nitrogen mustard, or by suppressor mutations. This strain also possesses *rfa* and *uvr*B mutations. The *rfa* mutation causes a deficiency in the enzymes that are responsible for the synthesis of the polysaccharide portion of the lipopolysaccharide coat. The *rfa* mutation causes an extensive loss of the bacterial cell wall and so increases the permeability of the cell to compounds possessing large, complex ring systems. The Δ*uvr*B mutation is a large deletion that eliminates this excision–repair system for DNA, and thus partially prevents repair of damaged DNA.

Strain TA1537 possesses a frameshift mutation, *his*C$_{3076}$, wherein there is an addition of a single base pair to the *his*C gene (2). It is reverted by compounds that delete a base pair from DNA. These include diethylsulfate, *N*-methyl-*N'*-nitro-*N*-nitrosoguanidine, and acridines. TA1537 also possesses *rfa* and Δ*uvr*B mutations.

Strain TA1538 also possesses a frameshift mutation, hisD$_{3052}$ (2). Here, however, two base pairs have been added to the *his*D gene. It is reverted by 2-nitrosofluorene, which is known to cause a loss of two base pairs from DNA, and by aromatic nitroso derivatives of amine carcinogens. It too possesses *rfa* and *uvr*B mutations.

Strains TA98 and TA100 are derivatives of strains TA1538 and TA1535, respectively (2). They are identical to the parent strains except for the addition of an R factor-containing plasmid, pKM101. The mechanism by which the presence of this plasmid increases the sensitivity of these strains to mutagenesis is not fully understood. It has been suggested that this plasmid, which also confers ampicillin resistance, enhances error prone repair of damage caused by the mutagenic agent.

Although these strains are immediately valuable in detecting compounds that are mutagenic directly, they are ineffective in detecting promutagens, compounds that require metabolic activation by NADPH-dependent microsomal enzymes. Bacteria lack these enzymes and so are incapable of effecting the metabolic transformations necessary for the conversion of promutagens to mutagens. To alleviate this deficiency, Ames, and others (3,4,5,6) have developed a mutagenicity assay that combines metabolic activation by liver microsome preparations with the standard *Salmonella* strains in vitro. Using this assay, a variety of compounds, such as aflatoxin B$_1$, benzo(a)pyrene, acetylaminofluorene, benzidine, and dimethylamino-*trans*-stilbene, are converted by metabolic activation to potent frameshift mutagens. It is believed that the amino-, dimethylamino-, and acetylamino- groups of amine carcinogens are converted to nitroso-, hydroxylamino-, and hydroxylacetylamino- derivatives. These derivatives are known activation products of liver metabolism and potent frameshift mutagens. The same is true of polycyclic hydrocarbons, which are converted to epoxides. These mutagens have a ring system sufficiently planar for stacking intercalation with DNA base pairs that could result in frameshift mutation. It has also been found that the potency of a frameshift intercalator is increased by orders of magnitude if the ring system contains a side chain that could covalently link to DNA.

The *Salmonella*/Mammalian-Microsome Mutagenicity Assay (Ames Test)

The *Salmonella*/mammalian-microsome mutagenicity assay, or Ames test as it is commonly referred to, is a test system that can be set up and used routinely in most laboratory settings equipped with microbiological facilities. Although the test seems rather straightforward, care must be taken to standardize the procedures used in a given laboratory to ensure that consistant results can be obtained on a routine basis.

Solubilizing the Test Material

The first step in conducting an Ames test is to select an appropriate solvent in which the test material can either be dissolved or uniformly dispensed. Whenever possible, water or buffer should be used. If the test material is not water soluble, then dimethylsulfoxide (DMSO) should be tried next. If neither H_2O nor DMSO is a suitable solvent, then acetone, and ethanol should be attempted. Dr. Ames laboratory has published a list of solvents that are compatible with the test system (*1*). Any time a new solvent is used for the first time, a number of questions must be asked. (1) Does the solvent show any indication of reacting with the test material? (2) Is 50–100 μL of the solvent toxic to the tester strains? (3) How does the solvent affect the activity of the metabolic activation system?

One should avoid solvents that chemically react with the test material since one might then inadvertently be testing reaction products instead of the originally intended material. Although, whenever possible, a totally nontoxic solvent should be selected, some solvent toxicity to the tester strains can be tolerated if no other alternative solvents are available. If fewer than 10^7 cells/plate survive solvent exposure, the test system may be compromised and misleading results may be obtained. The effect of the solvent on the metabolic activation system can be measured by adding the solvent at the time of plating to the positive controls requiring activation. A solvent that does not affect the microsomal activity should be selected if at all possible. If reduced microsomal activity is observed and no alternative solvent is available, then this should be kept in mind when the results of the Ames test are evaluated.

Dose Range Selection

Once a suitable solvent has been determined, then an effective dose range should be selected over which to test the chemical in the Ames test. In order to select the dose range, it will be necessary to expose one or more

TABLE 1
Preliminary Toxicity Study TA100 Revertants/Plate

Test article Concentration μg/plate	+S-9[a]			−S-9[b]		
	Viable counts	Revertants	Background lawn	Viable counts	Revertants	Background lawn
0	300	125	1	280	140	1
0.3	280	128	1	282	142	1
1.0	295	127	1	290	138	1
3.3	305	122	1	270	135	1
10	301	120	1	195	130	1
33	285	131	1	90	100	2
100	230	130	1	50	60	2
333	175	110	2	15	10	4
1,000	100	72	3	0	0	5
3,333	0	0	5	0	0	5
10,000	0	0	5	0	0	5

[a]Dose range selected with S-9 = 10–1000 μg.
[b]Dose range selected without S-9 = 2–200 μg.

of the tester strains (TA100 should be sufficient) to a wide range of test article concentrations up to 5–10 mg/plate and to evaluate the results for evidence of toxicity. In order to obtain the most information regarding the toxicity of the test material, determinations of the viable count, the revertant recovery, and the background lawn condition should be made at each test article dose level both with and without a metabolic activation system. The presence of the microsomal enzymes will often reduce the toxicity of the test material or, less frequently, will increase the toxicity of the test material.

Toxicity is evidenced by a reduction in viable counts, a reduction in revertant recovery, and/or the thinning or disappearance of the background lawn. Any one or all of these signs may be apparent at any time, as shown in Table 1. A reduction in viable counts is usually observed before any reduction in revertants or background lawn. After reviewing the resulting data, if possible, a top concentration should be selected that causes an obvious reduction in revertants per plate. The remaining dose levels should span at least a 100-fold range of concentrations and not be separated by a dilution of greater than 1:5. The dose range with S–9 may be different than without S–9. This approach increases the likelihood that weak mutagens will be detected.

The Mutagenesis Assay

The day before the assay is to be conducted, fresh nutrient broth cultures should be set with each of the tester strains to be used. The inoculated cultures should be incubated with shaking at 37°C and should be harvested in late log phase. Allowing the cultures to incubate into the stationary phase of growth can result in reduced responsiveness of the tester strains to some mutagens. The harvested cultures should be stored at 4°C until their use in that day's assays.

Each culture should be checked for the presence of the *rfa* wall mutation, and the plasmid-containing strains should also be checked for the presence of the plasmid. To check each culture, an aliquot of each should be plated and a disk containing crystal violet should be placed on the agar surface of each plate. An ampicillin-containing disk should also be placed on the agar surface of each plate inoculated with a plasmid containing strain. A 12–20 mm zone of inhibition around the crystal violet-containing disk after 24 h incubation at 37°C indicates the presence of the *rfa* wall mutation. No zone of inhibition around the ampicillin disk after incubation indicates the presence of the pKM101 plasmid. The microsomal enzyme mix (S-9 mix) should be prepared immediately before its use in the assay. For routine screening purposes, 0.1 mL of liver homogenate should be added per mL of S-9 mix. During its use in the assay, the S-9 mix should be stored on ice and frequently mixed by gently swirling the flask in which it is contained. The test material should be prepared immediately before its use in the assay to minimize loss of potency or integrity. It is preferable to serially dilute the test material to provide the four to six dose levels normally used in an Ames test. Plating a constant volume of test material, such as 50 µL from each of the appropriate dilution tubes, is preferable to plating different volumes from one test material stock solution. This ensures that any solvent effects will be the same at all dose levels.

Once the S-9 mix and test material are prepared, remove the tester strains from their 4°C storage location and commence plating. The sequence of events required in the plating procedure are critical to obtaining consistent data. Under no circumstances should the tester strain or the S-9 mix be allowed to sit in the molten top agar for extended periods of time. A good working sequence for plating is to add test material to three tubes, if plating in triplicate (two tubes if plating in duplicate) then tester strain and finally the S-9 mix. Always add the materials in the same sequence and then plate them in the same sequence. Each three-tube set should take no more than 30–45 s from the time the first component is added to the first tube to the time the third tube is plated. Establishing a set plating procedure and adhering to it is essential to obtaining consistent results.

Care should be taken so as to not carry any test material back into the S-9 mix or the tester strain working stocks. This could happen if care is not taken to ensure that pipeting devices used to deliver the S-9 mix or the tester strains do not contact the overlay tube already containing an aliquot of the test material. Back contamination as described above could result in unexplained toxicity or mutagenicity patterns if the test material was either strongly toxic or mutagenic. Once plating of a test material has begun, it should continue with as little interruption as possible until all tester strain/S-9 combinations have been completed. This approach will minimize any effects that test material or S-9 liability could have on the experimental results.

It is important that, after the top agar and test material have been overlayed onto the minimal bottom agar, the poured plate be placed upon a level surface so that the overlay will be of uniform thickness once it has solidified. Plating on uneven surfaces can result in gradient effects where localized areas of toxicity or mutagenicity will occur in the top agar. This can result in spurious colony counts, making interpretation of the resulting data very difficult.

After all of the experiment has been plated, the plates should be inverted and placed in a ventilated 37°C incubator for 48 h. If the incubator is not properly vented, volatile test materials can produce spurious toxic or mutagenic effects, invalidating any experiment housed in the incubator.

Selection of Positive Controls

The number and type of positive control chemicals selected will depend upon the application for which the Ames test is being used. If a particular class of chemicals is being studied in a series of experiments, then it would be wise to select positive controls that are similar in structure/ activity to the class of chemicals being tested. However, in the routine screening of unknown chemicals, it is important to select a standard set of positive control chemicals and establish as data base for each tester strain/ positive control combination with which to monitor the sensitivity of each tester strain and each batch of S-9 mix in each experiment. A minimum set of positive controls should include one direct acting mutagen for each tester strain and one promutagen plated on at least one tester strain. This approach will ensure that each tester strain as well as the S-9 mix are performing as expected. If time and materials are not limiting, then one direct acting and one promutagen for each tester strain should be used. This will allow for a more thorough monitoring of the test system.

Counting the Experiment

After the 48 h incubation period, the resulting colonies should be counted and the results recorded appropriately. If the plates cannot be counted soon after the 48 h incubation period, they should be stored at 4°C until they can be counted.

Care should be taken to ensure that the colonies being counted are in fact revertants. The background lawn should be checked on each plate. If it is absent or has been severely reduced, then the macroscopic colonies observed might not be true revertants, but could be "phenotypic revertants" that have been able to scavange excess histidine present in the top agar to support their growth. If these colonies are picked and streaked on histidine-free agar they will not be able to grow.

If one of the currently available electronic automated colony counters is used to count revertant colonies, it should be carefully calibrated, as recommended by its manufacturer, before being so used. If the test material precipitates in the top agar, it will probably be necessary to hand-count each plate. Otherwise, the colony counter might also count the precipitate, thus giving greatly inflated colony counts.

Routine check-out of the colony counter is essential to ensure that the sensitivity of the instrument is consistent from one experiment to the next. This is especially important if the positive control plates are counted with an automated colony counter. Fluctuating sensitivity of the colony counter can cause positive control values to appear to vary from historical expectations.

Preincubation Methodology

A variation of the so-called standard Ames plate incorporation assay, is the preincubation assay. This approach is different from the plate incorporation assay in that instead of the reaction components (test material, tester strain, and/or S-9) being added to 2.0 mL of molten top agar immediately before plating, the components are first added to a culture tube where they are incubated for 20–30 min at an appropriate temperature, after which molten top agar is added and the mixture is then plated as described in the previous section. This approach greatly enhances the interaction of the test material with the tester strain and/or the S-9 mix. This procedure can sometimes detect the mutagenic activity of materials that would otherwise be negative in the Ames test. (8). Good candidates for use in the preincubation assay would be volatile materials, materials that break down rapidly in aqueous environments, or materials that apparently require more intimate interaction with the activation system. Some nitrosamines are more readily detected using the preincubation methodology. The mutagenic activity of formaldehyde has been demonstrated using the preincubation method (9). This material had previously been reported as negative in plate incorporation assays. When using the preincubation

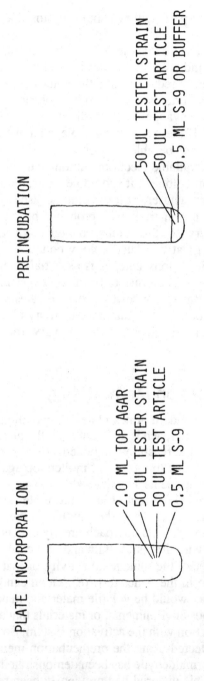

Fig. 1. Methodology for plate incorporation and preincubation assays.

method, one should keep in mind that solvent effects are much more exaggerated than with the plate incorporation method. This results from the relatively higher concentration of solvent in the reaction tube during the preincubation period than that found when the components were added directly to 2 mL of molten top agar immediately before plating in the plate incorporation assay. A similar problem can exist with very toxic test materials. The mutagenicity of the test material can be masked by the enhanced toxicity of the test material during the preincubation period. This toxicity is diminished in the plate incorporation approach because of the dilution or buffering effects of the top agar. Experience will show that there is no hard rule, however. Success with one or both methods will depend upon the relative mutagenicity/toxicity/test material lability, solubility, and so on.

Applications

Because of its versatility, the Ames test can, with appropriate modifications, be used to evaluate an almost limitless variety of test materials from complex industrial formulations or environmental samples to body fluids from laboratory animals or humans. Testing uncharacterized complex mixtures should be approached with caution. The presence of potent mutagens in a mixture of several other chemical components can be masked by the toxicity of one or more of the other nonmutagenic components. If this situation is suspected, fractionation of the test material is recommended. In this way, separation of the toxic component or components from the mutagenic component or components may be accomplished. The mutagenic component or components may then be detected in one or more of the subfractions. Evaluating body fluids such as urine can provide valuable information regarding the genotoxic potential of test materials or their matabolites. This approach involves dosing the animals in an appropriate manner and then collecting the urine of the treated animals and either testing it directly in the Ames test or first extracting the urine by various chromatography techniques and then testing the extract.

The *Escherichia coli* Tryptophan Reversion Assay

The *Escherichia coli* tryptophan reversion mutagenicity assay has been used widely for genetic testing (*11,12,13*). The strains most commonly used are the tryptophan auxotrophs WP$_2$ and WP$_2$ *uvr*A and WP$_2$ *uvr*A/

pkM101. Historically, this test system has been used to complement the Ames *Salmonella* test system. This was because of the observation that prior to the introduction of the pκM101 plasmid into tester strains TA1535 and TA1538 (to form tester strains TA100 and TA98, respectively) some chemicals such as nitrofurans were active only in the *E. coli* test system. Since the development of TA98 and TA100, however, few mutagens are detected only in the *E. coli* test system and not the *Salmonella* test system.

The *E. coli* test system should not be used alone in blind testing programs because of its reduced sensitivity to frameshift mutagens.

The procedures used in conjunction with the *E. coli* test system are essentially the same as those used throughout the *Salmonella* test system, including the use of microsome preparations from mammalian tissues.

Forward Mutation Assays

This section is not intended to be an extensive review of the literature concerning the *E. coli* and *Salmonella* forward mutation systems, but is intended to give the reader a basic understanding of the theoretical basis and the experimental design of the forward mutation system and of its possible role in screening for environmental mutagens.

Several bacterial forward mutation assays have been developed in recent years (*14,15,16,17*). The ideal bacterial forward mutation assay would be one that would retain the great sensitivity of the reverse mutation assays, but would require only one tester strain, instead of several, to detect all classes of gene mutations.

As pointed out earlier, the *Salmonella* tester strains used in the Ames test each possess a specific mutant base pair or sequence of base pairs that have caused the loss of activity of the histidine biosynthetic enzyme product of the gene in which they reside. To regain the function of that gene product, a back mutation must occur at the site of the lesion. The "target" for the would-be mutagen is therefore very small and very specific. One must remember that base substitution mutations can be directly reverted only by base substitution mutagens. Likewise, frameshift mutations can be reverted only by frameshift mutagens. For this reason, two or more tester strains must be utilized in reverse mutation assays in order to detect both of these classes of gene mutations. In addition, some known mutagens require specific target base sequences in order to be detected as mutagens: 9-aminoacridine specificity for *Salmonella* tester strain TA1537 rather than TA1538 is a good example. The nagging question is: "How many mutagens go undetected in bacterial reverse mutation assays because the target lesion is not the appropriate base sequence?'' Theoretically, this problem should be alleviated in the ideal forward mutation assay since the "target" is in fact the entire DNA sequence of the gene coding for the specific enzyme and not just one or a few base pairs within that gene. With the greatly increased size of the "target," the probability of detecting a wider array of mutagen types could be enhanced.

The bacterial forward mutation systems generally utilize either *Salmonella* or *E. coli* indicator strains and use drug resistance or altered growth potential in the presence of certain carbon sources as endpoints. Unlike the reverse mutation assays that select for mutations occurring at previously mutated target sites, the forward mutation assay selects for mutations that have occurred in normal or wild-type DNA sequences, and that result in an altered gene function that can be detected as a recognizable phenotype under the appropriate selective conditions.

The system chosen as an example of a bacterial forward mutation system is mutation to 8-azoguanine (8-AG) resistance. This system has been described by Skopek et al. (*15*).

When preparing to conduct this type of assay, one should follow the same basic procedures and philosophy in handling the tester strains, test samples, and liver homogenate preparations as described for bacterial reverse mutation assays.

Appropriate preliminary dose range-finding studies should always be conducted in order to select the appropriate range of dose levels over which to test the potential mutagen. The following flow chart is a summary of the procedures used to induce and select for 8-AG resistant mutants.

Combine the following in a glass culture tube

Log phase cells

+

Small aliquot of
test chemical dilution

+

S-9 mix (when used)

↓

Incubate at 37°C
for 1–2 h

↓

After treatment period, centrifuge the cultures and resuspend
in phosphate-buffered saline (PBS) to a final cell concentration of ~1.0 × 10⁷/mL

To determine # of 8-AG-resistant (8-AG^R) cells, approximately 1.0 × 10⁶ cells are overlayed in soft agar on minimal bottom agar containing 50 μg/mL 8-AG	To determine the number of viable cells surviving treatment, aliquots of the appropriately diluted PBS culture are over-layed in soft agar in minimal bottom agar without 8-AG
Incubate at 37°C for 36–48 h	Incubate at 37°C for 36–48 h
Count colonies	Count colonies

The fraction of 8-AG^R mutants can be calculated as follows:

$$8\text{-AG}^R \text{ Fraction} = \frac{\text{Number of colonies on 8-AG-containing plates}}{\text{Number of colonies on plates without 8-AG} \times 10^{-4}}$$

Appropriate concurrent solvent and positive controls should always be included with each day's assays.

Using the approach described above, Skopek et al. (18) tested 16
known mutagens in the five standard Ames *Salmonella* tested strains and
in a TA1535 histidine revertant and its pκM101 plasmic-containing derivative. Histidine reversion was measured in the five standard strains and
resistance to 8-AG was measured in the two derived strains. The 16
chemicals included both base substitution mutagens and frameshift
mutagens and some that required metabolic activation and some that did
not. The authors basically concluded that the forward mutation assay and
the reverse mutation assay were equisensitive to this group of mutagens.
Other workers using other bacterial forward mutation systems have found
varying results when comparing their forward mutation systems to the reverse mutation systems. Although the actual sample size is quite small, it
does not appear that any current bacterial forward mutation system can
replace the Ames *Salmonella* reverse mutation assay. The utility of these
forward mutation systems should be judged only after having used them
to test a large number of coded mutagens and nonmutagens. Perhaps
these systems will be useful in supplementing the results obtained in the
standard bacterial reverse mutation assays.

References

1. Ames, B. N., McCann, J. and Yamasaki, E., *Mutation Res.* **31**, 347 (1975).
2. Maron, D. M., and Ames, B. N., *Mutation Res.* **113**, 173 (1983).
3. Ames, B. N., Lee, F. D. and Durston, W. E., *Proc. Natl. Acad. Sci. USA* **70**, 782 (1973).
4. Ames, B. N., Durston, W. E., Yamasaki, E. and Lee, F. D., *Proc. Natl. Acad. Sci. USA* **70**, 2281 (1973).
5. Franz, C. N. and Malling, H. V., *Mutation Res.* **31**, 365 (1975).
6. Gletten, H., Weekes, U. and Brusick, D., *Mutation Res.* **28**, 113 (1975).
7. Miller, E. C. and Miller, J. A., The Mutagenicity of Chemical Carcinogens: Correlations, Problems, and Interpretations in *Chemical Mutagens: Principles and Methods for Their Detection,* ed. A. Hollaender, vol. I, Plenum Press, New York, 1971, pp 83–119.
8. Maron, D., Katzenellenbogen, J. and Ames, B. N., *Mutation Res.* **88**, 343 (1981).
9. Yahagi, T. M., Degawa, M., Seino, Y., Matsushima, T., Nagao, M., Sugimura, T., and Hashimoto, Y., *Cancer Letters,* **1**, 911 (1975).
10. Haworth, S., Lawlor, T., Mortlemans, K., Speck, W. and Zeiger, E., *Environmental Mutagenesis* **5**, (Supp. 1) 1 (1983).
11. Bridges, B. A., *Laboratory Practice* **21**, 413 (1972).
12. Green, M. H. L. and Muriel, W. J., *Mutation Res.* **38**, 3 (1976).
13. Venitt, S. and Crofton-Sliegh, C., *Mutation Res.* **68**, 107 (1979).
14. Mohn, G. R. and Ellenberger, J., The Use of *Escherichia coli* K-12/343/113 (λ) as a Multipurpose Indicator Strain in Various Mutagenicity Testing Procedures, in *Handbook of Mutagenicity Test Procedures,* B. Kilbey, et al., eds. Elsevier, Amsterdam 1977, pp 95–118.
15. Skopek, T. R., Liber, H. L., Krolewski, J. J. and Thilly, W. G., *PNAS* **75**, 410 (1978).
16. Ruiz-Vazquez, R., Pueyo, C. and Cerda-Olmedo, E., *Mutation Res.* **54**, 121 (1978).
17. Vithayathil, A. J., McClure, C. and Myers, J. W., *Mutation Res.* **121**, 33 (1983).
18. Skopek, T. R., Liber, H. L., Kaden, D. A. and Thilly, W. G., *PNAS* **75**, 4465 (1978).

Chapter 12

Yeast Assays in Mutagen and Carcinogen Screening

David J. Brusick

Introduction

The yeasts offer tremendous versatility in genetic screening. It is probably safe to say that more different genetic endpoints can be detected in yeast than any other single test species.

Yeasts represent a class of organisms known as lower eukaryotes. This means that the cell structure of yeasts has similarities with animal cells, but retains characteristics related to plant and bacterial cells. One of those characteristics that seems to be critical in the application of yeasts to genetic screening is the cell wall/cell membrane complex. The cell wall of yeast cells is relatively thick and plant-like and may inhibit molecular transport. In addition, the yeast cell membrane does not have the same molecular composition as animal cells and is rather selective regarding the types of molecules that can be transported into and out of the cells. Consequently, yeasts often appear rather insensitive to the mutagenic activities of chemicals that show strong responses in bacteria and tests using mammalian cells.

Yeasts are also known to possess a rather well-developed cytochrome oxidase metabolic capability that produces metabolic products (4). However, adaptation of exogenous S9 mix to yeast tests has met with only limited success (2, 3, 8).

Although less is known about the biochemical pathways of DNA repair for yeasts than for bacteria and possibly animal cells, it is known that they are relatively complex and effect the processes of mutagenesis.

Part of the versatility of yeasts rests with the fact that these microorganisms can be easily maintained in the haploid (N) or diploid (2N) condition and that the ability to maintain the cells in the diploid state opens up several opportunities for testing not available with other microorganisms (9). Although direct cytogenetic analysis is not possible because of the small size of yeast chromosomes, it is possible to study chromosome phenomena in yeast such as crossing-over and chromosome loss, as well as specific locus mutation in both the forward and reverse direction. Table 1 summarizes several of the tests that can be conducted in yeast.

Description of Selected Yeast Assays

Tests to Detect Forward Mutation

There are two relatively routine methods to measure forward mutation in yeast. One method uses *Saccharomyces cerevisiae* and the other *Schizosaccharomyces pombe*.

The *Saccharomyces cerevisiae* strain S288C (α, p^+, can^s), a haploid organism, permits the detection of forward mutations at an arginine-specific permease locus. A mutational block in this permease locus renders the cell resistant to an arginine homlog, canavanine sulfate ($can^s \rightarrow can^r$). The S288C prototropic haploid strain is used to measure the induction of mutations by chemicals that can cause a mutational block in the permease locus. The ratio of canavanine sensitivity to canavanine resistance is considered as an index to measure the mutagenicity of the test chemical. A description of the method is given in reference 1.

The *Schizosaccharomyces pombe* strain P1 (SP *ade* 6-60, *rad* 10-198, h⁻) is a haploid organisms that grows as a red culture caused by the *ade* 6-60 mutation. This mutation produces a block in adenine biosynthesis that produces a red pigment within the cell. A mutation at any one of five genetic loci that control biochemical steps of adenine biosynthesis preceding the *ade* 6 gene product will stop the synthesis of adenine before the red intermediate molecule and result in white-colored colonies. Both base-pair substitution (BPS) and frame-shift (FS) mutations can be detected in this assay; a description of the test is given in ref. (5).

TABLE 1
A Comparison of Screening Techniques Employing Yeasts

Test	Organism	Haploid (H) or Diploid (D)	Strain	Genetic damage detected	Reference(s)
Mutations	S. cerevisiae[a]	H	S288CU	Forward mutation from canavanine[s] to canavanine[R]	1
	S. pombe[b]	H	P1	Forward mutation at five genes preceding all ade-6 in purine biosynthesis	5
	S. cerevisiae	H	S138/S211	Reverse mutation in two met[−] indicator strains	3
	S. cerevisiae	H	XV185-14C	Reverse mutation at his-1, hom-3, and org-4 loci	6
Mitotic recombination	S. cerevisiae	D	D$_3$, D$_5$, D$_7$	Mitotic recombination involving ade alleles	9,11
Mitotic gene conversion	S. cerevisiae	D	D$_4$, D$_7$	Mitotic gene conversion at trp-5 loci	9
Aneuploidy	S. cerevisiae	D	D$_6$	Detects loss of chromosome XII	7

[a]Saccharomyces cerevisiae.
[b]Schizosaccharomyces pombe.

Tests to Detect Reverse Mutation

Reverse mutation in yeast can be studied using plate assays similar in design to the Ames test (see ref. *3* for a discussion).

Mutant cells are added to the surface of a selective agar medium along with the test chemical and S9 mix. Revertant cells can form colonies capable of growing on the selective medium after 3–4 days incubation.

Two systems have been used to examine numerous compounds. One is a single strain XV 185-14C containing several mutant alleles (*his* 1-7, *hom* 3-10, and *org* 4-17). The *his*‾ allele can be reverted by BPS agents and the *hom*‾ allele by FS agents (*6*). The second test employs two different mutants S138 (*met*‾) and S211 (*met*‾). S138 responds to FS agents and S211 to BPS agents (*3*). Although these tests respond well to direct acting mutagens, neither system works well as a plate test with S9 mix. A positive control agent for the activation plate assay which seems to work consistently is steriogmatocystin. Recent methods recommend a long (18 hour) preincubation exposure before plating.

Tests to Detect Mitotic Recombination and Mitotic Gene Conversion

Strains D_3, D_4, D_5, and D_7 were constructed by Zimmermann to detect these genetic phenomena (*9, 10*). Strain D_7 is capable of detecting both endpoints simultaneously and will be used as the illustration for this type of screen (*11*). D_7 produces white colonies under normal culture conditions.

Though the reciprocal recombination, which involves the exchange of genetic material between two nonsister chromatids during mitosis, is a nonmutational genetic event, it results in the homozygosity of recessive genes similar to a mutagenic effect. This homozygosity could bring about expression of deleterious phenotypes that are an indication of chromosomal and, hence, DNA alteration. The phenotypic expression of reciprocal recombination in yeast strain D_7 is red-pink colonies representing the homozygosity of the two recessive *ade*-2 alleles-(-*ade* 2-40 and *ade* 2-119). Mitotic gene conversion, is again a nonmutational genetic event. At the two-strand stage of nondividing cells of this diploid strain, the nonreciprocal recombination forms red or pink colonies; and at the four-strand replicative stage during cell division, gene conversion brings about red-white colonies, pink-white sectored colonies, or all red or all pink colonies.

1. Mitotic crossing over can be detected visually in this strain as pink and red twin-sectored colonies caused by the formation of homozygous cells of the genotype *ade 2-40/ade 240* (deep red) and *ade-2-119 ade 2-119* (pink) from the hetero allelic condition *ade 2-40/ade 2119* that forms white colonies.

2. Mitotic gene conversion is monitored by the appearance of tryptophan independent colonies from tryptophan-dependent colonies. The alleles involved are *trp 5-12* and *trp 5-27* derived from strain D_4.

A full description of the development of sector colonies is given by Zimmermann (9).

Strain D_7 is homoallelic *ilv* I-92 and can detect reverse mutation at either mutant allele or by allele nonspecific suppressor mutation. The mutation assay in D_7 appears to be capable of detecting BPS agents.

Test Method to Detect Aneuploidy (Chromosome Loss)

The yeast strain used in this technique is a diploid eukaryotic organism in which the induction of mitotic chromosome loss (aneuploidy) can be detected. It is believed that this test is a measure of nondisjunction.

Chromosome nondisjunction during mitosis in diploid cells leads to aneuploid cells. Nondisjunction is not only caused by mutagens, but also by agents interfering with the function of the spindle apparatus. Mitotic nondisjunction is a rare event and is detected in this *Saccharomyces cerevisiae* strain by the expression in mitotic segregants of coupled, recessive markers in otherwise heterozygous diploid cells (7).

Saccharomyces cerevisiae strain D_6 is a diploid yeast strain with the following genotype.

Chromosome III $\underline{his^4 \quad a}$

$\underline{+ \quad \alpha}$

Chromosome VII $\underline{ade^3 \quad leu1 \quad trp5 \quad cyh2 \quad met13}$

$\underline{+ \quad \quad + \quad + \quad + \quad +}$

Chromosome XV $\underline{ade2\text{-}40}$

$ade2\text{-}40$

The strain D_6 as shown carries a series of recessive and coupled markers on chromosome VII and when plated on the appropriate growth medium produces red colonies that are sensitive to the presence of 2 μg/mL cycloheximide in the growth medium. Loss of chromosome VII carrying the wild-type alleles, presumably by nondisjunction, results in the production of white (*ade* 3) colonies resistant to cycloheximide. The resistant, white colonies are then tested by replica plating on minimal media lacking the amino acides, leucine, tryptophan, or methionine to verify that both arms of chromosome VII were indeed lost.

Summary

Yeasts are versatile organisms and are extremely useful for genetic analysis. As screening organisms, they have somewhat limited application because of their resistance to a broad range of chemical classes, especially those containing the polycyclic hydrocarbon and aromatic amine carcinogens. The other problem concerns the lack of a good exogenous mammalian metabolic system. Recently, investigators have attempted to utilize the rather extensive intrinsic metabolic capabilities of yeast by conducting tests with growing cell cultures over extended treatment times. Although these modifications in methodologies have been helpful, significant problems in metabolic activation still exist (see ref. *8*).

The results of correlation studies with yeasts using a broad range of mammalian carcinogens shows a good correlation with most direct-acting agents, but an overall low correlation because of the absence of activity with many procarcinogens. At the present time, one of the most promising tests involving yeasts is the test for nondisjunction (aneuploidy) using diploid strain D_6. Strain D_6 is almost the only viable assay for aneuploidy which can be conducted on a routine screening basis.

Several good reviews of yeast test methods and comparative data analyses have been published (see ref. *3, 5, 8, 9*).

References

1. Brusick, D. J., *J. Bacteriol.* **109,** 1134 1972
2. Brusick, D., and Andrews, H., *Mutation Res.* **26,** 492 (1974).
3. Brusick, D. J., and Mayer, V. W., *Environ. Health Perspect.* **6,** 83 (1973).
4. Callen, D. F., and Philpot, R. M., *Mutation Res.* **45,** 309 (1977).
5. Loprieno, N., Use of Yeast as an Assay System for Industrial Mutagens, in *Chemical Mutagens: Principles and Methods for Their Detection,* Vol. 5,

Hollaender, A., and deSerres, F. J., eds., Plenum, New York, 1978, pp. 25–53.

6. Menta, R. D., and von Borstel, R. C., Mutagenic Activity of 42 Encoded Compounds in the Haploid Yeast Reversion Assay, Strain CV 185–14C, in *Evaluation of Short-Term tests for Carcinogens,* deSerres, F. J., and Ashby, J., eds., Elsevier/North-Holland, Amsterdam, 1981, pp. 414–423.

7. Parry, J. M., and Zimmermann, F. K., *Mutation Res.* **36,** 49 (1976).

8. *Summary Report on the Performance of Yeast Assays,* in *Evaluation of Short-Term Tests for Carcinogens,* deSerres, F. J., and Ashby, J., eds., Elsevier/North-Holland, Amsterdam, 1981, Chapter 7, pp. 68–76.

9. Zimmerman, F. K., Detection of Genetically Active Chemicals Using Various Yeast Systems, in *Chemical Mutagens: Principles and Methods for Their Detection, vol. 3, Hollaender, A., ed., Plenum, New York, 1973, pp. 209–239.*

10. Zimmermann, F. K., *Mutation Res.* **31,** 71 (1975).

11. Zimmermann, F. K., Kern, R., and Rasenberg, H., *Mutation Res.* **28,** 381 (1975).

Chapter 13

Mouse Lymphoma Cell Assays

Paul E. Kirby

Theory and Background

Since Chu and Malling (*1*) and Kao and Puck (*2*) first demonstrated that chemical mutagens could induce mutations in hamster cells in vitro, investigators have developed and refined in vitro systems that are capable of detecting chemically induced mutations (*3–8*). The benefits of using in vitro test systems for screening chemicals for mutagenic activity, compared to in vivo test systems, are economy and greatly improved speed of assay.

Most of the in vitro test systems are based on the ability to distinguish a mutant phenotype from a nonmutant phenotype by placing the cells in a medium that selects for one or the other. The number of mutant cells contained in a population can be quantified, and by comparing the number of mutants contained in a culture treated with a mutagenic agent versus a nontreated or solvent-treated culture, one can determine the number of induced mutations.

In addition, many chemicals designated as promutagens must be metabolically converted to an active form before their mutagenicity can be expressed via in vitro test systems. Most mammalian tissues are capable of activating promutagens, but since the liver is the major site of microsomal enzymatic activity, many investigators have used extracts from this organ to activate chemicals. Ames et al. (*9*) demonstrated that liver extracts could activate promutagens that were then detectable in the *Salmonella* (Ames) assay. Umeda and Saito (*10*) and Krahn and

Heidelberger (*11*) adapted this system for use in detecting mutagenic activity of promutagens in mammalian cells in vitro and Clive (*12*) adopted a similar system using rat liver S9 induced with a mixture of Aroclor 1242 and Arocolor 1254.

Clive and coworkers (*13*) selected the L5178Y mouse lymphoma cell line for developing a mutagenesis assay because several desirable characteristics were possessed by these cells. The cells grow in suspension culture, which makes it easy to obtain samples and split cultures, as opposed to cells that must be partially digested by enzymes to remove them from the surface on which they are growing. In addition, suspension growth gives the cells the ability to grow in soft agar, which allows colony formation and facilitates the enumeration of mutants. These cells also have a cloning efficiency that approaches 100% in soft agar, and a relatively short generation time of 10–12 h that yields colonies large enough for counting with an automatic colony counter 10–12 d after the initial seeding. This cell line recovers well from cryopreservation and grows in medium supplemented with horse serum. This is economically advantageous.

Clive and coworkers had originally used the hypoxanthine-guanine phosphoribosyl transferase (HGPRT) loci of L5178Y cells for detecting chemically induced mutations. However, there were inherent problems with this system using the selective agents available at that time (*13*). Specifically, the purine analog 8-azaguanine and 6-mercaptopurine, were evaluated for use in this system. They found that the number of wild-type cells killed by 8-azaguanine was dependent on the concentration of cells plated. A greater proportion of wild-type cells survived as a number of cells plated was increased. Since this was totally unacceptable, 6-mercaptopurine was evaluated as a suitable selective agent.

The concentration of 6-mercaptopurine (500 μg/mL) required to kill wild-type cells was effective over a range of 10^4–10^7 cells plated, so apparently it did not have the problem of 8-azaguanine. However, further investigation using 6-mercaptopurine showed that the killing and eventual lysis of wild-type HGPRT cells released substrates that were lethal to the HGPRT mutants. The greater the number of HGPRT cells killed, the lower the number of mutants that survived. This clearly showed 6-mercaptopurine to be an unacceptable selective agent, and at this point Clive et al. decided to evaluate the thymidine kinase locus for use in detecting chemically induced mutations.

The Thymidine Kinase Locus

Most mammalian cells possess two biochemical pathways in which thymidine monophosphate (TMP) is formed for eventual incorporation into DNA. These are the Thymidylate Synthetase (TS) and Thymidine Kinase (TK) pathways (Fig. 1).

The TS pathway, which is the main pathway, is dependent upon the metabolism of folic acid for the conversion of uridine monophosphate (dUPM) to thymidine monophosphate (dTMP), and it is because of this dependence on folic acid metabolism that the TS pathway can be shut down by exposing cells to the antifolic acid agent, methotrexate. Methotrexate competitively binds with the enzyme, dihydrofolic acid reductase, that catalyzes the reduction of dihydrofolic acid (DHFA) to tetrahydrofolic acide (THFA). Thus, the addition of methotrexate to cultures shuts down folic acid metabolism, resulting in the shut down of the TS pathway.

The TK pathway is a scavenger pathway in which endogenous or exogenous thymidine (TdR) is converted to dTMP through the action of the enzyme thymidine kinase. Cells that have TK capability can be selectively killed over cells that lack this capability by adding 5-bromodeoxyuridine (BUdR) or trifluorothymidine (TFT) to the culture medium. BUdR is converted through TK activity to BUdR monophosphate, which is a dTMP analog that kills the cell when incorporated into DNA. TFT apparently works by a different mechanism. It is phosphorylated through the TK system, and the phosphorylated TFT then kills the TK component cell by irreversibly inhibiting thymidylate

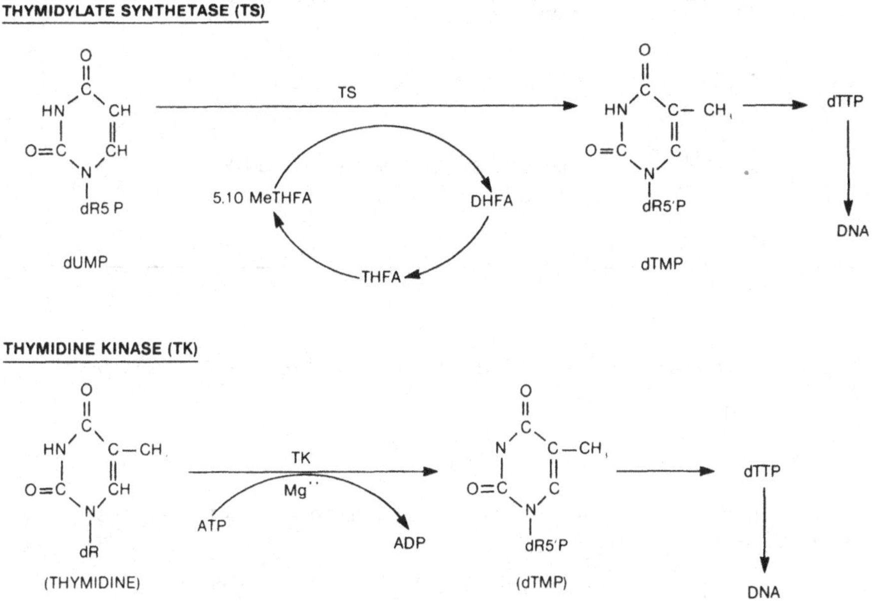

Fig. 1. Pathways of thymidine triphosphate synthesis.

synthetase A, thus shutting down the TS pathway. Since TFT does not require incorporation into DNA to be effective, it kills the sensitive cells prior to dividing, whereas BUdR allows the cell to divide several times and form microcolonies before they are killed.

Based on the principles discussed above, one can, through the manipulation of the culture medium, select for either TK-competent or TK-incompetent cells (Figs. 2 and 3). Cells heterozygous at the TK locus (TK+/−) have available both the TS and TK pathways, whereas TK-incompetent cells have only the TS pathway. If the thymidine analogs BUdR or TFT are added to the culture medium, TK+/− cells phosphorylate them by the TK pathway and the TK+/− cells are killed. Since TK−/− cells do not have the ability to phosphorylate BUdR or TFT, they survive in medium containing BUdR or TFT. On the other hand, TK+/− cells survive in medium containing methotrexate, and TK−/− cells are killed. Since methotrexate shuts down the TS pathway of dTMP formation, TK−/− cells cannot survive whereas TK+/− cells can utilize the TK system for the formation of dTMP.

The L5178Y TK+/−assay that monitors the forward mutation rate from TK+/− to TK−/− makes use of the ability to selectively kill TK−/− cells to prepare starting cultures.

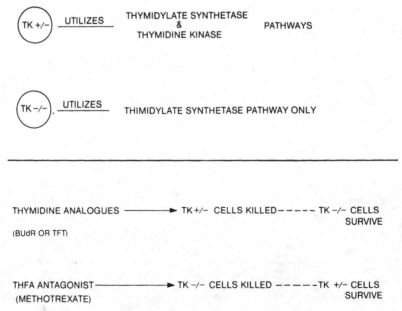

Fig. 2.   Selection for TK +/− and TK−/− cells.

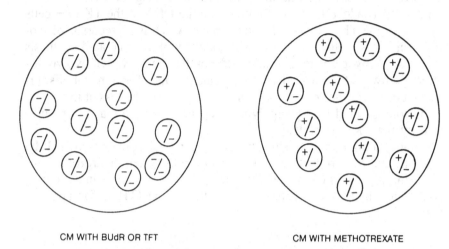

Fig. 3.   Colony formation in selective cloning medium (CM).

Test System Description

Test chemicals are evaluated for potential mutagenic activity in the L5178Y TK+/−assay by exposing populations of TK+/− cells to the chemical in question and, after a suitable expression period, determining whether the number of TK+/− mutants contained in treated cultures is significantly greater than that of control cultures. TK−/− cells are selectively grown in a soft agar medium containing TFT that kills the TK+/− cells.

Cell Preparation

It is important when performing assays from which conclusions are drawn based on comparisons of treated and control culture results, that the background frequency of the endpoint is as low as possible. L5178Y TK+/− clone 3.7.2C is the recommended cell line (*14*). In the L5178Y TK+/− system, the frequency of TK−/− mutants in a population of TK+/− heterozygotes is readily controlled by exposing them to THMG medium (Thymidine, Hypoxanthine, Methotrexate, and Glycine). Since methotrexate is an antagonist of folate metabolism, the TK−/− cells in the population are killed.

Folate metabolism is also vital to the synthesis of purines, the pyrimidine thymine, and the conversion of serine to glycine. Thus, thymidine, hypoxanthine, and glycine must also be included in the selective medium to prevent the loss of folate metabolism from killing the TK+/− cells. Thymidine is added for incorporation into the DNA of the TK+/− cells by way of the TK pathway. Hypoxanthine, which is a precursor of inosinic acid, is supplied since the main pathway of inosinic acid synthesis requires tetrahydrofolate. Inosinic acid can then be converted by two different pathways to either adenine or guanine. Since folate metabolism is also required for the conversion of serine to glycine, the loss of this activity is compensated for by supplying exogenous glycine that can be utilized by the TK+/− cells.

Since a lag period exists between the removal of cells from THMG medium and the production of sufficient levels of tetrahydrofolate, the cleansing process is completed by placing the TK+/− cells in a medium containing thymidine, hypoxanthine, and glycine (THG) for approximately 24 h.

Treatment and Expression Period

The mutation assay consists of exposing populations of L5178Y TK+/− cells to the test chemical for 4 h both with and without exogenous metabolic activation. The activation systems routinely used are Aroclor-induced rat liver S9 preparations. At the end of the exposure period the test chemical is removed from the cultures by centrifugally pelleting the cells, pouring off the supernatant, and performing two rinses with culture medium. The cultures are allowed to grow for an expression period of 2 or 3 d with population adjustments at 24 h intervals to maintain them in log phase growth.

Selection of TK−/− Mutants

At the end of the expresion period, cells from each culture are cloned in soft agar (cloning) medium, which allows them to grow into discrete macroscopic colonies that, after a sufficient incubation period, can be counted by hand or with an automatic colony counter. In addition to selecting out the TK−/− cells of a population, the percentage of viable cells in each population is approximated by cloning a specific number of cells from each culture in nonselective cloning medium (Fig. 4). (More detail will be given in the next section.) After determining the number of TK+/− colonies per restrictive medium (TFT) plate and the number of colonies per nonrestrictive medium (viable count, VC) plate, one can deduce the TK−/− mutant frequency per viable cell for each culture.

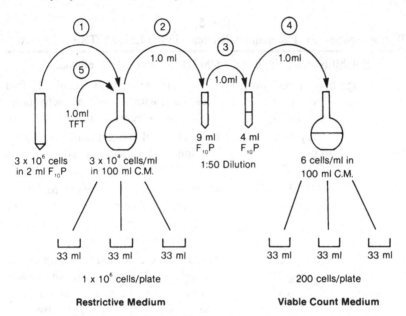

Fig. 4.   Illustration of cell dilution and plating in the cloning process.

If 100 TK$-/-$ colonies are counted in a plate seeded with one million cells, then one could conclude that the TK$-/-$ mutant frequency is $100/10^6$ cells plated. However, if 50% of the cells seeded were dead, as evidenced by only 100 colonies forming from 200 cells seeded in a viable count plate, the mutant frequency would be $200/10^6$ viable cells.

By determining the mutant frequency per viable cell, the possibility of having "false-negative" results arising from a reduction in the actual number of TK$-/-$ mutants because of toxic effects is eliminated. If a control and a treated plate each contained 50 TK$-/-$ colonies per million cells plated, one might conclude that the test chemical had not induced any increase in TK$-/-$ mutants; however, if the viable counts for the control plate were 200 colonies out of 200 cells seeded and the treated plate were 50 out of 200 seeded, there would be a fourfold increase in the mutant frequency per surviving cell of the treated culture over that of the control culture.

Experimental Design

In order to evaluate a chemical for mutagenic potential in the L5178Y TK$+/-$ system, one must select a solvent for dissolving the chemical and delivering it to the target cells, perform a range-finding experiment to de-

Fig. 5.

Testing Scheme for Evaluating Chemicals in the L5178Y TK+/− Assay

I	Solubility determination	DMSO, acetone, H_2O, ethanol
II	Range finding experiment dosing 37°C 5% CO_2	7 doses, 10,000 to 0.01 µg/mL, 10-fold dilutions with and without activation plus two solvent controls
	Day 1 adjustment 37°C 5% CO_2	Determine cell concentrations for each culture and if necessary, adjust them to 0.3×10^6 cells/mL
	Day 2 adjustment	Determine cell concentrations for each culture and discard. Determine suspension growth and relative suspension growth for each
III	TK+/− assay dosing 37°C 5% CO_2	Based on results of range finding experiment, 16 cultures with and without activation, treated over a range that produces 0–100% toxicity, plus two solvent controls
	Day 1 adjustment 37°C 5% CO_2	Determine cell concentrations for each culture and, if necessary, adjust them to 0.3×10^6 cells/mL
	Day 2 adjustment and cloning	Determine cell concentrations for each culture, and adjust those which will be cloned. Clone cultures exhibiting between 0 and 100% suspension growth.
	10–12 Day incubation period at 37°C with 5% CO_2 in air	
	Day 10–12 enumeration of colonies	Count the colonies by hand or with an automatic colony counter and determine mutant frequencies, induced mutant frequencies and % total growth

termine the proper dosing for use in the assay, perform the assay, and evaluate the results (Fig. 5).

Dimethyl sulfoxide (DMSO), acetone, water, and ethanol are the four solvents that have been used routinely in this and other systems. DMSO, acetone, and ethanol at levels of 1% final concentration are nontoxic and do not affect the spontaneous mutant frequency of the L5178Y TK+/− cell line. Care must be taken in selecting the solvents to insure that the test chemical is not reactive with the solvent. If a chemical is only partially soluble in any of these four, one may be able to increase the deliverable doses by diluting the chemical in culture medium.

Range Finding

Most chemicals that are positive in this system are detected when tested at doses that produce some degree of lethality. In order to obtain a rough estimate of the maximum dose required to achieve a toxic response, a range-finding experiment is performed. A typical range-finding test consists of preparing cell cultures in disposable centrifuge tubes, treating the cultures over a broad range of doses, and determining the cell population density approximately 24 and 48 h after the initial dosing.

Preparation of Tube Cultures

To begin the range finding test, one prepares a homogenous cell suspension containing 1×10^6 cells mL in medium that is 50% fresh medium (FoP) and 50% conditioned medium retained from the stock culture. A 6 mL volume of the suspension is dispensed to each culture tube, the cultures are gassed with 5% CO_2 in air, and then placed in a shaker incubator or on a roller drum at 36°C until treatment.

Preparation of S9 Mix

The cultures treated in conjunction with exogenous activation receive 4 mL of S9 mix. The S9 mix is prepared just prior to the beginning of the treatment process and it is maintained on ice until used.

To prepare it, 6.0 mg NADP and 11.25 mg isocitric acid (trisodium salt)/mL of S9 mix are dissolved in a volume of cold FoP equal to three-fourths of the desired final volume. The pH of this solution is adjusted to approximately 6.8 by adding 1.0N NaOH until the color of the solution approximates that of a normal bottle of FoP. This solution is filter sterilized, and freshly thawed sterile S9 homogenate (one-quarter the desired final volume of S9 mix) is added. The time span between preparation and use should not be allowed to exceed 30 min.

Test Article Dilution and Treatment of Cultures

Since some known chemical mutagens lose activity when in solution (15), all test articles and positive controls should be solubilized and dilution samples prepared just prior to treatment. For performing a range finding experiment one might select doses ranging from 10,000 μg/mL to 0.001 μg/mL with a tenfold reduction between doses or, in order to narrow the range further, perform intermediate dilutions resulting in doses such as 10,000, 5,000, 1,000, 500. . . . . . μg/mL.

To reiterate, immediately after the test article dilution has been performed, the tube cultures should be treated. A 4mL volume of FoP or S9 mix and 100 λ of the appropriate dilution sample is added to each tube culture and the cultures are gassed with 5% Co_2 in air. Cultures receiving 100λ of solvent only are used as controls. After the cultures have been treated, they are placed on a roller drum apparatus spinning at a rate sufficient to keep the cells thoroughly suspended (25 rpm works well) for the four hour exposure period. To avoid inactivation of light sensitive compounds, the test solutions should be prepared under amber lighting and the cultures should be kept in darkness during the exposure period.

After 4 h the test article is removed by centrifuging the cultures at 1000 rpm for 10 min and decanting the supernatant. The cells are washed twice in 10 mL of $F_{10}P$, resuspended in 20 mL of $F_{10}P$, gassed with 5% CO_2 in air, and placed on a roller drum apparatus at 37°C and a speed of approximately 25 rpm.

Cell Culture Adjustment During the Growth Period

Since the test article-induced toxic effect is quantified by comparing the growth of treated cultures with that of cultures receiving only solvent, samples of each culture are taken approximately 24 and 48 h after treatment to determine the cell population densities. At the 24 h mark the cultures are adjusted to 0.3 x 10^6 cells/mL.

The cell population density of each culture is determined by: (a) thoroughly mixing the contents of each tube by vortical action, (b) aseptically removing a 1.0 mL sample and placing it in 9.0 mL of 0.1% trypsin, (c) incubating the sample for 10 min at 37°C, (d) making counts with an electronic particle counter, and (e) calculating the number of cells/mL.

The cultures are adjusted by retaining a volume of each culture that, when diluted to a final volume of 20 mL with fresh $F_{10}P$, will contain 0.3 x 10^6 cells/mL.

$$\text{Volume of culture to retain} = \frac{(\text{Desired cell concentration}) \times (\text{Desired final volume})}{(\text{Current cell concentration})}$$

After adjustment, each culture is gassed with 5% CO_2 in air and replaced on a roller drum apparatus at approximately 25 rpm and 37°C.

Quantification of Toxicity

The toxic effect by the test article is quantified by calculating the Suspension Growth and Relative Suspension Growth for each culture. The Suspension Growth is simply a determination of the number of times the population of each culture has doubled. This is calculated by the following formula:

$$\text{Suspension growth} = \left(\frac{\text{Day 1 concentration}}{\text{Initial concentration}}\right) \times \left(\frac{\text{Day 2 concentration}}{\text{Day 1 adjusted concentration*}}\right)$$

The Relative Suspension Growth is simply the Suspension Growth of each culture expressed as a percent of the solvent control's Suspension Growth and is calculated as follows:

$$\text{Relative suspension growth} = \frac{\text{Treated culture suspension growth}}{\text{Solvent control suspension growth}} \times 100$$

An example of typical data resulting from a range finding test is presented in Table 1. One usually finds that there is a span from total kill to 100% growth with no intermediate values. This of course depends on the selected magnitude of gradation between doses.

Having established a range over which cultures can be treated to produce from 0 to 100% kill, one can now proceed with the assay.

The Mutagenesis Assay

Since one wants to evaluate a test chemical in this system over a range of doses that produces from approximately 0 to 90% kill in the test cultures, it is best to treat cultures over a broad range of doses, and after determining the toxic response from suspension growth data, selecting the desired cultures for cloning. In other words, enough cultures should be treated so that a few are totally killed, a few exhibit 100% Relative Suspension Growth, and many fall within the range from 0 to 100% kill. In this way one can select for cloning, based on suspension growth data, the cultures which are within the desired toxic range.

---

*This will be 0.3×10^6 cells/mL if adjustment is required. If adjustment is not necessary, it will equal the Day 1 concentration, which will reduce the equation to: (Day 2 concentration)/(Initial concentration).

TABLE 1
L5178Y TK+/− Range-Finding Data

Dose, μg/mL	Day 1 concentration, cells/mL	Day 2 concentration, cells/mL	Suspension growth	Relative suspension growth, %
10,000	0.040	0.020	0.07	0
1,000	0.040	0.050	0.07	0
100	0.250	0.310	1.03	4
10	1.350	1.510	22.7	101
1.0	1.400	1.498	23.3	104
0.1	1.320	1.521	22.3	100
0.01	1.360	1.488	22.3	100
0.001	1.290	1.470	21.1	94
Solvent control	1.380	1.500	23.0 ⎫ 22.4	
Solvent control	1.320	1.482	21.7 ⎭	

Preparation of Cultures, S9 Mix, and Treatment of Cultures

The preparation of the cultures and S9 mix is exactly as described previously for the range-finding experiments. The only difference is that the Mutagenesis Assay is performed on a much larger scale. The dilution of the test article and treatment is also performed as previously described for the range finding experiment.

Expression Period

A 2-d expression period is routinely used for the L5178Y TK+/− assay.* Samples are taken from each culture for cell population determinations at approximately 24 and 48 h as described for the range-finding experiment, and the cultures are adjusted to 3×10^5 cells/mL. At the 48 h period (day 2 of expression), the cultures are adjusted to 3×10^5 cells/mL in 10 mL of $F_{10}P$ in preparation for the cloning process.

---

*Some test chemicals may induce a greater number of TK−/− mutants if the cultures are allowed to express for a longer period of time. However, chemicals having weak mutagenic activity may be missed if a longer expression period is used because the TK−/− mutants may be diluted out to a nondetectable level by faster growing TK+/− cells.

Cloning

The cloning process, illustrated in Fig. 4, is the process by which the number of mutants existing in a population is quantified and the percent of viable cells in a population is estimated. The schema of Fig. 4 may look quite simple, but when working with a large number of cultures and with cells and agar-containing medium that are temperature sensitive, the timing of the process is critical.

The process of cloning can be broken down into the following steps.

1. Preparation of cloning medium.
2. Adding cells to the restrictive media flask.
3. Dilution of the cells and addition to the viable count flask.
4. Addition of the restrictive agent.
5. Plating the contents of the flasks.

It may at first appear ludicrous to consider some of the processes, such as the addition of cells to a flask to constitute a major step, but it is essential that the investigator be aware of many factors involved in these processes that can affect the quality of the experiment.

Step 1. Preparation of Cloning Medium

As anyone will attest who has worked with agar-containing medium and eucaryotic cells, attention to detail regarding temperature is essential. If the medium cools to 37°C or below, it begins to gel and if cells are placed in medium that is much above 37°C, they become less viable.

Cloning medium is prepared immediately prior to beginning the cloning process. Two hundred mL is required for each culture to be cloned and it is wise to prepare in total 300 or 400 mL extra in case of spills or breakage.

For each 100 mL of cloning medium, the following components are mixed:

Horse serum (heat inactivated)	20 mL
100× sodium pyruvate stock	1.0 mL
F_0P	70.5 mL
Purified agar	8.5 mL

The contents are warmed to 44°C in a water bath, and then 8.5 mL of a 4% agar* solution (~56°C) is added and the contents are thoroughly mixed. The final agar concentration should be approximately 0.34%.†

The cloning medium is maintained at 44°C and dispensed in 100 mL aliquots into the restrictive medium and viable count flasks which have been prewarmed to 37°C. Upon filling, the flasks are immediately placed in a shaker incubator (37°C) and the contents are allowed to equilibrate to 37°C prior to adding the cells.

Step 2. Adding Cells to the Flask

At this point of the experiment, the cultures selected for cloning should have been adjusted to 3×10^5 cells/mL in 10 mL of $F_{10}P$ gassed with 5% CO_2 in air and placed on a roller drum (25 rpm) at 37°C until the investigator is ready to begin the cloning process.

After the cloning medium in the flasks has equilibrated to 37°C, the cells in the tube cultures can be added to those designated for restrictive medium. The cells are pelleted by centrifugation at approximately 1000 rpm for 10 min and then the supernatant, except for 2 mL, is carefully removed by aspiration. The cells are resuspended in the remaining 2mL and then added to the appropriate flask. Since L5178Y cells tend to grow in clusters rather than single cells, it is of utmost importance that the clusters be broken apart before adding the cells to the cloning medium. If doublets, triplets, or any other quantity of cells greater than one per cluster are cloned, they will only form one colony instead of the two or three or more colonies that would be found if they had been disassociated. This can greatly affect the cloning efficiency observed in the viable count plates. The disassociation can be accomplished by vigorous vortexing and mixing, or one can aspirate the cells in medium and expel them back into the tube. Repeating this several times will effectively disassociate the cells. The cells and medium are then added to the 100 mL of cloning me-

---

*In our laboratory we have recently changed from using Noble Agar (Difco) to Purified Agar (Ibid). The latter is quality controlled by Difco for compatibility with cell cultures.

†This is the concentration we are using in our laboratory as of this writing, but any laboratory using this assay should determine the optimal for their system under their laboratory conditions. This is easily done by cloning cells (200 cells/plate) in a range of agar concentrations (i.e., 0.30%, 0.31%, 0.32% . . . 0.39%, 0.40%) and determining the concentration that gives the optimal cloning efficiency after 10–12 days incubation at 37°C and 5% CO_2 in air. One will find that the lower concentrations result in a cloning medium that is too loose and therefore does not allow the formation of discrete colonies. Microscopic observation will show thousands of cells streaming throughout the medium. The higher concentrations of agar will be too firm and will not allow the cells to readily divide, thus reducing cloning efficiency. One should obtain results that, when graphed approximate a normal distribution. The percent agar concentration chosen should of course be the one that lies under the peak.

dium, the tube is rinsed with 10 mL of cloning medium from the flask, and the flask is placed in the shaker incubator for 15 min to allow thorough mixing and the creation of a homogeneous cell suspension.

Step 3. Cell Dilution and Addition to the Viable Count Flask

This process is a fairly straight forward serial dilution, as outlined in Fig. 4, but one must work in a timely manner always keeping the contents of the flask at 37°C. If they cool much below this, the cloning medium will begin to clump. The numbers 1 through 5 in circles in Fig. 4 indicate the sequence of events. Step 1 was just described above. After the cells have been mixed in the first flask for 15 min, one takes a 1 mL sample and does 1:10 and 1:5 dilutions in $F_{10}P$ medium and then adds 1 mL to the flask designated as the viable count flask. This effects a 1:5000 dilution of the contents of the restrictive medium flask, resulting in approximately 600 cells in the viable count flask. The flask is again placed in a shaker incubator for 15 min to allow thorough mixing.

Step 4. Addition of the Restrictive Agent

After the 1 mL sample of cells has been removed from the restrictive medium flask, the restrictive agent trifluorothymidine (TFT) can be added. A 1 mL volume of a freshly thawed 100× stock solution of TFT is added so that the final concentration is sufficient to kill the TK+/− cells and not have any ill effects on the TK−/− cells. At present a final concentration of anywhere from 1.0 to 4.0 µg/mL is being reported.*

After the addition of TFT the flask is again placed in a shaker incubator for 15 minutes to effect thorough mixing.

Step 5. Plating the Contents of the Flasks

After proper mixing, the contents of each flask can be put into petri plates in preparation for incubation. It is important that each plate receive equivalent amounts† and this can be assured by pipeting the contents into the petri plates.

The plates are placed in cold storage at 40°C for 20 min and then in an environment of 5% CO_2 in air and 37°C for 10–12 d of incubation. It is important to check the cultures for the appearance of white colonies within the first 5 d of incubation. It normally takes at least 7 d for L5178Y

*Anyone desiring to implement this assay system should perform titer experiments to determine the effect of TFT concentration on the growth of TK −/− and TK +/−cells and, based on their results, select the concentration of TFT that works best in their own laboratory.

†In case a plate is lost because of contamination or spillage, the average results obtained from the remaining two should be representative of the expected average results from three plates.

cells to grow to a macroscopic size and therefore the appearnce of colonies prior to 7 d can usually be attributed to yeast contamination. If a yeast contaminant is allowed to remain for the entire incubation period, one may have difficulty distinguishing it from L5178Y colonies.

Enumeration of Colonies

After the 10–12 day incubation period, the colonies can be enumerated by either counting them with the naked eye or by using an automatic colony counter. Counting with the naked eye can be performed by placing a dot on the lid of the petri plate over each colony as it is counted and clicking off the counts on a digitometer.

Several brands of automatic colony counters are available that can be used for counting L5178Y colonies. The key to using any one of these instruments is that it must be adjusted and calibrated to duplicate manual counts. Once an instrument has been demonstrated to reproduce manual counts, it can be used routinely for counting colonies.*

After the number of colonies per plate has been determined for the assay, one can store the plates at 4°C until the data has been evaluated.

Data Evaluation

Mutant Frequency

The data can be collected on a form such as that represented in Table 2. The number of colonies for the restrictive medium plates and the viable count plates is entered for each given dose, and the averages are computed. The frequency of TK$-/-$ mutants per quantity of surviving cells is determined for each culture by the following formula:

$$\text{Mutant frequency per } 10^4 \text{ survivors} = \frac{\text{Average No. of TFT colonies}}{\text{Average No. of VC colonies}} \times 2$$

and the induced-mutant frequency is determined by subtracting the mutant frequency observed in solvent control cultures from that observed for a culture treated with a given dose of the test chemical:

Induced mutant frequency = Mutant frequency of treated cultures −
Average mutant frequency of solvent controls

*It is important that these instruments be checked and calibrated often to ensure that electronic drift has not caused undue variation in the counting process.

TABLE 2
L5178Y TK+/− Mouse Lymhoma Mutagenesis Assay
Cloning Data

Study Number				Study Director				Experiment Number		
Test Article Identity				Solvent				Metabolic Activation		
Test Article Conc.	No. of Colonies/TFT Plate 1	2	3	Avg. #/ Plate	No. of Colonies/V.C. Plate 1	2	3	Avg. #/ Plate	Mutant* Frequency	Induced Mutant* Frequency
Solvent 1										
Solvent 2										
A										
B										
A										
B										
A										
B										
A										
B										
A										
B										
A										
B										

Plates Counted By: _____   Calculations Performed By: _____
        (Signature & Date)   (Signature & Date)

* Per 10^4 surviving cells

Toxicity

The toxic effect of treatment with various doses of a test chemical in the L5178Y TK+/− assay is evaluated by two functions: (1) the suspension growth of each culture over the 2-day expression period in relation to the solvent control cultures and (2) the cloning growth of each culture in relation to that of the solvent control cultures.

Suspension growth is calculated by:

$$\text{Total suspension growth} = \frac{\text{Day 1 cell concentration}}{0.3 \times 10^6 \text{ cells/mL}} \times$$

$$\frac{\text{Day 2 cell concentration}}{\text{Day 1 adjusted cell concentration}} \times \frac{\text{Day 3 cell concentration}}{\text{Day 2 adjusted cell concentration}}$$

and the relative suspension growth is calculated as follows:

$$\% \text{ Control suspension growth} = \frac{\text{Treated culture suspension growth}}{\text{Average suspension growth of controls}} \times 100$$

The relationship of the cloning efficiency of treated cultures to that of the controls is expressed as

$$\% \text{ Relative cloning growth} = \frac{\text{Average VC of treated cultures}}{\text{Average VC of solvent controls}} \times 100$$

and the % of total growth of treated cultures is expressed as a function of the culture suspension and clonal growth as follows:

$$\% \text{ Total growth} = \frac{(\% \text{ Suspension growth}) (\% \text{ Cloning growth})}{100}$$

The resulting data from an L5178Y TK+/− assay therefore gives the investigator data about both mutation frequency and the toxic effects the test chemical had on the target cells.

In evaluating test data, one must first evaluate the validity of the assay and then determine if the results meet the criteria for a negative, positive, or equivocal response. There are several points that must be considered in regard to assay validity. They are:

1. Did the control cultures exhibit the normal rate of suspension growth.
2. Did the control cultures have the appropriate cloning efficiency (50% or better).
3. Did the control cultures exhibit a spontaneous mutant frequency within the normal range (0.2–$1.0/10^4$ survivors).
4. Did the positive control treated cultures exhibit induced mutant frequencies within the expected range.
5. Was a sufficient level of toxicity achieved in the cultures treated with the test article. (It is desirable to have at least one culture with between 10–30% survival.)
6. Were all of the other parameters associated with the assay within their normal range.

Once an assay has been judged valid, the criteria listed below may be used as guidelines for evaluating the response.

Positive: If one or more of the cultures exhibiting 10% or more total growth has a mutant frequency greater than twofold that of the solvent control cultures, and the response is dose-dependent.

Negative: If all of the cultures have mutant frequencies less than twofold that of the solvent control cultures, and there is no indication of a dose-dependent increase in mutant frequency.

Equivocal: (a) There is a dose-dependent response, although none of the cultures have mutant frequencies greater than twofold background.
(b) One or more cultures have mutant frequencies greater than twofold background, but there is no indication of dose dependence.

When attempting to apply these criteria to a particular set of data, one must be aware that they are to be used only as guidelines. It is impossible to formulate criteria that will cover every variation. Therefore, the conclusions drawn from a particular set of data must often be based on the scientist's evaluation. However, if the results of an assay are difficult to interpret, a repeat assay is recommended. By selecting alternative doses based on the first assay's results, the investigator may be able to produce clearly interpretable results.

References

1. Chu, E. H. Y., and Malling, H. V., *Proc. Nat. Acad. Sci.* **61,** 1306 (1968).
2. Kao, F. T., and Puck, T. T., *Proc. Nat. Acad. Sci.* **60,** 1275 (1968).
3. Clive, D., Flamm, W. G., Machesko, M. R., and Bernheim, N. J., *Mutation Res.* **16,** 77 (1972).
4. Sato, K., Slesinski, R. S., and Littlefield, J. W., *Proc. Nat. Acad. Sci. USA* **69,** 1244 (1972).
5. Albertini, R. J. and DeMars, R.,J., *Mutation Res.* **18, 199 (1973).**
6. Hsie, A., W., Brimer, P. A., and Mitchell, T. J., and Gosslee, D. G., *Somatic Cell Genet.* **1,** 383 (1975).
7. Knapp, A. G. A. C., and Simons, J. W. I. M., *Mutation Res.* **30,** 97 (1975).
8. Thilly, W. G., *J. Tox. Environ. Hlth.* **2,** 1343 (1977).
9. Ames, B. N., Durston, W. E., Yamasaki, E. Y., and Lee, F. D., *Proc. Nat. Acad. Sci. USA* **70,** 2281 (1973).
10. Umeda, M., and Sato, M., *Mutation Res.* **30,** 249 (1975).
11. Krahn, D. F., and Heidelberger, C., *Mutation Res.* **46,** 27 (1977).
12. Clive, D., Johnson, K. O., and Batson, A. G., The L5178Y TK+/− Mouse Lymphoma Assay: Protocols. Handout at the first annual "Mouse Lymphoma Workshop" held at the Burroughs Wellcome Co., Research Triangle Park, N.C., 1978.
13. Clive, D., Flamm, W. G., and Patterson, J. B., Specific-Locus Mutational Assay Systems for Mouse Lymphoma Cells, in *Chemical Mutagens: Princi-*

ples and Methods for Their Detection, Hollander, A., ed., Vol. 3, Plenum Press, New York, 1973, pp. 79–103.

14. Clive, D., Johnson, K. O., Spector, J. F. S., Batson, A. G., and Brown, M. M. M., *Mutation Res.* **59,** 61 (1979).

15. Jensen, E. M., LaPolla, R. J., Kirby, P. E., and Haworth, S. R., *J. Natl. Cancer Inst.***59,** 941 (1977).

Chapter 14

Chinese Hamster Ovary Mutation Assays

David J. Brusick

CHO System

CHO cells are widely used in cell biology, biochemistry, and genetic studies. Their widest application in genetic analysis is probably as target cells for in vitro cytogenetic analysis. The cells are readily available, grow with high cloning efficiency (> 80%), and have a reproducible generation time of 12–14 h (3). The relatively low number of morphologically distinct chromosomes facilitates cytogenetic studies. Table 1 summarizes the characteristics of this cell line.

The original application of CHO cells to mutation induction was made by Puck and Kao (7). Chu and Mallng (2) performed similar mutagenicity studies in V-79 cells, another hamster-derived cell line, at the same time. Much of the methodology described in this section is directly applicable to V-79 as well as CHO cells.

The CHO gene mutation assay, in its present form, is a result of the work of Hsie et al. (3). The selective system used in the CHO assay utilizes purine analogs to select for resistant cells that are presumed deficient in the enzyme hypoxanthine-guanine phosphoribosyl transferase (HGPRT). Selective agents that are typically used include 6-thioguanine (TG) and 8-azaguanine (AG).

The HGPRT pathway is part of a salvage pathway in the biosynthesis of DNA (1). The HGPRT structural gene is presumed to be

227

TABLE 1
Characteristics of CHO Cells[a]

---

1. Exhibit a stable karyotype over 20 years with a modal chromosome number of 20, which as a distinctly recognizable morphology.

2. Have a colony-forming capacity of nearly 100% in a defined growth medium.

3. Grow well in either monolayer or suspension with a relatively short population doubling time of 12–14 h.

4. Are genetically and biochemically well-characterized, with many genetic markers available, including auxotrophy, drug resistance, temperature sensitivity, and so on.

5. Respond well to various synchronization methods, including the mitotic detachment procedure that facilitates cell cycle study.

6. Are useful in somatic cell hybridization experiments because they readily hybridize with different cell types, including human cells; when the CHO–human cell hybrid is formed, there is subsequent rapid, preferential loss of human chromosome, which facilitates the assignment of marker genes to specific chromosomes or linkage groups in the human karyotype.

7. Quantitatively respond to various physical and chemical mutagens and carcinogens with high sensitivity.

8. Adapt to mutation induction either through coupling with a microsome activation system or through host (mouse) mediation.

9. Are capable of monitoring induced mutation to multiple gene markers, chromosome aberration, and sister chromatid exchange in the same mutagen-treated cell culture.

---

[a]From Ref. (4).

located on the X chromosome, which results in either an HGPRT +/o hemizygote in male (XY) cells or HGPRT +/o functional hemizygote because of X inactivation in female (XX) cells.

Loss of HGPRT activity resulting from mutation renders the HGPRT −/o cell resistant to 6-thioguamine or 8-azaquamine, and DNA is synthesized by de novo pathways.

The spontaneous background frequency of HGPRT mutants in the CHO line is in the range of 10^{-6} to 10^{-5} mutants/cell.

The most notable disadvantage of this test method is th absence of a published data base for testing with an activation system. Although the S9 mix can be coupled with the assay, routine procedures for bioactivation testing have not been published. Thus, an extensive portion of the CHO data base has been developed with direct-acting chemical mutagens. The data has been reviewed by Thilly and Liber (8) and Hsie et al. (4). The results of these tests (on a total of fewer than 20 compounds) shows a good correlation with carcinogenic responses. The published data base for this assay, however, is expanding rapidly.

Methods

The CHO assay evaluates the mutagenic potential of test articles in a specific-locus forward mutation assay using the CHO-K1 Chinese hamster cell line.

HGPRT is a cellular enzyme that allows cells to salvage hypoxanthine and guanine from the surrounding medium for use in DNA synthesis. If a purine analog such as TG is included in the growth medium, the analog will be phosphorylated via the HGPRT pathway and incorporated into nucleic acids, eventually resulting in cell death. A single-step forward mutation from $HGPRT^+$ to $HGPRT^-$ in the functional X chromosome will render the cell unable to utilize hypoxanthine, guanine, or TG supplied in the culture medium. Mutants are as viable as wild-type cells in normal medium because DNA synthesis proceeds by *de novo* synthetic pathways that do not involve hypoxanthine or guanine as intermediates. The basis for selection of the $HGPRT^-$ mutants is the lack of any ability to utilize toxic purine analogs (e.g., TG), which enables only the HGPRT mutants to grow in the presence of TG. Cells that grow to form colonies in the presence of TG are therefore assumed to have undergone mutation, either spontaneously or by the action of a test article, to the $HGPRT^-$ genotype (*1*).

Indicator Cells

The hypodiploid CHO-K1 cell line was originally derived from the ovary of a female Chinese hamster (*Cricetulus griseus*). The cell clone used by most laboratories, CHO-K1, was selected by Dr. T. T. Puck (University of Colorado Medical Center, Denver, CO) for high clonability and rapid doubling time.

Stocks can be maintained in liquid nitrogen. Laboratory stock cultures should be periodically checked by culturing methods for the absence of mycoplasma contamination. To reduce the negative control frequency (spontaneous frequency) of $HGPRT^-$ mutants to as low a level as possi-

ble, cell cultures are exposed to conditions that select against the
HGPRT$^-$ phenotype and are then returned to normal growth medium for
3 or more days before use.

Media

The cells are maintained in a modification of Ham's Nutrient Mixture F12
(F12) supplemented with L-glutamine, penicillin G, streptomycin sulfate,
and fetal bovine serum (15% by volume), hereafter referred to as culture
medium. Medium used for reducing the spontaneous frequency of
HGPRT$^-$ mutants prior to experimental studies consists of culture medium supplemented with $5.0 \times 10^{-6}M$ thymidine, $1.0 \times 10^{-5}M$ hypoxanthine, $2.0 \times 10^{-4}M$ glycine, and $3.2 \times 10^{-6}M$ aminopterin.
Recovery medium after cleansing consists of the cleansing medium minus
aminopterin. Selection medium is prepared from culture medium that
lacks hypoxanthine, but contains 10 μg/mL of TG and fetal bovine serum
reduced to 5% by volume.

Control Articles

Negative Control

A negative control consisting of assay procedures performed on untreated
cells should be run in all cases. If the test article is not soluble in growth
medium, an organic solvent (normally dimethylsulfoxide) may be used.
The final concentration of solvent in the growth medium should be 1% or
less. Cells exposed to solvent in the medium are assayed as the solvent
negative control to determine any effects on survival or mutation caused
by the solvent alone.

Positive Control Article

4-Nitroquinoline-1-oxide (4NQO) is a stable chemical that is repro-
ducibly and highly mutagenic to CHO-K1 cells. This chemical may be
used at 0.03 μg/mL as a positive control article for nonactivation studies.
As indicated previously, activation methods for this test have not been
well defined.

Dose Selection

The solubility of the test article in deionized water and/or DMSO should
be determined prior to study. Then a wide range of test article concentra-

tions are tested for cytotoxicity, using twofold dilution steps. Cells are quantitatively seeded at 200 cells/dish, allowed to attach for 3–6 h, then exposed to a minimum of 10 dilutions of the test article for 2 h. The cells are then washed and incubated in F12 culture medium for 7 d to allow colony development. For the mutation assay, relative cytotoxicities expressed as the percent of colonies compared to the negative control are used to select 5 or 6 doses covering the range from approximately 0 to 90% reduction in colony-forming ability.

Treatment

The procedure described for this parameter is based on that reported by Hsie et al. (3), with modifications suggested by Myhr and DiPaolo (6), and is summarized as follows. The assay is initiated by exposing 2×10^6 cells in a 150 mm dish to the test article for 2 h. Concurrently, three 60 mm dishes containing 20 cells each are exposed in the same manner as the large dish. After treatment, the cell monolayers are washed and fresh culture medium added. The small dishes are incubated for 7–8 d to permit colony development and the determination of the toxicity of treatment. The large dish is incubated for 3 d to permit growth and expression of induced mutations. Then the culture is subcultured on day 3 and again on day 5 to allow for additional growth and expression time. The cultures are reseeded at 2×10^6 cells in a 150 mm dish at each subculture.

Normally, nine culture conditions are used to initiate the assay. These conditions consist of two vehicle control cultures, one positive control, and six treatment levels. In addition, an extra 150 mm culture is exposed to the high dose. Twenty-four hours after treatment a cell count is made, and if the count is greater than 1×10^6 cells, the assay should be terminated and reinitiated with an adjusted dose range.

At the end of the expression period (6–7 d), each culture is reseeded at 2×10^5 cells/100-mm dish (10 dishes total) in mutant selection medium. Also, three 100 mm dishes are seeded at 200 cells each in culture medium to determine the cloning efficiency of each culture. After incubation for 7–9 d, the ratio of TG-resistant colonies in the mutant selection dishes to the number of colonies in the cloning efficiency dishes are used to calculate the mutant frequency (e.g., mutants/10^6 surviving cells).

Assay Acceptance Criteria

An assay normally may be considered acceptable for evaluation of test results only if all of the following criteria are satisfied.

The average absolute cloning efficiency of the vehicle controls should be between 70 and 115%. A value greater than 100% is possible because of errors in cell counts (usually $\pm$ 10%) and dilutions during cloning. Cloning efficiences below 70% do not necessarily indicate substandard culture conditions or unhealthy cells. Assay variables can lead to artifically low cloning efficiencies in the range of 50–70% and still yield internally consistent and valid results. Assays with cloning efficiencies in this range may be acceptable, dependent on scientific judgment of the specific circumstances. All assays below 50% cloning efficiency should be considered unacceptable.

The background mutant frequency (average of the vehicle controls) is calculated. The normal range of background frequencies for assays performed with different cell stocks is 1×10^{-6} to 10×10^{-6}. Assays with backgrounds greater than 15×10^{-6} are not necessarily invlaid, but should be interpreted with caution.

For test articles with little or no mutagenic activity, an assay must include applied concentrations that reduce survival to approximately 10% to 15% of the average vehicle control or reach the maximum applied concentrations given in the evaluation criteria. A reasonable limit to testing for the presence of mutagenic action is about 85–90% killing of cells. There is no maximum toxicity requirement for test articles that clearly show mutagenic activity.

An experimental mutant frequency may be considered acceptable for evaluation only if the cloning efficiency is 10% or greater. This limit avoids factors larger than ten in the adjustment of the observed number of mutant clones to a unit number of cells (10^6) able to form colonies.

Mutant frequencies are normally derived from sets of ten dishes for the mutant colony count and three dishes for the viable colony count. To allow for contamination losses, an acceptable mutant frequency can be calculated from a minimum of five mutant selection dishes and two cloning efficiency dishes. The mutant frequencies for five treated cultures are normally determined in each assay. The toxicity of the test article is expected, on the basis of preliminary toxicity studies, to span the cellular responses of no observed toxicity to about 10% survival. An assay may need to be repeated with different concentrations to properly evaluate a test article.

The statistical tables provided by Kastenbaum and Bowman (5) may be used to determine whether the results at each dose level are significantly different from the vehicle control at the 95 or 99% confidence levels. This test compares variables distributed according to Poissonian expectations by summing up the probabilities in the tails of two binomial distributions. The 95% confidence level must be met as the minimum criterion for considering the test article to be active at a particular dose level.

The observation of a mutant frequency that meets the minimum criterion for a single treated culture within a range of assayed concentrations is not sufficient evidence to evaluate a test article as a mutagen. The following test results should also be obtained to reach this conclusion:

1. A dose-related or toxicity-related increase in mutant frequency should be observed. It is desirable to obtain this relation for at least three doses, but this depends on the concentration steps chosen for the assay and the toxicity at which mutagenic activity appears.

2. An increase in mutant frequency may be followed by only small or no further increases at higher concentrations or toxicities. However, a decrease in mutant frequency to values below the minimum criterion in a single assay is not acceptable to classify the test article as a mutagen. If the mutagenic activity at lower concentrations or toxicities is large, the test should be repeated.

3. If an increase of about two times the minimum criterion or greater is observed for a single dose near the highest testable toxicity, as defined in the Assay Acceptance Criteria section of this chapter, the test article can be considered mutagenic.

A test article can be evaluated as nonmutagenic in a single assay only if the minimum increase in mutant frequency is not observed for a range of applied concentrations that extends to toxicity causing about 10–15% survival.

References

1. Chu, E. H. Y., and Powell, S. S., *Adv. Human Genet.* **7,** 189 (1976).
2. Chu, E. H. Y., and Malling, H. V., *Proc. Natl. Acad. Sci. USA,* **61,** 1306 (1968).
3. Hsie, A. W., Brimer, P. A., Mitchell, T. J., and Gossless, D. G., *Somat. Cell Genet.* **1,** 247 (1975).
4. Hsie, A. W., Conch, D. B., O'Neill, J. P., San Sebastian, J. R., Brimer, P. A., Mackanoff, R., Riddle, J. C., Li, A. P., Fuseoe, J. C., Forbes, N., and Hsie, M. H., Utilization of a Quantitative Mammalian Cell Mutation System CHO/HGPRT, in Experimental Mutagenesis and Genetic Toxicology, in *Strategies for Short-Term Testing for Mutagens/Carcinogens,* Butterworth, B. E., ed., CRC Press, West Palm Beach, FL, 1977, pp. 39–54.
5. Kastenbaum, M. A., and Bowman, K. O., *Mutation Res.* **9,** 527 (1970).
6. Myhr, B. C., and DiPaolo, J. A., *Cancer Res.* **38,** 2539 (1978).
7. Puck, T. T., and Kao, F. T., *Proc. Natl. Acad. Sci. USA* **58,** 1277 (1967).
8. Thilly, W. G., and Liber, H. L., A Discussion of Gene Locus Mutation Assays in Bacterial, Rodent and Human Cells, in Strategies for Short-Term Testing for Mutagens/Carcinogens, Butterworth, B. E., ed., CRC Press, West Palm Beach, FL, 1977, pp. 39–54.

Chapter 15

Drosophila Assay Systems

David J. Brusick

Drosophila

Drosophila melanogaster is a common insect in nature that has proven to be an extremely valuable genetic tool. The initial work with *Drosophila* was performed by Morgan et al. (*3*). However, these early studies with *Drosophila* were primarily limited to genetic fine structure analysis and the mechanisms of chromosome rearrangement and distribution during meoisis. Induced mutation was first shown in *Drosophila* using X-irradiation by Muller (*6*). Later Auerbach et al. established that chemicals (e.g., nitrogen mustard, formaldehyde, and so on) were capable of inducing mutations in this organism (*1*).

Drosophila melanogaster offers many advantages for the detection of mutagens in a multicellular eukaryote. This organism has a short generation time (12–14 d) and a well-defined genetic system that allows rapid assays for a total spectrum of genetic damage ranging from gene mutations and deletions to heritable translocations and chromosome losses owing to breakage and nondisjunction. Extensive evidence has shown that *Drosophila* possess the enzymatic capacity to convert a wide variety of indirect mutagens to their active forms (*11*). In addition, mutagenic activity can be tested in specific germ cell stages by applying brooding analysis. For recent extensive reviews, see Vogel and Sobels (*9*) and Würgler et al. (*12*).

Correlative analysis of carcinogens that are mutagenic in *Drosophila* has been reviewed by Vogel (*10*). The sex-linked recessive lethal test in

Drosophila provides a reasonably good predictive tool both for direct acting and procarcinogens. Drosophila is particularly sensitive when assessing the mutagenic activity of water, soluble solids, and liquids, as well as gases. Although at one time *Drosophila* was thought to be refractile to aromatic amine and polycyclic hydrocarbon carcinogens, improved testing techniques have resulted in many chemicals of these classes, such as benz(a)pyrene and *N*-acetoxy-*N*-acetyl-2-aminofluorene, being shown active (*10*).

The test systems available in *Drosophila* cover the spectrum of genetic endpoints (i.e., point mutations, chromosome damage, nondisjunction, and mitotic recombination). However, the sex-linked recessive lethal (SLRL) assay is the most commonly performed *Drosophila* test and appears to be the most predictive for carcinogens. The SLRL test will be the primary source of discussion, therefore, in this section.

Drosophila stocks for conducting genetic tests are available from the *Drosophila* Stock Center located at Bowling Green State University, Bowling Green, Ohio.

Several alternative stocks are available for each of the types of assays, and selection of one over the other is most often based on individual preference. The care and handling of *Drosophila* flies does not require elaborate facilities and most laboratories could conduct tests with these organisms. A document, "The Drosophila Guide," that outlines the essential steps in handling fruit flies has been prepared (*4*). Familiarity with the methods described in this document is advisable before initiating *Drosophila* testing. Another publication that details more of the steps in performing genetic tests is "Drosophila as an Assay System For Detecting Genetic Damage" by Würgler et al. (*12*).

The most commonly used strains are Oregon-K, Oregon-R, Canton-S, and Berlin-K. Each strain possesses certain unique characteristics and sensitivities, but no single strain is considered superior. Lee (*5*) has developed engineered strains carrying useful genetic markers related to the test schemes, but these strains are more limited to research programs than for routine testing.

Sex-Linked Recessive Lethal Assay

Test Characteristics

Size of the Test

The spontaneous background of recessive lethals on the X chromosome of *Drosophila* ranges from 0.1 to 0.3%. Test strains showing a spontaneous frequency within this range are considered acceptable.

TABLE 1

Selection of the Population Size for *Drosophila* SLRL Assays[a]

If the spontaneous background for the tester strain is:	The number of flies examined in the control and the treated groups should be:	To detect a significant increase of:
0.10%	5667[b]	0.2%[c]
0.15%	6572	0.2%
0.20%	7000	0.2%
0.25%	8223	0.2%
0.30%	9200	0.2%

[a]Adapted from: Würgler, F. E., Graf, V., and Berchtold, W., *Arch. Genet.* **48**, 158 (1975).

[b]If two matings are to be used to cover (1) mature sperm (days 1–3) and (2) immature sperm (days 4–7), then the numbers sampled at each mating should be approximately half of the number shown.

[c]If two matings are used as described in footnote a, the level of sensitivity of each mating period will be sufficient to detect a significant increase of approximately 0.35%.

Though successive mating of treated males to new groups of females (brooding) has been used to identify cell-stage sensitivity to chemical mutagens, the EPA GeneTox Committee recommends that only post-meiotic cells (spermatids and mature sperm) be analyzed.

A selection of the number of flies (chromosomes) to be analyzed can be developed from data reported by Würgler in which the percent to be detected establishes the number of flies analyzed. This information is given in Table 1. The values in Table 1 identify the numbers of X chromosomes that should be evaluated to detect a 0.2% increase (roughly a doubling of the typical spontaneous background) in lethals.

Controls

It is advisable to use a concurrent negative control group equal in size to the treated group for routine testing. This means that if the spontaneous background for a particular test strain is 0.2%, an experiment conducted with a negative control and a single treatment level will consist of approximately 14,000 analyzed flies. Positive control experiments should be conducted periodically, but need not be performed concurrently with every study. Most studies can be performed using only a single test concentration if adequate toxicity testing is conducted prior to the SLRL assay for dose determination. In the preliminary toxicity testing, the parameters of lethality as well as induced sterility must be determined in order to establish a useable test exposure.

Statistical Analysis

The Kastenbaum-Bowman test (4) is typically recommended for statistical analysis of data. Data collected from the double-mating scheme should be analyzed both with and without pooling the broods.

Data Base

The GeneTox Program identified in Chapter 2 has reviewed the existing published data for results with the Drosophila Sex-Linked Lethal Assay. This review, to be published in "Mutation Research" in 1982, will form the data base for this assay.

Repair Deficient Insects

During the past several years, substrains of *Drosophila* have been isolated that are defective in one or more steps in repair pathways (2,7). These substrains are under examination as possible test organisms for routine screening. At the present time, no single substrain has shown a generalized increase in sensitivity to mutation induction.

Methods

Sex-Linked Recessive Lethal Test in *Drosophila melanogaster*

The sex-linked recessive lethal test in *Drosophila* provides a short-term in vivo mutagen screening system in a eukaryotic organism. The test measures the frequency of lethal mutations in approximately one-fifth the total genome of the fly. Accumulated evidence has indicated this test is the most sensitive among the different test systems available in *Drosophila melanogaster* (12).

Control Articles

Ethylmethane sulfonate (EMS) at $0.015M$ in 1% sucrose solution may be used as the positive control as a single, 24-h exposure on the final day of the dosing schedule. The males dosed should be of the same age and stock as those used for the test article. The solvent or vehicle used for the test article should be used as the negative control and administered concurrently with the test article.

Culture Conditions

Drosophila cultures are maintained at ~25°C in glass shell vials. The culture medium used may be Carolina Biological Instant *Drosophila* medium (Formula 4-24, without dyes). Flies are immobilized with filtered CO_2 for handling.

Test Article Administration

Although methods for inhalation of gases or injection of insoluble compounds in suspension are available, feeding is the simplest and will be described in this chapter.

Solubility Testing

Each test article should be tested for solubility; the primary choice for a solvent is distilled water. If a test article is insoluble in water it should be dissolved in ethanol, acetic acid, or acetone, and then diluted. The final concentration of solvent other than water should be $\leq 2\%$ of the feeding solution. Dimethysulfoxide (DMSO) has been shown to interfere with the metabolic activity in the endoplasmic reticulum and should be avoided as a solvent. Butter may successfully be used to suspend insoluble test agents.

Palatability and Toxicity Testing

A test for palatability and toxicity must be performed by preparing a test article in distilled water containing sucrose and any necessary solvents. The solution is then administered by the following method. A peice of chemically inert glass filter paper, lining a shell vial, is saturated with 1.5 mL of the test solution. Fifty adult males are then placed in each feeding vial and observed for feeding behavior and toxic effects. To ensure uptake it may be necessary to use concentrations of sucrose varying between 1 and 5% and to vary the feeding time between 1 and 3 days. It is useful at this point to include food coloring in the feeding solutions of certain vials, since the coloring is readily distinguishable in the gut and feces of *Drosophila* and it can therefore be easily determined whether the flies have ingested the test article. Vials containing the coloring agent should not be used for assessment of toxicity. Should it be necessary to extend the dosing period beyond 24 h, the test article must be reprepared and the flies transferred to a new feeding vial.

Fertility Testing

Once the solubility and toxicity have been established, a small pilot study should be conducted to determine the fertility of the treated males. Selected concentrations of the test article will be prepared, and the dosed males should be put through the same mating sequence as that to be used in the actual test to ensure that sufficient numbers of progeny will be available for analysis.

Collection of Males

To provide males of approximately uniform age for treatment, males from culture bottles in optimum condition that are produced from timed (1-day) egg samples are collected and held for a 2-day maturation period. The males, then between 2 and 3 d of age should be randomized prior to treatment. A sufficient number of healthy males for the test are transferred to a single empty bottle, mixed and parcelled into groups of 50. They may be held in empty vials for several hours before exposure, since this period of removal from a food supply will ensure immediate uptake of the feeding solution.

Mating and Scoring

The treated males are mated individually to sequential groups of three virgin *Basc* females. The brooding scheme to be employed consists of a sequence determined by the particular spermatozoa, spermatids, spermatocytes and/or spermatogonia. Each treated male is assigned a unique identification number that is written onto the vial and identifies the females inseminated by that male throughout the brooding sequence. In this way the progeny of each male are kept separate and the data recorded in such a way that the origin of each tested chromosome is known. This method will eliminate the possibility of false positives resulting from clusters of identical lethal mutations originating in one treated male.

The F_1 progeny of each culture are visually inspected to make certain the proper cross was made. The desired number of F_1 females are then pair-mated to their brothers. It is desirable to test an approximately equal number of F_1 females per treated male to avoid biasing the data.

In the F_2 generation, each culture vial (representing one treated X chromosome) is examined for the presence of males with wild type eyes. If this class of males is present, the culture is considered nonlethal and discarded. If this class is absent, the vial is marked as a potential lethal and set aside for further examination. The following criteria may be applied to cultures suspected of being lethal:

1. If 20 or more progeny are present and there are no wild type males, the culture is considered to carry a lethal mutation on the treated chromosome and further testing will not be required. The chance of missing a male carrying the treated X chromosome in a population of this size is $(\frac{1}{2})^5$ or < 0.05; or

2. If there are fewer than 20 progeny or if there is one wild type male, the culture should be retested by mating up to three of the females heterozygous for the treated and *Basc* chromosomes to *Basc* males. The progeny of these crosses are then scored for the presence of wild type males.

The *Basc* (*Muller-5*) mating scheme recommended for this test is shown below:

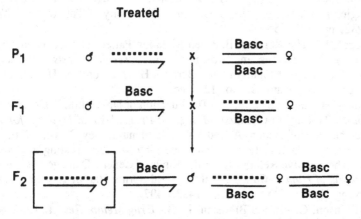

[ ] This class of male is absent if a lethal mutation occurred on its X chromosome.

---- Treated X chromosome

Data Analysis

When the data are compiled, the total number of X chromosomes tested should equal the sum of the lethal and nonlethal cultures. The frequency of X-linked recessive lethals is calculated as:

$$\frac{\text{Number of lethals}}{\text{Number of lethals + Number of nonlethals}} \times 100 = \% \text{ Lethal}$$

Statistical methods for data analysis are described in the text.

References

1. Auerbach, C., *Science* **158**, 1141 (1967).
2. Boyd, J. B., Golino, M. D., Nguyen, T. D., and Green, M. M., *Genetics* **84**, 485 (1976).
3. Demerec, M., *Biology of Drosophila*, Wiley, New York, 1950.
4. Demerec, M., and Kaufmann, B. P., *Drosophila Guide*, 7th edition, Carnegie Institution of Washington, Washington, DC, 1961.
5. Lee, W. R., Sega, A., and Bishop, J. B., *Mutation Res.* **9**, 323 (1970).
6. Muller, H. J., *Science* **66**, 84 (1927).
7. Smith, P. D., Dusenberg, R. L., Cooper, S. F., and Baumen, C. F., Examining the Mechanism of Mutagenesis in DNA Repair-Deficient Strains of *Drosophila melanogaster*. In, *Environment Mutagens and Carcinogens*, Sugimura, T., Kondo, S., Takebe, H., University of Tokyo Press, Tokyo 1982, pp. 147–155.
8. Vogel, E., The Relation Between Mutation Pattern and Concentration by Chemical Mutagens in *Drosophila*, in *Screening Tests in Chemical Carcinogenesis*, Montesano, R., Bartsch, H., and Tomatis, H., eds., IARC Scientific Publications, No. 12, Lyons, 1976.
9. Vogel, E., and Sobels, F. H., The Function of Drosophila in Genetic Toxicology Testing, in *Chemical Mutagens: Principles and Methods for Their Detection*, Hollaender, A., ed., vol. 4, Plenum, New York, 1976.
10. Vogel, E., Identification of Carcinogens by Mutagen Testing in *Drosophila:* The Relative Reliability for the Kinds of Genetic Damage Measured, in *Origins of Human Cancer*, Vol. C, Cold Spring Harbor Laboratory, Cold Spring Harbor, NY, 1977 pp. 1483–1497.
11. Wilkinson, C. F., and Brattsten, L. B., *Drug Metab. Rev.* **1**, 153 (1972).
12. Würgler, F. E., Sobels, F. H., and Vogel, E., Drosophila as Assay System for Detecting Genetic Changes, in *Handbook of Mutagenicity Test Procedures*, Kilbey, B. J., et al., (eds.) Elsevier, Amsterdam, 1977, pp. 355–373.

Section B

DNA Damage and Repair Assays

Chapter 16

Detection of DNA Damage and Repair in Bacteria

David J. Brusick

Introduction

During the initial correlation studies conducted with the Ames mutation assay in *Salmonella,* considerable attention was drawn to the apparent "false negative" responses. Within the context of this concern, several investigators have proposed that the Ames test should be supplemented with other bacterial techniques believed to identify the Ames "false" negatives. Two of the most commonly used tests in this regard measure the DNA-modifying activity of chemicals. These tests do not measure mutation, but rather use differential sensitivity between two bacterial strains, one of which cannot repair DNA damage, as a method of identifying genotoxic agents.

Bacteria DNA-modifying test methods, like the Ames test, can be performed as qualitative plate (spot) assays or as semiquantitative assays in which individual colony counts are used to determine survivals. The time required for these techniques is shorter than that for the Ames test, usually involving only a 24–30 h test period, and because only two strains are used in the test, the number of plates needed for a study is less than one-half that required for the typical Ames test.

Although published data indicate that several of those carcinogens that are not mutagenic in the Ames test can be successfully detected by the bacterial DNA damage and repair assays, the interpretation of test results from a DNA repair test, both mechanistically and as indicative of toxicity, remain the most significant limitations of these procedures. DNA repair tests presumably respond to damage to DNA, but cannot establish whether that damage will ultimately be involved in the production of a mutation.

E. coli DNA Repair Test

The methods for conducting the E. coli DNA repair test were published by Slater et al. (7) as a rapid detection system for mutagens and carcinogens. The initial description of the test consisted of a qualitative plate assay. Two strains of E. coli, one normal (pol A^+) and one deficient in DNA polymerase-I (pol A_1^-) are spread on the surfaces of two agar medium plates at similar densities. In the center of each plate, identical quantities of test material are added: (a) as a solution saturated on a filter paper disc, (b) as a solution or suspension to small wells made in the center of the agar plates, or (c) as soluble crystals directly to the surface of the agar. The plates are then incubated for 24 h at 37°C and examined for visible evidence of inhibition of growth. The size of the zone of inhibition around the test material is measured for both pol A^+ and pol A_1^- bacteria and compared (Fig. 1). The results of the test are generally interpreted as follows:

1. If there is no zone of inhibition around the test material in either plate, the test is considered a "no test" and the study is typically repeated at higher concentrations. If higher concentrations are not possible, the chemical can be evaluated in a modification of the tests that employs a liquid suspension exposure followed by direct survival colony counts (6).

2. If a zone of inhibition is present, but is equal in diameter for both pol A^+ and pol A_1^- strains, the compound is considered negative in the DNA repair test (i.e., the toxicity is not DNA-directed).

3. If there are zones of inhibition present and the zone for the pol A_1^- strain is larger than that for the pol A^+ strain, the test result is considered positive.

Detailed methods for the plate and liquid suspension versions of this assay are described in a comprehensive review by Rosenkranz and Leifer (6). This review article also compiles most of the published data for the test through 1979.

The limitations of the initial version of this assay involve the poor detectability of genetic chemicals that are insoluble and therefore do not diffuse through the agar (e.g., give rise to "no tests") and the lack of a

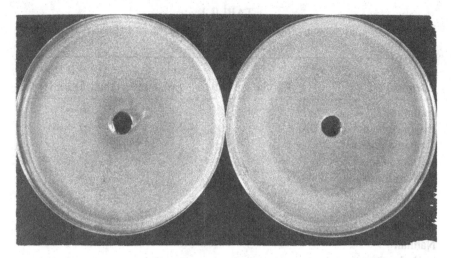

Fig. 1.   Two plates from the *pol* A$^+$/A$^-$ assay. The zone of inhibitions is larger for the *pol* A$^-$ strain indicating a toxic effect directed at the DNA. The presence or absence of active repair enzymes is clearly identified in this assay.

good method to incorporate an activation system (S9 mix) into the technique. Both of these limitations were solved to a degree by the use of a liquid suspension exposure and direct colony count. This modification, however, involves considerably more work than the plate test and does not totally compensate for the solubility problem.

The advantages of the test, as mentioned in the introduction, are those of short performance time, low cost, and most important the ability to detect some carcinogens missed by the Ames test. Examples of some of these chemicals are listed in Table 1. Correlation data for the DNA repair test versus carcinogenicity shows that a combination of the plate and liquid suspension versions detected approximately 74% of the carcinogens employed in the comparison of Rosenkranz and Leifer (6).

B. subtilis Rec-Assay System

The rec-assay using *Bacillus subtilis* was first described as a screening assay by Kada et al. (4). This organism is a gram-positive bacterium and is believed to be more permeable to many chemicals than *E. coli*, a gram-negative organism. The cell wall structures for gram-positive and gram-negative bacteria differ considerably.

The two strains of *B. subtilis* used in the rec-assay are M45 *Rec$^-$* (a recombinationless strain selected on the basis of its UV and gamma radia-

TABLE 1

Examples of Carcinogens That Can Be Detected in the *E. coli* DNA Repair Test
but Not in the Ames Test[a]

Chemical	Carcinogenicity	Ames test response	*E. coli* DNA repair test response
Auramine 0	+	−	+
Bis-(*p*-dimethylamine di-phenylamine)	+	−	+
p-Chloraniline	+	−	+
p-Rosaniline	+	−	+
o-Toluidine	+	−	+
Safrole	+	−	+
1,2-Dimethylhydrazine	+	−	+
Natulan	+	−	+
N-Hydroxyurethane	+	−	+

[a]Adapted from Rosenkranz and Leifer (6). It should be noted also that numerous examples exist in which the *E. coli* DNA repair test does not detect carcinogens detected by the Ames test. Therefore, the two tests can only be considered complementary. The Ames test should remain the test of choice among the test bacterial screens.

tion sensitivities) and H17 Rec^+. Differential killing between the two strains is used to screen for genotoxic agents.

The rec-assay, like the *E. coli* DNA repair system, consists of a rapid plate test method as well as a liquid suspension version (3). Instead of spreading the cells over the agar media in a lawn as is done for *E. coli*, the rec-assay plate test employs streaks of the H17 and M45 strains. Differential growth after 14 h at 37°C is qualitatively determined by the length of the streak and by the area of inhibition (Fig. 2). Interpretation of responses is the same as that used for the *E. coli* test. The limitations of this method are similar to the *E. coli* test and involve a significant loss of sensitivity for agents that are highly insoluble or those that require S9 metabolic activation in order to exhibit their genotoxicity.

Kada (2) reported that storage of the plates at 4°C overnight before incubating at 37°C would increase the sensitivity of the test to some chemicals by permitting an extended period of diffusion for chemicals of low stability.

Another version of the rec-assay plate test with reported enhanced sensitivity (as well as the inclusion of S9 mix activation system) uses *B. subtilis* spores as indicators rather than the vegetative cells (1). The spore rec-assay employs a lawn of spores and detects zones of inhibition much like those observed in the *pol* A^+/*pol* A_1^- test. The bacterial spores of-

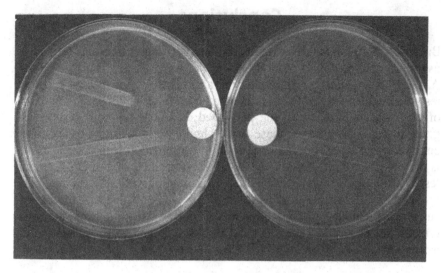

Fig. 2. Two plates from rec-assay. The two strains respond differently on the treated plate (left). The *rec⁻* strain shows a greater zone of inhibition than the *rec⁺* strain when subjected to the test material in the filter paper pad. The control plate (right) shows no difference in growth.

fer not only increased sensitivity, but also internal consistency since spore preparations can be stored for over a year without loss in viability. This allows one mass culture to be used for a large number of independent tests. The increased sensitivity of the spores may be a function of altered cell permeability in spores versus vegetative cells.

Detailed descriptions of the plate test and liquid suspension versions of the rec-assay are given in a review by Kada et al. (*3*). This review also provides a detailed compendium of pesticides and metal compounds tested in the rec-assay. A publication by Hirano et al. (1976) gives the results for a diverse group of 500 chemicals tested in the rec-assay. Again, it was evident that this assay alone does not show extremely good predictability for carcinogens.

The rec-assay can also detect certain genotoxic agents more efficiently than *E. coli* or the Ames test; however, it appears to be most effective as a screen for metal carcinogens. Suspected carcinogenic compounds such as beryllium ($BeSO_4$), cadmium ($CdCl_2$), chromium ($K_2Cr_2O_7$), and vanadium ($VOCL_2$) were detected in the rec-assay. Most of these carcinogens are negative in other microbial screens. Other carcinogens that have been detected in the rec-assay but not in the Ames assay include diethylstilbestrol, 1,2-dimethylhydrazine, patuline, safrole, thioacetamide, and thiourea (*3*).

Conclusions

Bacterial DNA repair assays may, under specific circumstances, play a useful complementary screening role to the Ames assay. The *E. coli pol* A^+/A_1^- assay and the *B. subtilis* rec-assay are two of these screening tests that have been carefully studied and used in tests with large numbers of chemicals. A review of the published data base for both systems is given in ref. *5*. Neither of these two techniques are sensitive or accurate enough to use alone, but may be useful in combination with other tests. It is not possible to determine in advance when the inclusion of DNA repair tests would be beneficial other than in screening batteries for metallic compounds. It appears that, for both of the DNA repair tests, the liquid suspension versions are most suitable for routine screening because of increased sensitivity and the amenability of the technique to S9 metabolic activation.

References

1. Hirano, K., Narui, K., Sadaire, Y., and Kada, T., *Mutation Res.* **53,** 200 (1978).

2. Kada, T., *Mutation Res.* **38,** 340 (1976).

3. Kada, T., Hirano, K., and Shirasu, Y., Screening of Environmental Chemical Mutagens by the Rec⁻ Assay System with *Bacillus subtilis,* in *Chemical Mutagens: Principles and Methods for Their Detection,* vol. 6, deSerres, F. J., and Hollaender, A., eds. Plenum, New York, 1980, pp. 149–173.

4. Kada, T., Sadaire, Y, and Tutkikawa, K., *Ann. Rep. Natl. Inst. Genet.* **21,** 72 (1970).

5. Leifer, Z., Kada, T., Mandel, M., Zeiger, E., Stafford, R., and Rosenkranz, H. S. *Mutation Res.* **87,** 211 (1981).

6. Rosenkranz, H. S., and Leifer, Z., Determining the DNA-Modifying Activity of Chemicals Using DNA-Polymerase-Deficient *Escherichia coli,* in *Chemical Mutagens: Principles and Methods for Their Detection,* vol. 6, de Serres, F. J., and Hollaender, A., eds., Plenum, New York, 1980, pp. 109–147.

7. Slater, E. E., Anderson, M. D., and Rosenkranz, H. S., *Cancer Res.* **31,** 970 (1971).

Chapter 17

Mammalian DNA Repair Assays

David J. Brusick

Theoretical Considerations

DNA repair is an important process in all organisms. Intracellular systems of different types appear to have developed very early in evolution since the fundamental biochemical pathways and enzymatic components associated with repair processes, such as photoreactivation and excision repair, are very similar in both prokaryotic, submammalian eukaryotic organisms, and mammals (1).

The importance of DNA repair as a barrier to genotoxic damage in vivo has not been fully assessed, but it appears to be critical in protection against mutation and cancer induction at "typical" environmental exposures. Studies have shown that some human diseases resulting in DNA repair deficiency are also characterized by increased cancer susceptibility in the affected individuals (Table 1). Cells from these individuals are also more sensitive to mutation induction and chromosomal breakage than cells from nonaffected "normal" individuals (4). A comparison of chemical-induced mutation frequencies in "normal" and repair deficient human cells is shown in Fig. 1. The presence of repair appears to result in a "threshold" or region of no detectable effect. Loss of DNA repair affects cell survival as well as mutation frequencies.

Analysis of DNA repair in mammalian cells both in vitro and in vivo can serve as a means to understand the parameters of genotoxic risk (i.e., how does DNA repair affect the dose–response curves of genotoxic

TABLE 1

Repair-Deficient Diseases and Cancer Susceptibility

	Xeroderma pigmentosum	Ataxia telangiectasia	Fanconi's anemia
Frequency			
Homozygotes ($-/-$)	1/300,000	1/40,000	1/300,000
Heterozygotes ($+/-$)	1/300	1/100	1/300
Cancer probability[a]			
Homozygotes than age	Skin cancer: >0.5 (melanoma > 0.1)	0.1 (Lymphoreticular: 0.06; leukemia: 0.02)	> 10-fold normal
Heterozygotes	Greater than normal in South	Greater than normal < 45 years, 50% greater mortality than average	Normal
Etiologic agent	Sunlight	?	?
Cell sensitivity	Ultraviolet and mimetics	X-rays, alkylating agents	Crosslinking agents
Repair deficiencies	One or more of excision, photoreactivation, and postreplication	Some cell strains defective in "X-ray" repair	Some cell strains defective in crosslink repair

[a]Approximate average cancer probabilities:
Skin cancer prevalence: 0.005.
Melanoma incidence: 6×10^{-5}/yr.
Lymphoreticular cancer: 13×10^{-5}/yr.
Leukemia ($t_{max} \sim 4$ years); 42×10^{-6}/yr.
From Setlow, R. B., in *Principles of Genetic Toxicology*, Brusick, D. J., ed., Plenum, NY, 1980.

THE EFFECT OF DNA REPAIR ON THE MUTATION
FREQUENCY IN HUMAN FIBROBLASTS

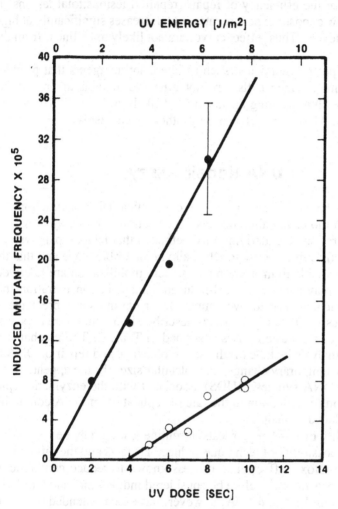

○ NORMAL HUMAN DIPLOID FIBROBLASTS
● XP4BE REPAIR DEFICIENT HUMAN DIPLOID FIBROBLASTS

An apparant no effect dose is observed in normal cells which is lost in cells
without the capacity to repair genotoxic lesions.

Fig. 1.   The sensitivity of normal and excision repair-defective human fibroblasts. The dose–response curve is shifted to the left (showing "no effect"
response) without DNA repair. From Brusick *Principles of Genetic Toxicology*,
Plenum Press, New York, 1980.

agents over the low dose range) and as a sensitive assay system capable of identifying chemicals that react with DNA to produce repairable lesions. The former function may well prove to be a critical component or risk estimates since the efficiency of repair (repaired lesions:total lesions) is almost 1 at low exposes exposure rates, but decreases significantly at high (MTD) dose levels. Thus, effect curves are not likely to be linear from the origin.

Some types of chemicals, such as intercalating agents that produce mutation in mammalian cells, are not effective at inducing repairable DNA damage. Intercalating agents are not likely to break DNA or produce adducts. They are mutagenic by other mechanisms.

DNA Repair Assays

A convenient method of estimating direct chemical/DNA interaction that leads to DNA molecular alterations is the detection of repair system stimulation. The rationale underlying this method is that DNA repair systems will be mobilized in response to DNA alkylation or breakage and that the techniques available to measure repair system mobilization are relatively sensitive and may detect chemical-induced damage at concentrations below those that will lead to overt mutation or chromosome breakage.

The types of DNA repair assays described in the literature appear to fall into one of the basic classes described in Table 2. The mechanisms involved in analysis include (a) the actual breakage and repair of DNA as evidenced by temporary changes in molecular size, (b) the appearance of unscheduled DNA synthesis (UDS) associated with the enzymatic repair processes, and (c) reduction in the rate of replication of DNA containing chemical-induced damage.

The utility of DNA repair tests in routine testing may be limited because of the possibility of technique-induced artifacts and the difficulty in defining a genotoxic effect via a process known to reduce genotoxicity. DNA repair tests must therefore be considered indirect indicators of DNA alterations. Both EPA and FDA, however, have recommended the use of DNA repair tests in certain circumstances.

The selection of a mammalian DNA repair assay should be based to some extent on the nature of the chemical(s) being evaluated and the capabilities of the testing laboratory. Most of the tests listed in Table 2 have been used to study fundamental mechanisms of DNA repair and have not been extensively employed in routine testing situations. The two UDS assays represent the "most used" tests and the UDS method with rat hepatocytes offers several advantages over the WI-38 cell assay (Table

3). The technique looking for changes in the rate of DNA replication is very rapid and may also prove to be an excellent screening tool. More studies comparing this method to the UDS models should be performed in multiple laboratories to establish its overall reliability and reproducibility. It is likely, however, that DNA repair tests will remain as confirmatory tests in multitest batteries and not primary tests.

Data Base

Most of the assay systems described in Table 2 have not undergone validation with large numbers of chemicals. Most of the test systems have, however, been studied with a few well-known genotoxic agents such as nitrosamides, alkylsulfates, and some nitrogen mustards. And most of the tests respond to these agents, but those responses cannot be considered formal validation of the systems. The system that has been subjected to the most extensive set of chemicals is the UDS system in rat hepatocytes. A review by Williams provides both procedures and validation responses for approximately 40 substances (6). Recently, the hepatocyte UDS technique has been extended to an in vivo/in vitro assay in which hepatocytes are removed from animals exposed in vivo and then assayed for UDS in vitro (3). In vivo exposure has definite advantages in attempting to extrapolate the in vitro responses to the in vivo conditions.

Methods

The UDS assays employing rat hepatocytes appear to be the most applicable to carcinogen screening. The in vitro version of the test has been subjected to a reasonable amount of validation, it has been applied successfully in several different laboratories, and its capacity for metabolic activation/detoxication is well-suited to this application. The following study design is based on the method published by Williams (5).

Objective

The objective of this technique is to detect DNA damage caused by a test article, or an active metabolite, by measuring UDS in primary rat hepatocytes in vitro. The existence and degree of DNA damage can be inferred from an increase in nuclear grain counts compared to untreated

TABLE 2

General Classification of DNA Repair Assays Employing Mammalian Cells

Type of repair system	Examples	References
Alteration of DNA Integrity		
The basis for this type of test is that chemical-induced DNA damage will reduce the molecular size of DNA via breakage. A recovery (repair) period following exposure will result in reversal of the effect due to the repair process.	Alkaline elution tests which detect breakage by layering DNA for treated cells on membrane microfilters and eluting with alkaline buffer. The amount of DNA passing through the microfilter is presumed to be a function of the amount of DNA strand breakage.	Kohn and Grimek-Ewig, *Cancer Res.* **33**, 1849 (1974)
	Alkaline sucrose gradient tests that measure shifts in DNA molecular weight. DNA breakage will alter the sedimentation of DNA and this phenomena can be readily observed in new bands of DNA in the gradient.	Regan, Setlow, Francis, and Lijinsky, *Mutation Res.* **38**, 293 (1976)
Stimulation of Unscheduled DNA Synthesis (UDS)		
The basis for this type of test rests with assumption that chemical-induced DNA synthesis is not associated with scheduled cell division (i.e., repair synthesis). Repair synthesis (UDS) may be detected by scintillation or autoradiographic techniques.	Increased ³H-thymidine incorporation in human diploid fibroblasts (WI-38) arrested in G₁. Increased ³H-thymidine uptake can be detected by measuring the tritium incorporated in extracted DNA via scintillation analysis or by coating nuclear grains in photographic emulsion overlaying cell nuclei.	Stich, San, Lam, and Koropatrick, in *Origins of Human Cancer*, Hiatt, Watson, and Winsten, eds., Cold Spring Harbor Laboratory, New York, 1977, pp. 1499–1512.
	Increased ³H-thymidine incorporation in primary rat hepatocyte cultures. This	Williams, *Cancer Res.* **37**, 1845 (1977)

method exclusively employs the autoradiographic method.

Reduction in the Rate of DNA Synthesis

The basis for this type of test rests with the assumption that the rate of DNA synthesis in cells grown under very carefully controlled conditions will be reduced if chemical-induced DNA damage is present.

The test measures decreases in rates of synthesis of DNA in HeLa cells. ^{14}C-thymidine-labeled cells are exposed to a chemical and then pulsed with ^{3}H-thymidine. DNA damage prevents normal rates of incorporation of ^{3}H-thymidine into the new complementary molecule. Thus the synthesis rate for mutagen treated cells is lower than for the controls.

Painter, *Nature* **265**, 650 (1977)

Biochemical Analysis for Repair Products

The basis for this method is that DNA repair can be detected by the identification of DNA repair products (dimers, adducts, etc.) or by repair replication.

Repair replication in which repaired regions of DNA are identified as unlabeled segments of DNA within semiconservatively labeled DNA by isopyenic gradient centrifugation. Another method involves BUdR photolysis of repaired segments of DNA.

Painter and Cleaver, *Nature* **216**, 369 (1967)

During the repair process, the excision system removes the charged area. The presence of DNA adducts or nucleotide dimers is measured in cell-free extracts after chemical exposure. The presence of repair products is evidence for primary DNA damage.

Amacher and Lieberman, *Biochem. Biophys. Res. Comm.* **74**, 285 (1977)

TABLE 3
A Comparison of UDS Assays in WI-38 Cells and Rat Hepatocytes

| Characteristic | Target cell | |
	WI-38 fibroblasts	Rat hepatocytes
Metabolic activation	Requires exogenous source such as S9	Endogenous metabolism with enzymes in an *in vivo* "state"
Maintenance of cells in G_1 phase	Requires addition of hydroxyurea to prevent S-phase escape	Intrisic property of attached hepatocytes. Low background of S-phase nuclei ($>0.2\%$)
Source of cells	Cells must be purchased low passage number becomes important. Fibroblasts are of human origin	Cells readily available. Cells are primary and are epithelial in origin
Validation	Validated with direct-acting agents. Poor data base with chemicals requiring bioactivation	Validated both with direct acting and procarcinogens. Good correlation between positive responses and carcinogenic activity.
In vivo model available	No	Yes

hepatocytes. The types of detectable DNA damage are unspecified, but must be recognizable by the cellular repair system and result in the incorporation of new bases (including ^{3}H-TdR) into the DNA. The normal background of cells in S-phase for hepatocytes is less than 0.2%.

Materials

Indicator Cells

The hepatocytes can be obtained from adult, male, Fischer 344 rats (weighing 150–300 g). The cells are collected by perfusion of the liver *in situ* with a collagenase solution. Monolayer cultures are established on plastic cover-slips in culture dishes and used the next day for the UDS assay. Collection of the cells is described in detail in a later section.

Medium

The cell cultures are established in Williams' Medium E supplemented with 5% fetal bovine serum, 2 mM L-glutamine, 1 μg dexamethasone, 100 U/mL penicillin, 100 μg/mL streptomycin sulfate, and 150 μg/mL gentamycin. After the establishment period, the dexamethasone and serum components should be removed. This latter culture medium is referred to simply as WME.

Control Articles

Negative Control

A negative control consisting of assay procedures performed on untreated cells should be performed in all cases.

Positive Control Articles

Several chemicals known to induce UDS in rat hepatocyte primary cell cultures can be used as positive controls. For example 2-acetylaminofluorene (2-AAF) at $2.5 \times 10^{-4}M$ (50 μg/mL) is acceptable.

Dosing Procedure

The test article should be dissolved at the highest desired concentration in WME containing 1% serum. Lower concentrations should then be prepared by serial dilution with WME plus 1% serum. If the test article is incompletely soluble in WME, dimethylsulfoxide (DMSO) may be substituted as the solvent. Treatments can be initiated by replacing the medium on the cell cultures with WME (1% serum) containing the test article at the desired concentration.

Dose Selection

A preliminary cytotoxicity test must be initiated with a series of applied concentrations of test article, starting at a maximum concentration of 1000 μg/mL (or 1000 nL/mL) and diluting in twofold steps to about 0.06 μg/mL (0.06 nL/mL). Cells should be exposed for a period of 18 h, approximately 2 h after initiation of the primary cultures. After removal of the test article, cells are incubated an additional 2–4 h in WME. A viable cell count (trypan blue exclusion) is then obtained. Those treatments that reduced the number of viable cells below about 50%, relative to the negative control, should be eliminated from further testing.

Collection of Hepatocytes

The hepatocytes are obtained by perfusion of livers *in situ* for 4 min with Hanks' balanced salts (Ca^{2+}- and Mg^{2+}-free) containing 0.5 mM ethyleneglycol-bis(β-aminoethyl ether)-*N,N*-tetraacetic acid (EGTA), and HEPES buffer at pH 7.0. The WME with 100 U/mL of Type I collagenase is perfused through the liver for 10 min. The hepatocytes are obtained by mechanical dispersion of excised liver tissue in a culture containing the WME culture medium and collagenase. The suspended tissue and cells should then be filtered through sterile cheesecloth to remove cell clumps and debris. The filtrate is centrifuged and the cell pellet resuspended in WME containing 5% serum and 1 μM dexamethasone. After obtaining a viable cell count, a series of 35-mm dishes (each containing a 25-mm round, plastic coverslip) is inoculated with approximately 0.5×10^6 viable cells in 3 mL of WMe plus dexamethasone and 5% serum per dish.

An attachment period of 1.5–2 h at 37°C in a humidified atmosphere containing 5% CO_2 is used to establish the cell cultures. Unattached cells are then removed and the cultures refed with 2.5 mL WMe. Some of the cultures can be used for the preliminary cytotoxicity test, while the remaining cultures are incubated at 37°C until the next day for the UDS assay.

The UDS assay is initiated by replacing the media in the culture dishes with 2.5 mL WME containing 1% fetal bovine serum, 1 μCi/mL ^{3}H-thymidine, and the test article at the desired concentration. Each treatment, including the positive and negative controls, is performed on seven cultures, four of which will not receive ^{3}H-thymidine and are used for cytotoxicity measurements. After treatment for 18 h, the test article is removed and the cell monolayers washed twice with WME. The four cultures used to monitor the toxicity of each treatment are refed with WME and returned to the incubator. The other three cultures from each treament are refed with 2.5 mL WME containing 1 μCi/mL of ^{3}H-TdR and incubated for an addition 3 h of labeling. The labeling is terminated by washing the cultures with WME containing 1 mM thymidine. The toxicity of each treatment is monitored by performing viable cell counts on two cultures 2–4 h after treatment and on two cultures about 20–24 h after treatment.

The nuclei in the labeled cells are swollen by placement of the coverslips in 1% sodium citrate for 10 min. Then the cells are fixed in acetic acid:ethanol (1:3) and dried for at least 24 h. The coverslips are mounted on glass slides (cells up), dipped in Kodak NTB2 emulsion, and dried. The coated slides should be stored for 10 days at 4°C in light-tight boxes containing packets of Drierite. The emulsions are then developed in D19, fixed, and stained with Williams' modified hematoxylin and eosin.

The cells can then be examined microscopically at approximately 1500× magnification under oil immersion. UDS is measured by counting nuclear grains and subtracting the average number of grains in three nuclear-sized areas adjacent to each nucleus (background count). This value is referred to as the net nuclear grain count. The coverslips should be coded to prevent bias in grain counting.

Evaluation Criteria

The net nuclear grain count should be determined for 50 randomly selected cells on each coverslip. Only normal-appearing nuclei should be scored, and any occasional nuclei blackened by grains too numerous to count should be excluded as cells in which replicative DNA synthesis occurred rather than repair synthesis. If the actual count for any nucleus is less than zero (i.e., cytoplasmic count is greater than nuclear count), a net value of zero should be used in the calculation of the mean value. The mean net nuclear grain count is determined from the triplicate coverslips (150 total nuclei) for each treatment condition.

Several criteria have been formulated on the basis of published results.

The test article may be considered active in the UDS assay at applied concentrations that cause:

1. An increase in the mean nuclear grain count to at least six grains per nucleus in excess of the concurrent negative control value, and/or

2. The percent of nuclei with six or more grains to increase above 10% of the examined population, in excess of the concurrent negative control, and/or

3. The percent of nuclei with 20 or more grains to reach of exceed 2% of the examined population, and/or

4. Statistical analysis.

References

1. Hanawalt, P. C., Friedberg, E. C., and Fox, C. F., eds., *DNA Repair Mechanisms*, Academic Press, New York, 1978.

2. Larsen, K. H., Brash, D., Cleaver, J. E., Hart, R. W., Maher, V. M., Painter, R. B., and Sega, G. A., *Mutation Res.* **98,** 287 (1982).
3. Mersalis, J. C., and Butterworth, B. E., *Carcionogenesis 1:64-625,* 1980.
4. Paterson, M. C., Environmental Carcinogenesis and Imperfect Repair of Damaged DNA in *Homo sapiens*: Causal Relationship Revealed by Rare Hereditary Disorders, in *Carcinogens: Identification and Mechanisms of Action.* Griffin, A. C., and Shaw, C. R., eds. Raven Press, New York, 1979, pp. 251-276.
5. Williams, G. M., *Cancer Res.* **37,** 1845 (1977).
6. Williams, G. M.: The Detection of Chemical Mutagens/Carcinogens by DNA Repair and Mutagenesis in Liver Cultures, in *Chemical Mutagens,* Vol. VI. deSerres, F. J., and Hollaender, A., eds., Plenum Press, New York, 1980, pp. 61-79.

Section C

Cytogenetic Assays

Chapter 18

Cytogenetic Assays

Aberrations and SCE Techniques

David J. Brusick

In Vitro Cytogenetics

Cytogenetic analysis can be performed on almost any cell line with the following characteristics: (1) stable karyotype, (2) ability to grow in culture, (3) reproducible cell cycle, (4) compatible with an S9 metabolic activation system.

Stable Karyotype

The stable karyotype permits recognition of induced damage. If the lines are not stable and subject to spontaneous fluctuations in chromosome numbers or ploidy, evaluation of chemical-induced damage becomes impossible. These lines might be suitable for SCE analysis, however.

Growth in Culture

The requirement for growth in culture medium relates to the necessity of analyzing cells treated in different stages of the cell cycle. Cells in different stages of the cell cycle have variable sensitivity to genotoxic effects (Table 1). The majority of mutagens are believed to be S-phase dependent

265

Table 1
Stages of a Typical Mammalian Cell[a]

Events	G₁ Stage	S Stage	G₂ Stage	M Stage
	GAP₁	Synthesis of DNA	GAP₂	Mitosis:
Relative DNA content	1	1–2	2	2–1
Common types of aberrations observed[b]	Chromosome breaks	Mixed	Chromatid breaks	
	Rings			
	Translocations		Quadriradials	
	Deletions			
	Dicentrics		Triradials	
	Fragments		Fragments	
Relative sensitivity to genotoxic effects	Low	High	Moderate	Low

[a] Shown as relative lengths of the total cell cycle period for in vitro conditions.
[b] These aberrations are the types observed when the exposed G₁, S, or G₂ cells are scored at the first metaphase (M1). If the cells are scored at M2 or M3 the aberration types are mixed and lose identity with the cell stage.

since most aberrations appear to be induced during S-phase or require an intervening S-phase between treatment and expression.

Reproducible Generation Time

This characteristic relates to the previous characterization in that cell cycle stages cannot be predicted without a reasonable well-characterized growth rate. SCE staining requires an understanding of the cell cycle rate associated with the target cells.

Compatibility with an S9 Activation System

Many chemical mutagens are not active in their parental form and require metabolic activation. Many cell lines used as target cells for cytogenetic studies are not metabolically competent for a broad range of chemicals which may require metabolic activation and must therefore be augmented with an S9 mix during exposure to the test material. Cell lines commonly used in in vitro cytogenetics such as the CHO line are compatible with the standard S9 mix described by Ames et al. (1); however, PHA-stimulated human lymphocyte cultures are rather sensitive to the toxic properties of S9 mix making activation studies with these cells difficult but not impossible.

Advantages and Limitations of In Vitro Cytogenetic Assays

In vitro cytogenetics has a specific place in genetic toxicology testing, but is possibly more susceptible to testing artifacts than other in vitro tests. The reason for this is associated with the fact that as cells begin to die from the cytotoxic effects of chemical or physical agents, the chromosome integrity of the cells becomes fragile and damage begins to appear. This damage may be the result of membrane disruption, osmotic shock, and severe pH imbalance and should not be confused with responses generated by true genotoxic chemicals. Thus, careful selection of dose levels and test conditions are extremely important in conducting in vitro cytogenetic studies. Without stringent quality control conditions, in vitro results may not be validly extrapolated to the in vivo state.

Another disadvantage believed to be associated with cytogenetic studies is the inherent test insensitivity. The induction of many types of chromosome aberrations appears to be the result of multiple DNA "hits," whereas gene mutations are believed in most cases to follow single "hit" kinetics. If so, then one would expect to see point mutation induction at lower dose levels than required for the production of gene mutation. In *Drosophila* the dose response data for sex-linked recessive lethal (measured gene mutation) and dominant lethal (chromosome aberrations) induction appears to support this hypothesis (*12*). This might produce a technique-related "false negative" result if only cytogenetic testing is employed in the screening processing. The phenomenon is represented in the hypothetical response curves shown in Fig. 1. In this illustration, the dose level required to demonstrate significant chromosome aberration induction (Dose C) is too toxic for good survival of the organism and the chemical appears to be negative when in fact, there is significant, but undetected, induction of gene mutation at lower doses of A and B.

One facet of in vitro cytogenetics, SCE induction, may solve a portion of this problem since SCE induction kinetics seem to resemble

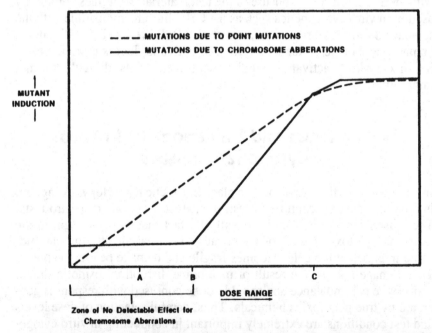

Fig. 1. Hypothetical dose–response curve illustrating a situation in which chromosomal analysis yields negative data for a mutagenic chemical. The test agent may be assumed negative if concentration "B" represents the maximum tolerated dose. If higher concentrations such as "C" can be tested then either point mutation or cytogenetic assays would be reliable.

Table 2
The Associations Between Mutation, SCE, and Chromosome Aberration
Induction In Vitro

Chemical tested	Induces gene mutation	Induces SCEs	Induces chromosome aberration
Formaldehyde	+	+	+/−
Benzene	−	−	+
Benz(a)pyrene	+	+	−
Sodium azide	+/−	+/−	−
Cytosine arabinoside	?	−	+
Ethanol	−	−	−
Caffeine	+/−	+/−	+/−
Hydroxyurea	?	−	+
Mitomycin C	+	+	+
Aflatoxin B$_1$	+	+	+
Cyclophosphamide	+	+	+
Adriamycin	+	+	+
Triethylene melamine	+	+	+
Acetone	−	−	−
Diethylstilbestrol	+	−[a]	+
Sodium nitrite	−	+	+
Sodium ascorbate	−	+	+

[a]Positive results have been observed under special treatment conditions (*13*).

gene mutation induction more closely than aberration induction (*3*). Therefore, an in vitro cytogenetic evaluation combining SCE and aberration analyses should provide a reasonably comprehensive survey. Some examples of this relationship are shown in Table 2. The results shown suggest a general concordance between mutation and SCE induction across a range of mutagens, but is not consistent enough to totally substitute the SCE assay for a mammalian cell gene mutation test.

Several cell lines, such as CHO, L5178Y, or WI-38, and primary cell sources, such as peripheral lymphocytes, are commonly used for in vitro cytogenetics analysis. Of these cell sources, the Chinese hamster ovary (CHO) line is probably the most frequently selected for routine screening. Its availability, ease of growth, short generation time, and relatively low chromosome number are but a few of the desirable qualities. This line is amenable to analysis for chromosome aberration as well as SCEs.

Methods for Chromosome Aberration Analysis

The objective of an in vitro chromosome analysis is to establish whether the test article or available metabolites can interact with cells to induce visible chromosomal breaks, rearrangements, or changes in chromosome numbers (4). Chemically induced DNA lesions may result in breaks in chromatin that are either repaired by the cell in such a way as to be undetectable, or they may result in visible damage. Aberrations result as a consequence of mistakes in repair processes that fail to rejoin DNA strain breaks, or rejoin the breaks in abnormal configurations (5).

Scoring for aberrations occurs when cells enter mitosis for the first time (M1 cells) after chemical exposure. Aberrations are sensitivity scored in M1 cells before they are lost during the cell proliferative process or converted into complex derivatives during subsequent cell cycles. In the case of the CHO cells used here, most dividing cells examined 10–12 h after treatments are in M1 phase.

Medium and Cell Cultures

CHO cells can be grown in McCoy's 5a medium supplemented with 10% fetal calf serum (FCS), L-glutamine, penicillin, and streptomycin. Cultures are set up approximately 24 h prior to treatment by seeding 8×10^5 cells/75 cm^2 plastic flask in 10 mL of fresh medium.

Test Compound

The test compound should be dissolved in an appropriate solvent such as culture medium, water, ethanol, acetone, or dimethylsulfoxide. Serial dilutions should be carried out so as to achieve desired final concentrations by addition of 0.1 mL test solution/10 mL culture medium.

Control Articles

Solvent Controls

Solvent controls contain the solvent for the test article, e.g., water, ethanol, acetone, and dimethylsulfoxide, at the same concentration used in test cultures.

Positive Controls

Known mutagenic and chromosome breaking agents should be used. The following examples are acceptable.

• No metabolic activation required: Triethylenemelamine (TEM) at 1.0 μg/mL.

• Metabolic activation required: Many mutagens do not act directly, but must be converted to active intermediates by enzymes found in microsomes. An example is cyclophosphamide (CP) that can be used at a final concentration of $2-5 \times 10^{-4}M$.

The Metabolic Activation System

The in vitro metabolic activation system comprises rat liver microsomal enzymes and an energy-producing system necessary for their function (NADP and isocitric acid). The enzymes are contained in a preparation of liver microsomes (S9 fraction) from rats treated previously with an inducing agent (Arochlor 1254).

S9 Reaction Mixture Employed for Activation

Component	Final concentration in culture flasks, amount/mL
NADP (sodium salt)	2.4 mg
Isocitric acid	4.5 mg
Homogenate (S9 fraction)	15 μL

Toxicity and Dose Determination

The solubility, toxicity, and concentrations for the test compound are determined prior to screening by examining the survival of CHO cells exposed to a wide range of concentrations of the test article. The concentrations selected for the cytogenetics assay in CHO cells should include a concentration that produces a 30–50% reduction in cell survival, and up to five lower doses. After chemical treatment and incubation for a total of 10–12 h, cells are removed from flasks by trypsin and the proportion of dead cells is determined by trypan blue dye uptake.

Cell Treatment

Assay Without the Metabolic Activation System

One day after culture initiation, approximately 3×10^6 cells are treated with the test article at predetermined doses for the remaining culture period of 10–12 h. Colcemid is added for the last 2–3 h of incubation ($2 \times 10^{-7}M$ final concentration) to accumulate dividing cells, and metaphase cells are collected by mitotic shake-off (11). The cells are swollen with 0.075M KC1 hypotonic solution, then washed three times in fixative (methanol:acetic acid, 3:1), dropped onto slides, and air-dried.

Assay with the Metabolic Activation System

Cells are incubated at 37°C for 2 h in the presence of the test article, the S9 reaction mixture, and growth medium without fetal calf serum (FCS). The short incubation time is used because prolonged exposure to the S9 mixture is toxic to cells; also enzyme activity is lost rapidly at 37°C. Serum is omitted to avoid the possible inactivation, by binding to the serum proteins, of short-lived, highly reactive intermediates produced by S9 enzymes. After the 2-h exposure period, cells are washed at least twice with buffered saline and normal growth medium containing 10% FCS is added. Incubation is continued for a further 8–10 h, and thereafter the procedure is that described above.

Staining and Scoring of Slides

Slides are stained with 5% Giemsa at pH 6.8 for subsequent scoring of chromosome aberration frequencies. At least one hundred cells are scored per dose. For control of bias, all slides are coded prior to scoring and scored "blind." The complete list of aberrations scored is:

Chromatid gap	Pulverized chromosome	Chromatid break
Pulverized chromosomes	Chromosome gap	Pulverized cell
Chromosome break	Complex rearrangement	Chromatid deletion
Ring chromosome	Chromatid fragment	Dicentric chromosome
Acentric fragment	Minute chromosome	Triradial
Quadriradial	Endoreduplication	Greater than 10 aberrations

Gaps are not usually counted as significant aberrations. Open breaks may be considered indicators of genetic damage, as are configurations resulting from the abnormal repair of breaks such as multiradials, rings, and multicentrics.

Evaluation Criteria

The following factors are taken into account in evaluation:

- The estimated number of breaks involved in production of the different types of aberrations observed.
- The frequency of cells with more than one aberration.
- Any evidence for increasing amounts of damage with increasing dose, i.e., a positive dose response.

Statistical analysis employs the Student t-test to compare the aberration frequency in treated cells with solvent and negative controls (2). The difference is considered significant where $p < 0.05$.

Methods for SCE Induction

Sister Chromatid Exchange

The frequency of sister chromatid exchanges (SCEs) is a very sensitive indicator of exposure of the genetic material to chemical mutagens. The SCE test simply involves treating cultured CHO cells with a test compound, growing the cells with 5-bromodeoxyuridine (BrdU) for about a day, and making chromosome preparations that are stained for detection of SCE.

The chromosomes of dividing cells consist of two identical halves, or sister chromatids. To see exchanges between these (SCEs), a staining technique is used to differentiate between the chromatids. This is achieved by growing cells in the presence of BrdU; after two cell cycles, one chromatid contains twice as much BrdU as the other and reacts differently to certain stains. Based on this method, one chromatid will stain intensely while its pair, or sister, is pale.

Medium and Cell Cultures

CHO cells for this assay can be grown in McCoy's 5a medium supplemented with 10% fetal calf serum (FCS), L-glutamine, penicillin, and streptomycin. cultures are set up approximately 24 h prior to treatment by seeding 8×10^5 cells/75 cm^2 plastic flask in 10 mL of fresh medium.

Test Compound and Control Articles

Immediately before use, a stock solution of the test compound should be prepared in a suitable solvent such as culture medium, distilled water, dimethylsulfoxide, acetone or absolute ethanol. Serial dilutions should be carried out so as to achieve desired final concentrations by addition of 0.1 mL test solution/10 mL culture.

Solvent Controls

Solvent control cultures contain the same concentration of solvent as the test cultures.

Positive Controls

Known mutagenic and chromosome breaking agents should be used. Examples of both are given below.

- No metabolic activation required: Triethylenemelamine (TEM) can be used at 0.25 μg/mL.
- Metabolic activation required: Cyclophosphamide can be used at 2.6 μg/mL.

Toxicity and Dose Determination

The toxicity and doses for the test compound should be determined prior to screening.

See *Toxicity and Dose Determination* for chromosome aberration induction for a description of these methods.

Cell Treatment

Assay Without the Metabolic Activation System

One day after culture initiation, approximately 3×10^6 cells are treated with the test article for 2 h. Then, 5-bromo-2′-deoxyuridine (BrdU; 10 μM final concentration) are added to the culture tubes, and incubation continued in the dark for 26–30 h. Colcemid is added for the last 2–3 h of incubation (2×10^7 M final concentration), and metaphase cells will be collected by mitotic shake-off (11). The cells should be swollen with 0.075M KCl hypotonic solution, then washed three times in fixative (methanol:acetic acid, 3:1), dropped onto slides, and air-dried.

Assay with the Metabolic Activation System

Cells are incubated at 37°C for 2 h in the presence of the test article and the S9 reaction mixture, in growth medium without fetal calf serum (FCS). After the 2-h exposure period, cells are washed at least twice with buffered saline, and normal growth medium containing 10% FCS and 10 μM BrdU will be added. Incubation is continued for a further 26–30 h, and thereafter the procedure is that described above.

The Metabolic Activation System

The in vitro metabolic activation system is the same as that described in the chromosome analysis protocol.

Staining and Scoring of Slides

Staining for detection of SCE is accomplished by a modified fluorescence plus Giemsa (FPG) technique (6,8). Slides are stained for 10 min with Hoechst 33258 (5 μg/mL) in phosphate buffer (pH 6.8), mounted with the same buffer and exposed at 55–65°C to "black-light" from 15-W tubes for the amount of time required for differentiation between chromatids. Finally, slides are stained with 5% Giemsa for 10–20 min and air-dried.

M2 cells should be scored for the frequency of SCE per cell. At least fifty cells should be scored per dose.

For control of bias all slides will be coded prior to scoring and scored "blind."

Evaluation Criteria

If an increase in SCE is observed, one of the following criteria must be met to assess the compound as positive:

Two-fold increase: Approximately a doubling in SCE frequency over the "background" (solvent and negative control) levels, at a minimum of three doses.

Dose response: A positive assessment may be made in the absence of a doubling if there is a statistically significant increase at a minimum of three doses *and* evidence for a positive dose response.

In some cases, statistically significant increases are observed with neither a doubling or a dose response. These results are assessed according to repeatability, the magnitude of the response, and the proportion of the dose levels affected.

Statistical analysis employs a *t*-test (2) to compare SCE frequencies in treated cultures with negative and solvent controls.

Data Bases

The GeneTox program described previously has reviewed both the SCE and in vitro chromosome aberration data bases (9,10).

A recent review by Perry (7) contains most of the reported SCE responses. In most of these studies S9 activation systems were used, and, in general, the SCE/carcinogenic correlation is good. The correlation between in vitro cytogenetic responses and carcinogenic activity of chemicals lacks a good evaluation because of the often poor quality of in vitro studies. When more rigid controls and test protocols are applied, the rate of false responses has been reduced and the correlation looks considerably more impressive.

Overall Assessment

There are many approaches to in vitro cytogenetic analyses, each with its own particular advantages and limitations. It is difficult to identify a single system which consistently provides unequivocally accurate answers. The in vitro cell lines such as CHO are probably the most useful for routine screening because of the suitability to S9 application. The analysis of chemicals for clastogenicity and SCE induction in CHO cells with an S9 activation system generates responses with a good correlation to the chemicals carcinogenic activity. More false positives are likely to be encountered than false negatives because of the possibility for artifact production when test conditions are not carefully controlled.

References

1. Ames, B. N., McCann, J. and Yamasaki, E., *Mutation Res.*, **31**, 347 (1975).
2. Bancroft, H., *Introduction to Biostatistics*, Hoeber-Harper, 1957.
3. Carrano, A. U., Thompson, L. H., Lindl, P. A. and Minkler, J. L., *Nature*, **271**, 551 (1978).
4. Chromosome Methodologies in Mutagen Testing: Report of the *Ad Hoc* Committee of the Environmental Mutagen Society and the Institute for Medical Research. *Toxicol. Appl. Pharmacol.*, **22**, 269 (1972).
5. Evans, H. J., *International Review of Cytology*, **13**, 221(1962).
6. Goto, K., Maeda, S., Kano, Y., and Sugiyama, T., *Chromosoma*, **66**, 351 (1978).
7. Perry, P., Chemical Mutagens and Sister-Chromatid Exchange, in *Chemical Mutagens: Principles and Methods for Their Detection*, Volume 6, F. J. deSerres and A. Hollaender, eds., Plenum Press, New York, pp. 1–39, 1980.
8. Perry, P. and Wolff, S., *Nature*, **251**, 156 (1974).
9. Preston *et al.*, *Mutation Res.*, **87**, 143 (1981).
10. Latt et al., *Mutation Res.*, **87**, 17 (1981).
11. Terasima, T. and Tolmach, L. J., *Nature*, **190**, 1210 (1961).
12. Vogel, E., The Relation Between Mutation Pattern and Concentration by Chemical Mutagens in Drosophila, in *Screening Tests in Chemical Carcinogenesis*, Montesano, R., H. Bartsch, and L. Tomatis, eds., Lyon (IARC Scientific Publications No. 12), 1976.
13. Wolff, S., Sister Chromatid Exchange as a Test for Mutagenic Carcinogens, in *Cellular Systems for Toxicity Testing*, Volume 407, G. M. Williams, V. C. Dunkel, V. A. Ray, eds., The New York Academy of Sciences, New York, pp. 142–153, 1983.

Section D

Transformation Assays

Chapter 19

In Vitro Transformation Assays Using Mouse Embryo Cell Lines

Balb/c-3T3 Cells

John O. Rundell

In Vitro Transformation of Balb/c-3T3 Cells

Balb/c-3T3 cells have been widely applied to the routine testing of chemicals for their in vitro transforming potential. Although a number of 3T3 cell clones have been described, few are useful in the context of morphological transformation and all of those that are presently available were originally isolated by T. Kakunaga (7). The lineage of these cells has been discussed earlier, but it is important to realize that the majority of chemical screening studies have been conducted using Kakunaga's clone 1-13 and therefore the methods described in the following sections apply specifically to this clone.

Clone 1-13 of Balb/c-3T3 cells multiply in culture until a monolayer is achieved and then cease further division; i.e., they exhibit density-dependent inhibition of replication or "contact inhibition." These cells, if injected into Balb/c or athymic mice, do not produce tumors (7,11), although tumorigenicity can be demonstrated among a variety of Balb/c-3T3 clones under conditions of solid surface implantation (4). However, clone 1-13 cell populations treated in vitro with chemical carcinogens may give rise to cellular foci of differential growth and morphology superimposed on the cell monolayer. When these foci of transformed cells are isolated, and the cells grown to larger numbers and transplanted into appropriate host animals, sarcomatous tumors develop (*7,11*). Thus, the appearance of foci of morphologically altered cells is associated with the process of the cellular acquisition of malignant properties and this observation forms the basis for the use of these cells in chemical screening for carcinogenic potential.

Materials and Methods

Target Cells

As previously mentioned, the Balb/c-3T3 cells presently used in 3T3 cell transformation assays were derived by Takao Kakunaga (*7*) from Aaronson and Todaro's 3T3 clone A-31 (*1*). Transformable A-31 subclones were also isolated by DiPaolo (*5*) and Quarles and Tennant (*10*) in independent experiments, but these cells were subsequently lost and therefore will not be considered further here. A number of different A-31 subclones were distributed by Kakunaga including A31-11, A31-13, and 714, and results using these subclones have been reported (*6–9, 11–13*). A31-13 (1-13), or a derivative of it, has been used by Sivak during the course of the recently reported NCI-sponsored comparative studies (*6*), and in several industrial research and toxicology laboratories, including our laboratory at LBI. At the same time, a variety of new A-31 subclones have been developed in Dr. Kakunaga's laboratory and certain of these have been distributed to US and European investigators (T. Kakunaga, personal communication). Thus, several different transformable subclones of A-31 appear to be in use and since each may exhibit unique biological qualities, the general study design described by Kakunaga (*7*) may require modification if applied to subclones other than 714 or 1-13.

Cell Culture Methodology

3T3 1-13 cells exhibit a doubling time of approximately 18 h when cultured in Eagle's Minimal Essential Medium (EMEM) supplemented with 2 mM L-glutamine and 10% selected fetal bovine serum (FBS). Under those culture conditions, their maximum cell density is approximately 5.1×10^4 cells/cm^2 decreasing to near 2.5×10^4 cells/cm^2 under conditions of liquid holding. When plated at low density, for example, 5–10 cells/cm^2, their absolute cloning efficiencies range between 30 and 50%. An initial plating density of ~360 cells/cm^2 is generally used in the dishes seeded for use in the transformation assay (7,11–13). Assuming a 50% plating efficiency and a final saturation density of about 2.5×10^4 cells/cm^2, between 6 and 8 cell generations elapse between the time of plating and the occurrence of density-dependent inhibition of growth. The significance of this is that a minimum of two to three cell divisions have been shown to be required for the "fixation" of the cellular events that lead to the expression of the transformed phenotype (8), and that development and recognition of the morphologically transformed phenotype is dependent upon the formation of the "confluent" monolayer. In this regard, both the final saturation density and the time required to attain this density can be influenced by culture conditions. Though less stringent than the Syrian hamster embryo assay system, standardized culture conditions are of great importance to establish and maintain when conducting the 3T3 cell transformation assay. This is nowhere more important than in the handling of stock cultures, in that the frequency of the appearance of spontaneously transformed foci in the transformation assay is directly influenced by stock culture history. In this regard, maintenance of stock 3T3, 1-13 cell cultures under conditions of liquid holding results in an increase in spontaneous transformation frequencies apparently because of the selective advantage of the rare transformant in the "contact inhibited" monolayer. Conversely, even under conditions of stock culture logarithmic growth, spontaneous transformed cells accrue in the population, thus limiting the useful life of any given culture. To control the spontaneous transformation frequency, it is necessary to maintain subconfluent conditions (i.e., maintain logarithmic growth) among 1-13 target cell populations and to evaluate, for any given subclone, its relation to passage level.

Reagents

Beyond considerations of stock culture husbandry, the conditions for the development of the transformed morphology in 1-13 cells is much less stringent than that for SHE cells. In this regard, selection of FBS lots for use in the assay is relatively simple, and this fact greatly increases the ease with which this assay can be established. The major consideration in FBS screening for this system is support of clonal growth. In this regard, we have found that sera that support a high cloning efficiency at low concentrations (2–5% v/v) without toxicity at high concentrations (15–20% v/v) are particularly appropriate for 1-13 cells. Most investigators employing 1-13 cells use Eagle's Minimal Essential Medium (EMEM) without supplementation, except for L-glutamine, FBS and, perhaps, an antibiotic. The FBS concentrations is usually reduced during the course of the assay in keeping with the observations of Kakunaga (7) for 3T3 cells and Bertram (3) for 10T½ cells.

Balb/c-3T3, 1-13 Cell Culture

The general growth and culture characteristics of 1-13 cells have been described earlier and given the requirements for maintenance of stock culture logarithmic growth, no unusual procedures are required for the use of these cells. Stock cell populations may be readily cryopreserved using 9–10% DMSO in the freezing medium without resort to automated cell freezers. In our laboratory, ampules containing about 1×10^6 cells are routinely frozen using a stepwise method consisting of 2-h-long cycles at $-20°C$ and $-80°C$ followed by storage over liquid nitrogen. Cell recovery using this method approximates the cloning efficiency of these cells (30–50%) and stock cultures are readily established from single ampules. Nonetheless, an adequate period of growth should be provided before use of the target cells in the assay to allow for recovery from the freeze-thaw insult.

Experimental Design

Aside from considerations of test chemical chemicophysical properties, significant questions regarding the dose selection for the 3T3-cell transformation assay exist. As has been previously discussed, at least two schools of thought are apparent regarding dose selection criteria. According to one idea, dose selection should be predicated on an upper limit criterion whose central feature is application of a type of arbitrary exclusion rule. An example of the use of an arbitrary criterion may be found in the recently published results of the NCI Carcinogenesis Testing Program (6), wherein Sivak elected to limit the maximum tested dose of "nontoxic" test chemicals to 100 µg/mL (the highest dose level used in the preliminary toxicity test). In contrast to this approach, we employ a dose selection criterion that is based exclusively on the empirically determined response characteristics of the 3T3 target cell population. The basis for this are our findings that the maximum transforming activities of a variety of model carcinogens were resolved over a similar and narrow range of cell survivals, whereas noncarcinogens and carcinogens requiring metabolic activation were inactive when tested over the same range of relative survivals (11). These observations showed that the limiting 3T3-cell survivals for the transformation assay lie between 10 and 20% and that the sensitivity of the assay was optimal when test chemical doses were selected around the limiting survival value (*11*). Application of these conditions to routine testing is straightforward in that test chemical cytotoxicity is the only variable requiring analysis for purposes of dose selection. Accordingly, using a clonal growth assay, we analyze the toxicity of a given test chemical over a concentration range that results in survivals ranging from an apparent 0 to 100% (i.e., resolving, within the confidence limits of the experimental conditions, the chemicals complete cytotoxicity profile).

Using these survival data, we select doses for the transformation assay so that the highest dose selected causes survivals in the 10–20% range. Lower doses are chosen along the ascending survival curve so that their separation reflects the steepness of the curve. Operationally, the preliminary cytotoxicity assay is conducted using triplicate dishes seeded with 200–300 3T3 cells for each condition. The test chemical is diluted in the appropriate solvent (e.g., acetone, ethanol, DMSO, culture medium) so as to form a series of 15 concentrations in twofold dilution steps and then added to the 3T3 cell cytotoxicity cultures, resulting in a series of final concentrations in the test cultures, usually ranging between 1.0 mg/mL and 0.061 µg/mL. After 3 d of treatment, the test chemical is removed from the cytotoxicity assay cultures and incubation continued for an additional 4–5 d to allow for colony growth. The cytotoxicity cultures are then fixed and stained, the surviving colonies are counted in both treatment and control sets, the relative survivals for each treatment condition are calculated, and doses are selected from a semilogarithmic plot of the resultant survival data.

Although various approaches to the problem of dose selection have been employed, the methods used for the transformation assay *per se* have generally followed those first described by Kakunaga (*7*).

Twenty-four hours prior to treatment with the test chemical, a series of 25-cm^2 tissue culture flasks or ~28 cm^2 (60 mm) tissue culture dishes are seeded with 350–400 3T3 cells in EMEM. The number of replicate cultures employed by various investigators varies between 12 and 20, but larger number of cultures may be necessary to accomodate the attrition caused by contamination or to compensate for the toxicity of treatments, such that the number of cells surviving the treatments are similar over the tested concentrations of the test chemical. In this regard, Sivak has calculated that ~20 culture vessels are required in a replicate set to determine a statistically significant doubling in the number of transformed foci (*12*), but this calculation assumes equal survivals among the treated populations and thus may be inappropriate for sample size determinations.

After 24 h incubation to allow for target cell attachment and recovery from the trauma associated with the plating process, the cultures are treated for 72 h with the preselected doses of test chemical, washed, refed, and the incubation continued with biweekly refeedings. The concentration of FBS is usually reduced by a factor of about ½ soon after termination of chemical treatment, in keeping with previously published observations (3, 7). After a total incubation period of 28–31 d, the cultures are fixed, stained with 10% aqueuous Giemsa, and scored for the appearance of foci of morphologically transformed 3T3 cells.

The criteria used for scoring of the Balb/c-3T3 morphologically transformed phenotype have been described (7). Briefly, at the end of the 4-week incubation period, cultures of normal cells yield a uniformly stained monolayer of flat closely packed cells. In contrast, transformed cells form a dense mass (focus) that stains deeply and is superimposed on the surrounding monolayer of normal cells. Transformed foci of 3T3 cells exhibit several variations in their morphological features. Some foci consist of a dense, multilayered zone of cells exhibiting a random, crisscrossed orientation of fibroblastic cells at the focus periphery and extensive invasiveness into the contiguous monolayer. 3T3 cell foci exhibiting these morphological features are sometimes referred to as "Type III" foci and, as was previously discussed, scoring may be limited to this morphological type (6). However, other focus morphologies appear in both treated and untreated cultures, including foci consisting of more rounded cells with little peripheral criss-crossing, but with extensive piling-up of cells at the focus center. Flat foci, exhibiting little or no piling-up, but with a criss-cross pattern of overlapping cells throughout the colony, may also be observed. Foci of these latter two types are sometimes referred to as "Type II" foci and these, along with small foci consulting of highly ordered cells, may not be scored. Because the central feature of the transformed morphology is random cellular orientation, and because there is no published evidence supporting the concept that there are significant biological differences between "Type III" and "Type II" foci for 3T3 cells, we score on the basis of the lack of cellular orientation alone (see Chapter 4 for a discussion of the transformed phenotype and the basis for selective scoring.)

The spontaneous transformation frequency of the 3T3 cells used in our laboratory ranges between 0 and ~1.0 focus/60 mm dish with an arithmetic mean of approximately 0.3 focus/dish. This mean frequency compares well with the normal spontaneous frequency range of 0.11–0.40 focus/dish for another subclone of A31-13 cells reported by Sivak (6). These spontaneous frequency values are important in the evaluation of assay results for a given test chemical because qualitative estimates of chemical activity are made in comparison to the spontaneous control value. As was previously pointed out, control of the background (spontaneous) frequency by use of stringent techniques of cell husbandry is extremely important in the construction of assay evaluation criteria, particularly in that the maximum transformation frequencies resolved for model compound treatments are limited by the toxicity of treatment as well as by the intrinsic transforming potential of the tested chemical. As a consequence, where the induced frequencies are close to the spontaneous value, statistical resolution may depend upon the reproducibility of the observation and this is critically dependent upon control of the variance in the spontaneous frequency.

To arrive at a qualitative estimate of a test chemical's transforming potential, we employ Bailey's Modification of Student's t-test (2). The criteria employed in our laboratory were developed during the course of our studies of approximately 30 model carcinogens and noncarcinogens. In general, we consider that a response at a single dose that just obtains the 95% confidence level in a single assay as insufficient evidence for activity. However, if the 95% or a higher level of confidence is observed for a given dose in two independent assays, then the results are interpreted as positive evidence for chemical activity in the assay. Results attaining the 99% confidence level over one or more doses, or the 95% confidence level with clear evidence of a dose-related response, are similarly interpreted.

Other assay evaluation methods have been used and these are exemplified by the criteria used by Sivak (6, 12) in which it was tacitly assumed that a doubling in the mean number of transformed foci for a given treatment was significant if the experiment was conducted so that the observed increase could have attained the 95% confidence level.

References

1. Aaronson, S. A., and Todaro, G. J., *Science* **102**, 1024 (1968).
2. Bailey, N. T. J., *Statistical Methods in Biology*, Wiley, NY, 1959.
3. Bertram, J. S., *Cancer Res.* **37**, 514 (1977).
4. Boone, C. W., and Jacobs, J. B., *J. Supramolecular Struct.* **5**, 131 (1976).
5. DiPaolo, J. A., Takano, K., and Popescu, N. C., *Cancer Res.* **32**, 2686 (1972).
6. Dunkel, V. C., Pienta, R. J., Sivak, A., and Traul, K. A., *JNCI* **67**, 1303 (1981).
7. Kakunaga, T., *Int. J. Cancer* **12**, 463 (1973).
8. Kakunaga, T., *Int. J. Cancer* **14** 736 (1974).
9. Little, J. B., *Cancer Res.* **39**, 1474 (1979).
10. Quarles, J. M., and Tennant, R. W., *Cancer Res.* **35**, 2637 (1975).

11. Rundell, J. O., Guntakatta, M., and Matthews, E. J., Criterion development for the application of Balb/c-3T3 cells to routine testing for chemical carcinogenic potential, in *Short-Term Bioassays in the Analysis of Complex Environmental Mixtures, III,* Waters, M. D., Sandhu, S. S., Lewtas, J., Claxton, L., Chernoff, N., and Nesnow, S., eds., Plenum Press, NY, 1983, pp. 309–324.

12. Sivak, A., Charest, M. C., Rodenko, L., Silveria, D. M., Simons, I., and Wood, A. M., Balb/c-3T3 cells as target cells for chemically induced neoplastic transformation in *Adv. Mod. Environ. Tox.,* Vol. 1, *Mammalian Cell Transformation by Chemical Carcinogens,* Mishra, N., Dunkel, V., and Mehlman M., eds., Senate Press, NJ, 1981.

13. Sivak, A., and Tu, A. S., Factors influencing neoplastic transformation by chemical carcinogens in balb/c-3T3 cells, in *The Predictive Value of Short Term Screening Tests in Carcinogenicity Evaluation* Williams, G. M., et al., eds. Elsevier/North-Holland, NY, 1980.

Chapter 20

In Vitro Transformation Assays Using Mouse Embryo Cell Lines

C3H/10T½ Cells

John O. Rundell

In Vitro Transformation of C3H/10T½ Cells

C3H/10T½ C18 cells ("10T½") have been employed in a variety of studies aimed at elucidation of the mechanism of cell transformation and, like 3T3 cells, have also been applied to the problem of chemical screening. This cell line was isolated from cultured C3H mouse embryo cells by Heidelberger and his colleagues (12, 13) and the 10T½ cells in use by various investigators can be traced directly to this laboratory. 10T½ cells and 3T3 cells exhibit a number of common characteristics, with the result that the assay protocols developed for the two cell lines are quite similar. For example, both cell lines are subject to post-confluence inhibition of replication ("contact inhibition") and, in both cases, model carcinogen treatments result in the formation of foci of transformed cells superimposed on the contiguous monolayer of normal cells. As was the case for 3T3 cells, cells isolated from transformed 10T½ foci are transplantable. However, unlike 3T3 cells, the neoplastic potential of transformed 10T½ isolates appears to be linked to the degree of their initial expression of the morphologically transformed phenotype. Nonetheless, the basis for the use of 10T½ cells is similar to that previously described for SHE and 3T3 cells; the development of the transformed morphology is linked to the expression of cellular neoplastic qualities and therefore test material induction of the transformed phenotype is thought to be a reflection of the material's carcinogenic potential.

Materials and Methods

As described above, 10T½ cells were first described by Heidelberger's group (*12, 13*) and their present application to chemical screening is based on the subsequent observations of the developer's laboratory (*2, 4, 8, 11*), as well as studies conducted by other investigators using cells obtained directly from Heidelberger (*1, 3, 5–7, 9, 14*). To this author's knowledge, only clone 8 of 10T½ cells has been distributed and, thus, published 10T½ transformation assay data has been obtained for a single clone using a nearly-common study design.

Cell Culture Methodology

10T½ cell populations double with an interval of 15–16 h when grown in Eagle's basal medium (BME) supplemented with 10% v/v heat-inactivated fetal bovine serum and 2 mM L-glutamine (*13*). The saturation density of these cells is about $3–4 \times 10^4$ cells/cm^2 (*13*). The cloning efficiency of 10T½ cells ranges between 10 and 30% when plated at 5–10 cells/cm^2.

Most investigators have employed a 36 cells/cm^2 initial plating density for the transformation assay (*5, 12*), with the result that about 13 cell generations elapse before the maximum saturation density is obtained (assuming a 30% plating efficiency; see ref. *12*). Plating at higher densities (e.g., 360 cells/cm^2) has been shown to result in a marked reduction in the induced transformation frequency (*5*). This may be because of a requirement for cell division prior to fixation of the cellular events necessary for the expression of transformation, as has been shown for 3T3 cells by Kakunaga (*10*).

As is described elsewhere for 3T3 cells, cell husbandry is extremely important to the conduct of the 10T½ cell transformation assay. Thus, as with 3T3 cells, liquid holding on 10T½ cells results in the appearance of spontaneously transformed cells. This problem can be potentially avoided by maintaining logarithmic growth conditions among stock cultures, but even under these conditions, spontaneously transformed cells will ultimately appear, with the result that the useful life of any given stock culture is limited to relatively few passages.

Reagents

Cell culture reagent selection for 10T½ cells is relatively straightforward. Screening of plasticware and culture medium for toxicity and growth support is usually conducted using clonal growth as the endpoint. Though plasticware obtained from various suppliers is usually adequate, an occasional toxic lot will be encountered, and thus each lot should be screened before use. Similarly, the major suppliers of culture medium utilize similar formulations and quality control procedures and, thus, though few problems are generally encountered, media screening is also an important preliminary step in the use of 10T½ cells. Of greater importance is the selection of fetal bovine serum for use in the assay. The reason for this lies in the intrinsic lot-to-lot variability of this complex biological reagent both in terms of their content of essential (but undefined) growth factors and their in-process contamination with adventitious agents. We have found that sera lots that support 10T½ clonal growth over the 5–15% v/v concentration range are adequate for use in the transformation assay. However, the ability of these "adequate" sera to support optimal expression of the transformed phenotype is variable, and thus, sera screening should always be conducted against the transformation assay after preselection based on clonal growth support.

10T½ Cell Culture

Stock 10T½ cell populations can be readily cryopreserved without the use of programmed cell-freezing apparatus. Most investigators use DMSO (~10% v/v/) in the cell-freezing medium, but glycerol (also ~10% v/v/) may also be used. 10T½ cells are quite resistant to the damage caused by the freeze-thaw process and viable cell recoveries usually approach the cloning efficiency value even when cell freezing is conducted by direct freeze over liquid nitrogen. 10T½ cells are usually frozen at about $0.5–1.0 \times 10^6$ cells/freezer vial and enough stock cells can be obtained from a single vial to conduct several assays after a single passage.

Experimental Design

As has been previously described for the 3T3 cells transformation assays, dose selection is critical to the analysis of a test chemical's transforming potential in the 10T½ assay. However, unlike the case of the 3T3 assay, the basic consideration of the toxicity of treatment is somewhat complicated by the low initial cell densities normally used in the 10T½ assay. The reason for this lies at the level of the surviving cells' ability to form a monolayer when the surviving fraction is below about 0.5. For example, under control conditions (no added toxicity) the proportion of the plated cells surviving and therefore contributing to the population's growth and the formation of the monolayer is probably about 30% (300 cells/60 mm dish or about 11 cells/cm^2). If additional reductions in survival are imposed by chemical treatments, the number of viable cells remaining may fall to a level wherein discreet cell colonies, rather than a cell monolayer, will be formed. Thus, if the toxicity of treatment results is about 10% relative survival, then the effective plating efficiency and the plating efficiency after treatment (0.3 × 0.1 = 0.03), with the result that only about 30 of the initial 1000 cells plated/60 mm dish will survive. These cells will form colonies that may persist as discreet entities even after 4–6 weeks incubation. This parodoxical effect of the toxicity of treatment can be theoretically overcome by increasing the initial plating densities in experimental sets in proportion to the survivals predicted from a preliminary clonal toxicity assay.

However, in our experience with 3T3 cells, proportional plating results in a reduction in the recovery of transformed foci and Heidelberger's data would seem to suggest that a similar result might be expected for 10T½ cells (12). Accordingly, dose selection should ideally be accomplished so that the cell survival to the maximum tested dose is adjusted to assure formation of a monolayer. The available evidence points to a permissable range of between 30 and 50% and this is predicated on the observation that platings of as few as 3 cells/cm^2 will result in a confluent monolayer after 4–6 weeks incubation.

The methods for the conduct of the 10T½ assay are quite similar to those used for the 3T3 assay. The target cells are obtained by mild trypsinization from logarithmically growing stock cultures and plated at 1–2 × 10^3 cells/60 mm (28 cm^2) dish in 3–5 mL BME supplemented with 10% v/v heat-inactivated FBS and 2.0 mM L-glutamine. After 24 h incubation in a humidified 5% CO_2, 95% air, 37°C incubator, the cell cultures in replicate sets of 20 dishes/condition are treated with preselected doses of the test chemical. The treatments are continued for 24 h, after which time the test chemical is removed by aspiration, the cultures washed with balanced salt solution, refed, and incubation continued with refeeding on a twice-weekly schedule. In our laboratory, the concentration of FBS is reduced after the third or fourth refeeding to about 5% v/v (see ref. 3). After a total incubation period of approximately 6 weeks, the cultures are fixed with methanol, stained with 10% aqueous Giemsa, and scored for the appearance of transformed foci.

Three types of transformed foci have been described for 10T½ cells and the expression of these morphological types has been related to their oncogenic potential (*12*). The application of scoring criteria based on a resolution of these three types of transformed foci has immense potential impact on assay evaluation. The reason for this is that the distinction between types of morphologically transformed foci is quite subtle and therefore a considerable degree of subjectivity is involved in assay scoring. Comparisons of results for a given test chemical among investigators is thereby made difficult in a quantitative as well as in a qualitative sense. At the same time, these difficulties can be largely circumvented by independent confirmation of the expression of the malignant phenotype among various morphologies of foci by each laboratory. Such independent confirmation studies are, however, infrequently performed, and therefore the impact of subjectivity in 10T½ transformation assay scoring is difficult to quantify. In practice, then, investigators using the 10T½ assay score in relation to the criteria initially described by Heidelberger and his colleagues (*12*). These criteria were developed to distinguish between foci of Types III, II, and I, and were based on the observed transplantation frequencies of cells obtained from isolated foci of each type. Thus, about 85% of Type III foci yielded tumors upon transplantation into C3H mice, whereas no cells derived from Type I foci were transplantable. Type II foci were intermediate, yielding a transplantation frequency of about 50%. These types of foci differ from one another with regard to both their density (i.e., amount of cellular piling-up) and their orientation (i.e., degree of criss-crossing) (see ref. *12* for description and photomicrographs). Thus, Type II and Type III foci exhibit different degrees of the morphological attributes of the transformed phenotype, whereas Type I foci exhibit only evidence of moderate hyperplasia. Unlike 3T3 cells, but like SHE cells, little or no data describing a spontaneous frequency for 10T½ cell transformation has been published. The absence of a spontaneous frequency value raises important questions regarding both the performance and evaluation for the 10T½ assay. In this regard, investigators using this assay, in common with those employing the SHE cell transformation assay, have not generally utilized statistical criteria in the qualitative analysis of transformation frequenceis. In fact, because the spontaneous frequency in 10T½ cells was unresolved in the majority of published investigations, the appearance of one or two foci in a treatment group has been viewed as positive evidence of test chemical activity in the assay. Whether application of such a rule of the thumb criterion is appropriate in evaluations of 10T½ cell transformation awaits the results of assay response-characteristic studies and investigations into the question of the spontaneous transformation frequency.

References

1. Benedict, W. F., Banerjee, A., Gardner, A., and Jones, P. A., *Cancer Res.* **37**, 2202 (1977).
2. Bertran, J. S., and Heidelberger, C., *Cancer Res.* **34**, 526 (1974).
3. Bertram, S., *Cancer Res.*, **37**, 514 (1977).
4. Fernandez, A., Mondal, S., and Heidelberger, C., *Proc. Natl. Acad. Sci. USA* **77**, 7272 (1980).
5. Haber, D. A., Fox, D. A, Dynan, W. S., and Thilly, W. G., *Cancer Res.* **37**, 1644 (1977).
6. Haber, D. A., and Thilly, W. G., *Life Sci.* **2**, 1663 (1978).
7. Jones, P. A., Baker, M. S., Bertram, J. S., and Benedict, W. F., *Cancer Res.* **37**, 2214 (1977).
8. Jones, P. A., Benedict, W. F., Baker, M. S., Mondal, S., Rapp, U., and Heidelberger, C. *Cancer Res* **36**, 101 (1976).
9. Jones, P. A. Laug, W. E., Gardner, A., Nye, C. A., Fink, L. M., and Benedict, W. F., *Cancer Res.* **36**, 2863 (1976).
10. Kakunaga, T., *Int. J. Cancer* **14**, 736 (1974).
11. Mondal, S., Brankow, D. W., and Heidelberger, C., *Science* **201**, 141 (1978).
12. Reznikoff, C. A., Brankow, D. W., and Heidelberger, C., *Cancer Res.* **33**, 3239 (1973).
13. Reznikoff, C. A., Brankow, D. W., and Heidelberger, C., *Cancer Res.* **33**, 3231 (1973).
14. Terzaghi, M., and Little, J. B. *Cancer Res.* **36**, 1367 (1976).

Chapter 21

In Vitro Transformation Assays Using Diploid Syrian Hamster Embryo Cell Strains

John O. Rundell and Judith A. Poiley

In Vitro Transformation of Syrian Hamster Embryo Cells

Freshly prepared, diploid Syrian hamster embryo (SHE) cells, when plated at low density, will form colonies against a background of lethally irradiated homologous feeder cells (*1, 3, 5, 8–10*). These colonies exhibit a variety of cellular morphologies, but consist of highly ordered populations sometimes exhibiting contact inhibition and usually little or no evidence of perimarginal cellular crossing-over. In contrast, cells treated in vitro with chemical carcinogens may give rise to colony morphologies exhibiting evidence of cellular disorder, including significant perimarginal cell criss-crossing, characteristic of the transformed phenotype (*1, 9*). This morphological phenotype may occur in untreated cultures, but with extremely low frequency, and has been shown to be associated with the expression of malignant properties by carcinogen-transformed colony isolates (*4, 6, 8*). These observations form the basis for an assay system that has been applied to investigations into the mechanism of neoplastic transformation as well as the evaluation of chemicals for their genotoxic potential. The following sections describe the methodologies employed in these studies and are intended to provide investigators unfamiliar with cell transformation with the SHE assay's basic technical framework in relation to the 3T3 and 10T½ assays.

Materials and Methods

SHE cells may be freshly prepared for each assay (*1, 3, 5*), or alternatively, cryopreserved cell pools can be established so as to provide a uniform source of both target and feeder cells for use over an extended period of time (*10*). In either case, procurement of responsive cell populations is dependent upon identification of appropriate techniques, animals, and reagents for the initial preparation of the SHE primary cells.

Animals

The use of outbred Syrian hamster dams obtained from various laboratory animal suppliers has been reported (*1, 10*). No evidence of strain-dependent variance has been published and therefore it may be assumed that useful animals may be obtained from any of the several Syrian hamster breeders, although the presence of infective agents in the selected breeding colony can be problematic. Embryos for use in target and feeder cell preparation are usually obtained from animals in their thirteenth or fourteenth day of gestation. The use of first pregnancy animals is usually avoided when possible because such animals often yield few useful fetuses when compared to "proven breeders." Pregnant animals may be sacrificed by cervical dislocation or by use of anesthetics or CO_2 asphyxiation. The abdomen is normally washed with 70% ethyl or isopropyl alcohol, a midventral incision performed and the uteri resected. Healthy dams normally produce 11–15 fetuses with little or no evidence of fetal death or resorption. Abdominal and thoracic viscera are often inspected at necropsy for evidence of maternal disease, such as the presence of excess ascites, and compromised animals are then rejected. The fetuses are dissected from the uterine horns, their membranes removed, and erythrocytes and contaminating debris removed by saline wash. The crown–rump lengths of 13- and 14-d-old Syrian hamster fetuses usually range between 12–14 and 15–18 mm, respectively.

SHE Cell Primary Preparation

Most investigators decapitate and eviscerate the fetuses prior to their use in primary cell preparation. Fine tissue fragments are usually prepared from the collected fetuses so that the resultant fragments average near 0.2 mm in dimension. These fragments, often referred to as the tissue mince, are then transferred to a trypsinizing flask, washed once or twice in a balanced salt solution to further reduce erythrocyte contamination, and then washed again using the trypsin solution prepared for cell dissociation. The selection of trypsin is critical to successful production of useful primary cells and a variety of enzyme formulation have been employed.

The trypsin-mediated digestion or dissociation process presents a type of toxic insult and a balance between enzyme activity and toxicity has to be found in order to obtain a sufficient number of primary cells under conditions of minimal or controlled toxic selection. The useful primary cell population exhibits marked heterogeneity, which is a reflection of the balance between the tryptic dissociation of fetal cells and selective cell killing.

After the initial washes, the tissue fragments are again subjected to sequential trypsin treatments. The supernatant trypsin solutions contain the SHE primary cells and are usually collected into fetal bovine serum to inactivate residual tryptic activity, thus protecting the primary cells from excess enzyme activity. Several trypsinization and collection cycles may be conducted, the resultant cell suspensions pooled and, after centrifugal removal of the digestion enzyme, plated at about 0.13 million cells cm^2 in complete tissue culture medium (generally Dulbecco's Modification of Eagle's Minimal Essential Medium, DMEM). The primary cell yield from the tryptic dissociation of fetal tissue fragments normally ranges between 7.5 and 9.0 $\times$ 10^6 nucleated cells per fetus after two dissociation and collection steps. The primary cultures are usually incubated for 2–3 d until they are ~90% "confluent," after which they may be subcultured (secondary cultures) or cryopreserved according to published procedures (*1, 3, 10*). Many investigators discard cultures that show suboptimal growth or that do not exhibit the full range of morphological heterogeneity typical of SHE cell primary cultures. Such populations may, however, be retained and utilized as a source of feeder cells. The cell yield in the primary cultures usually approaches 0.13 million cells/cm^2 after 2 d growth, but yields as low as 0.075 million cells/cm^2 may be acceptable. The significance of these population density values lies in their relation to growth conditions and the ultimate saturation density of the primary cell population. The endpoint of the transformation assay is a type of morphological alteration that is best appreciated in fusiform cell populations. Thus, cultures that do not attain high saturation density (i.e., do not contain a high proportion of fusiform cells), may not develop the transformed phenotype after exposure to carcinogens.

Reagents

The development of the transformed phenotype in SHE cells is dependent upon the fetal bovine serum (FBS) used to supplement the growth medium. Many, perhaps most, lots of FBS are deficient in that they do not support SHE cell morphological transformaltion (12). The selection of culture medium and supplements in addition to FBS can also be of critical importance. In this regard, some investigators have found that the use of high glucose (4.5 g/L) and/or sodium pyruvate (usually 0.11 g/L) supplemented DMEM to be necesary for adequate SHE cell growth and expression of the transformed phenotype. The reagent requirements for the SHE cell transformation assay are quite stringent and demand systematic evaluation of FBS lots and media formulations to identify useful biologicals.

SHE Cell Culture

SHE cells are usually grown in DMEM and supplements to this medium may normally include sodium pyruvate, but the levels of this supplement, as well as the concentrations of sodium bicarbonate, glucose, and FBS, are usually determined using clonal and mass population growth and morphology as endpoints.

For purposes of describing cell culture methods, it is assumed that the SHE cell primaries were cryopreserved after 2–3 d culture. For use as target or feeder cells in the assay, the frozen cells are thawed and the cells (normally 2.5–5.0 million cells/vial) planted in growth medium.

After a few hours incubation, the culture medium is usually aspirated to remove the cell freezing supplement (e.g., DMSO or ethylene glycol) and refed. After an additional 2–3 d growth, approximately 6–8 million cells are generally obtained from each ~75 cm^2 culture dish. These cells may be collected by trypsinization, irradiated, and used directly as feeders or subcultured (usually 1:4 to 1:6) and the resultant tertiary cell population similarly utilized after an additional growth period.

For culture of the SHE target cells, a freezer vial containing 2.5–5.0 million cells is thawed, plated (usually in a 25 cm^2 dish), and refed after a few hours incubation. These SHE secondary target cells are usually used in the assay after about 24 h incubation. Longer growth periods for the target cell populations are usually avoided so that the cells do not senesce, and so that their metabolic characteristics are not dramatically altered in relation to the fetal tissues from which they were derived.

SHE cells normally exhibit low cloning efficiencies (CE) when plated at low densities; the observed CE is often near 1% of the plated cells. This low cloning efficiency places severe restraints on the design of SHE cell clonal growth assays, but these restraints can be largely removed by the use of lethally irradiated feeder cells. X-irradiated feeder cells are therefore commonly utilized for both SHE survival and transformation assays to improve the efficiency of colony formation. Irradiation of feeder cells is performed to prevent their colonization of the cytotoxicity or transformation assay dishes. The dose of X-irradiation used is usually 5000 rads, but the dose required is dependent upon the operating characteristics of the X-ray machine employed. At the same time, adequate cloning efficiencies can be obtained without the use of feeders. SHE secondary cells release easily and the conditions of trypsinization can be adjusted so as to prevent over trypsinization and the resultant losses in cell viability. Since complete recovery of the plated population is not necessary, control of the toxicity caused by trypsinization can result in cloning efficiencies on the order of 25% without the use of a feeder layer.

In any event, absolute cloning efficiencies in the presence of irradiated feeders should be in the range of 10–15% and efficiencies less than about 10% may be indicative of suboptimal conditions.

Experimental Design

A number of chemicophysical considerations are important in the testing of unknown chemicals, e.g., solubility, volatility, and stability. Because generalizations regarding the impact of these physical parameters are not readily formulated, the discussions that follow are based on observations made using typical model compounds [e.g., crystalline solids exhibiting well-described physical characteristics, such as benz(a)pyrene, 3-methylcholanthrene, N-methyl-N'-nitro-N-nitrosoguanidine, and so forth].

The solubility of the test chemical is of clear significance to the conduct of the assay and therefore solubility is generally evaluated in a series of prospective solvents. Among the more commonly employed solvents (assuming poor solubility in culture medium) are dimethylsulfoxide (DMSO), acetone, and ethanol. If one of these solvents is used, its final concentration in the cell culture is adjusted so that its presence does not contribute to the cytotoxicity of the chemical treatments; e.g., DMSO concentrations are generally well below 1% v/v. A clonal survival assay is used to estimate the cytotoxicity of the appropriately solvated test chemical. To do this, SHE target cells are plated at low density (250–500 cells/dish) onto an irradiated feeder layer. In our laboratory, fifteen dose levels of the test chemical, usually starting at 1 mg/mL (1 μL/mL for liquids) and decreasing in twofold dilution steps, are applied to replicate sets of SHE cell cultures. After 7–8 d incubation to allow for colony development, the fixed and stained cultures are examined to determine the number of colonies surviving the treatments. The doses to be applied in the transformation assay are then estimated from a plot of these survivals so that the highest dose chosen causes no more than an 80% reduction in colony-forming ability. Lower doses may also be selected and these are usually 1:2 or 1:4 dilution of the 20% survival concentation.

The assay procedures utilized by most investigators are based on those reported by DiPaolo (*1–5*) or Pienta (*9, 10*). Forty-eight hours prior to treatment, a series of ⁻28 cm^2 dishes are seeded with about 8×10^4 X-irradiated, feeder cells and incubated. The next day, each feeder cell culture is seeded with 300–500 target cells and incubation is continued. After an additional 18–24 h, a number of dishes are treated with various concentrations of the test chemical. A positive control, usually B(a)P or 3-MCA, and a solvent or culture medium negative control set are generally included to provide activity data for estimation of the assay's performance in relation to historical experience. The number of dishes (replicates) employed varies among investigators, but 12–20 dishes are generally set up for each treatment condition. The sensitivity of a given assay is profoundly influenced by the number of cells at risk. For example, B(a)P positive control treatments may result in the appearance of only 2–4 transformed colonies assay among 1000 colonies scored in a total of 20 dishes originally seeded with 500 target cells each. Reduction in the size of the replicate set to 12 or so dishes materially reduces the assay's sensitivity to the positive control treatment and increases the probability of a false-negative response in the test chemical treatment groups. The treated and control dishes are then incubated for an additional 7–8 d to allow for colony development and the expression of the transformed phenotype. The dishes are then fixed and stained and each colony examined at 20–100 diameters for evaluation of morphological transformation.

The criteria used for the scoring of morphological transformation of hamster cells have been described (*3, 9*). Briefly, normal or nontransformed colonies are characterized by an ordered, contact-inhibited morphology with little or no evidence of criss-crossing. In contrast, transformed colonies exhibit random orientation with evidence of crisscrossing at the colony periphery. The absence of cellular order coupled with the expression of crossing-over are the most significant criteria for transformation. In practice, however, the evaluation of the transformed phenotype is not unambiguous. The difficulties intrinsic to the process of scoring are largely a result of the heterogeneity of colony morphologies appearing in the negative control populations. These morphologies may be variously altered by chemical treatments and aberrant colonies may arise as a direct consequence of the toxicity of the treatment. Because of this, many investigators score the transformed phenotype in relation to the negative controls (3). Recently, Pienta has proposed a zonal scoring criterion for the SHE colony assay (9). This criterion may be applied without regard to the conditions of treatment and thus may be used as an absolute standard for scoring of the transformed phenotype in treated as well as in untreated cultures.

The spontaneous frequency of SHE cell transformation has generally been reported to be zero. Because of this, the appearance of a single transformed colony in one treated dish has often been interpreted as positive evidence of transforming potential (1, 3, 5, 6, 8–11). Although no general agreement regarding evaluation criteria for the SHE assay exists, Dunkel et al. (7) have applied somewhat more stringent criteria than those just described. Evaluations of the data arising from the NCI Carcinogenic Testing Program's evaluation of the SHE assay were predicated on (1) the presence of a dose response, and (2) the number of transformed colonies at a given dose. Accordingly, for a response to have been characterized as positive, one or more of the following conditions had to have been met:

1. The response was dose-dependent.
2. More than one dose induced transformed colonies with one dose resulting in at least two transformed colonies.
3. At least three transformed colonies were induced for a single dose.

Treatments that resulted in a single transformed colony were designated as questionable.

These criteria were apparently based on biological observations regarding the response characteristics of the assay system towards model carcinogens rather than on considerations of statistical significance. In this regard, it should be noted that there has appeared in the literature a statistical analysis of the SHE cell transformation assay (14). However, the question of the development of methods for the qualitative evaluation of results using this assay was not addressed, and therefore such evaluations continue to rely on biological considerations alone.

References

1. DiPaolo, J. A., *J. Nat. Cancer Inst.* **64,** 1485 (1980).
2. DiPaolo, J. A., and Donovan, P. J., *Expt. Cell Res.* **48,** 361 (1967).
3. DiPaolo, J. A., Donovan, P. J., and Nelson, R. L., *J. Natl. Cancer Inst.* **42,** 867 (1969).
4. DiPaolo, J. A., Nelson, R. L., and Donovan, P. J., *Science* **165,** 917 (1969).
5. DiPaolo, J. A., Nelson, R. L., and Donovan, P. J., *Cancer Res.* **31,** 1118 (1971).
6. Doniger, J., and DiPaolo, J. A., *Cancer Res.* **40,** 582 (1980).
7. Dunkel, V. C., Pienta, R. J., Sivak, A., and Traul, K. A., *J. Natl. Cancer Inst.* **67,** 1303 (1981).
8. Pienta, R. J., A transformation bioassay employing cryopreserved hamster embryo cells, in *Advan. Modern Env. Toxicol.,* Vol. 1, *Mammalian Cell Transformation by Chemical Carcinogens,* Mishra, N., Dunkel, V., Mehlman, M. eds., Senate Press, NJ, 1981.
9. Pienta, R. J., Lebherz, W. B., III, and Schuman, R. F., The use of cryopreserved Syrian hamster embryo cells in a transformation test for detecting chemical carcinogens, in *Short-Term Tests for Chemical Carcinogens,* Stich, H., and San, R. H. S., eds., Springer-Verlag, NY, 1981.
10. Pienta, R. J., Poiley, J. A., and Lebherz, W. B., III, *Int. J. Cancer* **19,** 642 (1977).
11. Poiley, J. A., Raineri, R., and Pienta, R. J., *J. Natl. Cancer Inst.* **63,** 519 (1970).
12. Schuman, R. F., Pienta, R. J., Poiley, J. A., and Lebherz, W. B., III., *In Vitro* **15,** 730 (1979).
13. Umezawa, K., Hirakawa, T., Tanaka, M., Katoh, Y., and Takayama, S., *Tox. Lett.* **2,** 23 (1978).

Section E

Short-Term In Vivo Carcinogenesis Assays

Chapter 22

Lung Tumor Assay

L. H. Smith and H. P. Witschi

Introduction

Several screening assays are available that allow testing of suspected carcinogens within a reasonably short time, are reproducible from laboratory to laboratory and allow estimates of relative potency. In vitro systems with prokaryotic and eukaryotic systems are most widely used. However, they do not take into account the response of an intact organism challenged by a carcinogen. An attempt to deal with this problem was made by developing short-term in vivo systems such as skin tumor induction in mice, breast cancer induction in female Sprague-Dawley rats, and lung tumor induction in mice (1). In 1975, Shimkin and Stoner published an excellent and incisive review paper that describes in detail how development of lung tumors in strain A mice may be used as a screening bioassay. The procedure is simple, reproducible, quantitative, comparatively short, and appears to have correctly predicted or confirmed the carcinogenic potential of many compounds. However, the lung tumor test has, to date, not been used widely and practically all available information on its use as a screening bioassay has been developed in one laboratory (2). The assay deserves to be studied more extensively and to be fully validated.

Rationale of Assay

The mouse lung tumor test is an in vivo bioassay that is used to detect the carcinogenic potential of chemicals. It is performed with strain A mice that have a high natural incidence of spontaneous lung tumors. Systemic administration of chemical carcinogens results in an increased incidence and multiplicity of the lung tumors. A test may be completed within 4–6 months and requires 60–100 animals per substance.

Basis Lung Tumor Test

Selection of Animals

Male or female strain A mice, about 6–8 weeks old are preferred. In experiments ranging over three decades it has been found that Strain A mice react very uniformly to a standard dose of the carcinogen urethane and usually develop one lung tumor per milligram of urethane injected intraperitoneally (ip).

Preliminary Toxicology

Prior to an assay, groups of five mice are injected (ip) with the test agent. The highest dose usually equals the acute single LD_{50} and three to four lower dose levels are serial 1:1 dilutions thereof. Three weekly injections are given for 2 consecutive weeks. The MTD is defined as the highest dose at which all five animals survive for 6 wk following the first injection of the test agent *(3)*.

Choice of Vehicle

The choice of the vehicle is dictated by the solubility of the test substance. Solutions are adjusted so that the desired dose is administered in 0.1 mL for each 10 g of animal weight. Alternately, mice may be given a fixed volume of solvent (0.1 or 0.2 mL) that contains the desired dose of substance calculated for an average body weight of the group.

Water-soluble substances are dissolved in sterile 0.9% NaCl solution. For water insoluble agents, tricaprylin (trioctanoin) has been the solvent of choice, but each lot of this vehicle should be tested for toxicity prior to its use in the tumor assay *(3)*. Corn oil is an acceptable alternative, provided the peroxide number is less than 10 mEq/kg of oil.

Bioassay: Treatment

Once the preliminary toxicity tests have been completed the assay can be started. The following is a slight modification of the procedure recommended by Shimkin *(2)*.

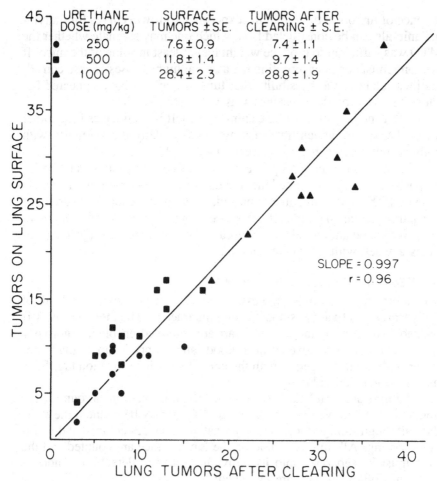

Fig. 1. Correlation between tumors visible on lung surface and in cleared lungs. Male strain A mice were injected ip with 250, 500, or 1000 mg/kg of urethane and killed 6 months later. Tumors were first counted on lung surface and recounted after clearing the lung (*10*).

Three dose levels are used for each test substance and each dose group consists of 30 randomly selected animals, housed under controlled conditions of humidity, temperature, and lighting. The high dose group receives the MTD, the medium dose group receives half the MTD, and the low dose group one-fifth of the MTD. The test substance is injected intraperitoneally three times a week (Monday, Wednesday, and Friday) for 8 weeks. The animals are checked daily and weights are recorded weekly or biweekly. Recording individual weights rather than an average cage or group weight can be, under certain conditions, a helpful determinant for judging the appropriateness of the dose levels used. Thus, in the absence of tumors at the end of the experiment, growth curves for individual animals can be constructed from which one may estimate whether the MTD was sufficient to produce weight loss at least in some of the mice. If not, one must consider repeating the assay at higher doses. These considerations relate to the possibility that tumors may not have appeared because the dose of the substance was not high enough.

After the last injection, the animals are left in their cages for another 4 months, during which time they are checked daily for mortality, with body weights being recorded every other week.

In each assay an appropriate number of control groups must be incorporated: one group treated the first day of the experiment with a single dose of 1000 mg/kg urethane to provide data on the response to urethane of a particular batch of animals. A second control group receives no treatment at all, and additional control groups consist of animals injected three times a week with the vehicle alone.

Bioassay: Termination and Scoring

Six months after beginning the assay, the animals are killed and 1 mL of Tellyesniczky's fixative is injected into the trachea. The thoracic cavity is opened and trachea, lungs, and heart are removed en bloc, vigorously rinsed in water to remove surface blood, and dropped into a small container with fixative together with the animal's ear identification tag. Each lung is stored individually.

Tumors are visible almost immediately after fixation as round white nodules raised above the pleural surface. They may be counted the same day, although storage for 24–48 h in fixative enhances contrast and facilitates scoring. All tumors visible on the lung surface are counted and the lung must be separated into its individual lobes to detect all tumors.

The following data are tabulated:

    1. Number of survivors in relation to the original group size.

    2. Tumor incidence, defined as the number of tumor-bearing animals per total number of surviving animals.

    3. Tumor multiplicity, defined as the average number of lung tumors per animal; i.e., the number of tumors found divided by number of animals per group. If, in a group of 10 animals, the number of tumors counted per animal were 0, 0, 0, 2, 6, 7, 1, 3, 0, 5, tumor multiplicity would be 2.4 ± 0.9 (SE: $n = 10$) tumors per lung.

Open Questions

Several unresolved questions need to be studied further. The suitability of other mouse strains needs to be determined. SWR mice, which are less expensive and easier to breed than strain A mice, could offer an acceptable alternative. Other strains (BALB/c, C57B1, C3H, and Sencar mice) are much more resistant to tumor induction by urethane and appear not to be sensitive enough.

No particular attention has been paid so far to the bedding of animals. Certain beddings (e.g., cedar wood shavings) may rapidly affect the activity of pulmonary mixed function oxidases (4). This makes it necessary to keep the same bedding in both control and experimental animals through each assay and from assay to assay. Different items such as bedding, the number of mice per cage, and protein content of the diet should be kept in mind when results from different laboratories are being compared.

Twenty to 30 animals per treatment group have been used in most assays. This figure is a compromise between keeping the number of animals reasonably manageable and obtaining sufficient data to permit a meaningful statistical analysis of tumor multiplicity among the different treatment groups (2, 5).

As in all chronic toxicity assays, dose setting often has some problems. Determination of the MTD with a total of 6 (3, 6) or 9 (7) injections is expedient and uses a minimum number of animals. However, selection of a MTD in this manner is not a guarantee that all animals will survive the lung tumor assay. Examination of a number of mouse lung tumor tests and our own experience show that often only a fraction of the animals survive the MTD determined in the preliminary toxicity studies (6, 7, 9).

As a vehicle for water-insoluble substances, tricaprylin, a defined chemical, appears to be preferable to corn oil, which is a mixture of several compounds. However, even highly purified preparations of tricaprylin can be toxic when given repeatedly. Tricaprylin toxicity is usually delayed and requires several weeks of treatment before becoming apparent, and the cumulative LD_{50} for an 8-week treatment is approximately 200 g/kg. The advantage of using a defined chemical having low toxicity must thus be balanced against using a mixture of chemicals having no detectable toxicity.

It is possible that not all tumors formed within a lung will reach the pleural surface within 4–6 months. Scoring surface tumors only could thus underestimate the number of tumors formed. When we compared tumors counted on the surface against tumors seen in the cleared lungs, we found a 1:1 relationship between surface tumors and tumors scored in the cleared lungs (unpublished data). The correlation coefficient was 0.96 and the average number of tumors seen on the surface was not significantly different from the number of tumors found in cleared lungs. Although theoretical considerations might call for scoring tumors in cleared lungs, practical observations do not warrant this time-consuming and expensive procedure in routine assays.

Finally, we need to consider when the animals should be killed. In several mouse strains given urethane, there is a steep initial increase in the number of tumors and this increase is often greater between 14 and 24 wk than it had been in the first 14 wk *(11–14)*. Based on these observations we suggest that animals should be killed 6 months after the beginning of treatment. A small increase in tumors seen after six months *(11, 12)* is not likely to increase the sensitivity of the assay. On the other hand, it would not seem advisable to kill animals earlier. It is conceivable, although not proven, that the effect of weak carcinogens, particularly at low doses, might become unequivocal only if animals are allowed to survive for 6 months rather than for 4.

Limitations and Sources of Error

There are two major problems with the lung tumor assay. One is that like all other screening procedures, it may produce false positive and, perhaps more important, false negative data. The second problem is interpretation of test data.

Data available in the literature show that 10 known human carcinogens *(15)* have been evaluated in the mouse lung tumor assay *(2, 9)*. Seven of these compounds were correctly identified as having carcinogenic potential in the lung tumor system and three were false negatives (Table 1). However, it is noteworthy that all of the three false negatives were with metallic compounds, one of which (As) has never been shown conclusively to be a carcinogen in experimental animals. For Cd and Cr the best available experimental evidence of carcinogenicity is the production of sarcomas at the site of injection, a finding the relevance of which is under discussion *(16)*. The International Agency for Research in Cancer reviewed a total of 296 chemicals tested through 1977. For 145 of them experimental evidence of carcinogenicity in animals tested was considered to be adequate *(15)*. Of the 145, a total of 19 had been tested in the lung tumor assay as well. Sixteen of these chemicals gave positive results (Table 1). The limited amount of data shows that the mouse lung tumor assay was quite accurate and that four out of six false negatives may be explained because they belonged to one particular class of compounds (metals) or were given in too low a dose [benz(a)anthracene].

The lung tumor assay has been used to rank carcinogens according to potency by calculating the dose of a given compound (μmol/kg) required to produce one lung tumor per mouse. In Table 2 the compounds are listed in increasing order of potency in the lung tumor test. It is interesting to compare these estimates of relative potency to a ranking system based on the Ames test *(17)*. Urethane is negative in the Ames test and

TABLE 1
Comparison of Lung Tumor Test with Other Data[a]

Human Carcinogens

Positive in tumor test	Negative in tumor test
Aflatoxin	Arsenite
Cyclophosphamide	Cadmium (acetate)
Melphalan	Chromium (sulfate)
Mustard gas	
Nickel (nickelous acetate)	
2-Napthlylamine	
Soot and tar	

Animal Carcinogens

Positive in lung tumor assay	Negative in lung tumor assay
Ortho-aminoazotoluene	Benz(a)anthracene
Aziridyl benzoquinone	Benzylchloride
Benzo(a)pyrene	Safrole
Chlorambucil	
Dibenz(a,h)anthracene	
Dibutylnitrosamine	
Diethylnitrosamine	
Dibenz(a,h)acridine	
Dimethyl nitrosamine	
Estradiol mustard	
Hydrazine	
Isonicotinic acid hydrozide	
Lead subacetate	
Nitrogen mustard	
Uracil mustard	
Urethane	

[a]Data on human and animal carcinogens from reference *15* and on lung tumor assay from references *2* and *9*.

hydrazine and methyl iodide are only weak mutagens, whereas in the lung tumor assay they are reasonably potent. On the other hand, AAF and N-OH-2AAF are highly potent in the Ames test, but rather ineffective in the lung tumor assay. At this point it is premature to draw any conclusions with regard to the merit and relevance of each ranking system. It is hoped that, as more data become available, it will be possible to compare a greater number of compounds.

TABLE 2

Comparisons of Estimates of Relative Potency for Production of Lung Tumors in Mice and Mutagenicity Assessed by the Ames Test

Lung tumor assay, μmol/kg of compound producing one tumor[a]		Ames test, nmol of compound necessary to produce one revertant[b]	
N-OH-2-acetylaminofluorene (OH-AAF)	13158	Urethane	Negative
2-Acetylaminofluorene (AAF)	11739	Hydrazine	Weak
Nitrosopiperidine (NP)	1343	Methyl iodide	Weak
Dibutylnitrosamine (DBN)	1225	Nitrosopiperidine	100.0
Methyl iodide (MI)	564	Diethylnitrosamine	100.0
Diethylnitrosamine (DEN)	370	Dimethylnitrosamine	50.0
Hydrazine (H)	122	Dibutylnitrosamine	6.67
Aflatoxin B1 (B1)	121	Melphalan	3.45
Dimethylnitrosamine (DMN)	35	Uracil mustard	2.5
Benzo(a)pyrene (BaP)	9.5	Nitrogen mustard	7.69×10^{-1}
Melphalan (ME)	4.0	Dibenz(a,h)anthracene	9.1×10^{-2}
Nitrogen mustard (NM)	3.0	3-Methylcholanthrene	1.72×10^{-2}
Uracil mustard (UM)	1.0	N-OH-2-AAF	2.08×10^{-2}
Dibenz(a,h)anthracene (DB)	1.0	2-AAF	9.26×10^{-3}
3-Methylcholanthrene (3MC)	0.9	Benzo(a)pyrene	8.26×10^{-4}
		Aflatoxin B1	1.42×10^{-4}

[a]Data from ref. (2).
[b]Data from ref. (17).

Analysis of a lung tumor test involves a comparison of tumor multiplicity between treated groups and corresponding vehicle control. According to Shimkin and Stoner (2), the following criteria should be fulfilled before it can be concluded that a particular test substance gave a positive response: (a) the number of lung tumors per mouse should be significantly higher in the treated group if compared by t-test to the appropriate control group; ideally, more than one tumor per mouse should be found; (b) there should be evidence for a dose–response relationship; (c) vehicle controls, untreated controls, and urethane-treated animals should have similar values as found in previous assays done under identical conditions.

When more data are available from several different laboratories, it may become necessary to redefine the criteria in relation to: (1) what consitutes a positive response, and (2) the best way to analyze the data statistically. However, it must be reemphasized, as pointed out by Shimkin and Stoner (2) that absence of a positive response in the mouse lung tumor assay is not proof of absence of carcinogenic potential and, most important, a positive response calls for further testing in other animal systems.

Advantages of the Assay

The lung tumor assay is a rapid screening test in whole animals and does not require lifetime exposure. Administration of a test compound to a whole animal will result in eventual metabolic activation or deactivation. Lung tumors are easily counted and collection of the data requires no special skill or training. A test involving seven to nine compounds (three dose levels per compound, 30 animals per group) together with the appropriate controls requires approximately one-quarter time of two persons and one supervisor for one-sixth year. Histopathology can be kept to a minimum. Costs to test a single compound may be only a fraction of a complete lifetime bioassay in whole animals and 5–10 times more than a conventional in vitro assay with a bacterial or mammalian cell system.

Conclusion

The lung tumor assay deserves to be considered as a potential in vivo screening test of value. The assay is easy to perform and it can be used to estimate relative potency of carcinogens. Lung tumors develop following administration of many different classes of chemical carcinogens, several of which, e.g., nitrosamines, are not readily detectable in skin tumor assays. In addition, lung tumor development is not limited to one sex as is the case for some tumors, e.g., mammary tumors in Sprague-Dawley rats. Scoring of lung tumors does not require special skills as for some assays, such as the altered foci induction in rodent liver (1). A positive lung tumor response may be induced by direct-acting carcinogens, reflect metabolic activation of a proximate carcinogen, interactions of the test agent with type II alveolar cells as putative targets, and those host-mediated factors that determine tumor expression. Although a negative lung tumor response will not be acceptable evidence for the lack of tumorigenic potential of a substance, a positive response justifies further investigation.

Acknowledgments

Research sponsored by the Office of Health and Environmental Research, US Department of Energy, under contract W-7405-eng-26 with the Union Carbide Corporation. By acceptance of this article, the publisher acknowledges the US Government's right to retain a nonexclusive, royalty-free license in and to any copyright covering the article.

References

1. Weisburger, J. H., and Williams, G. M., Chemical Carcinogens, in *Casarett and Doull's Toxicology,* Doull, J., Klaassen, C. D., and Amdur, M.D., eds., 2nd ed., Macmillan, New York 1980, pp. 84–138.
2. Shimkin, M. B., and Stoner, G. D., *Adv. Cancer Res.* **21,** 1 (1975).
3. Stoner, G. D., Shimkin, M. B., Kniazeff, A. J., Weisburger, J. H., Weisburger, E. K., and Gori, G. B., *Cancer Res.* **33,** 3069 (1973).
4. Malkinson, A. A., *Toxicol. Appl. Pharmacol.* **49,** 551 (1979).
5. Zweifel, J. R., *J. Natl. Cancer Inst.* **36,** 937 (1966).
6. Theiss, J. C., Stoner, G. D., Shimkin, M. B., and Weisburger, E. K., *Cancer Res.* **37,** 2717 (1977).
7. Theiss, J. C., and Shimkin, M. B., *Cancer Res.* **38,** 1757 (1978).
8. Poirier, L. A., Stoner, G. D., and Shimkin, M. B., *Cancer Res.* **35,** 1411 (1975).
9. Stoner, G. D., Shimkin, M. B., Troxell, M. C., Thompson, T. L., and Terry, L. S., *Cancer Res.* **36,** 1744 (1976).
10. Yuhas, J. M., *J. Natl. Cancer Inst.* **50,** 69 (1973).
11. Dyson, P., and Heppleston, A. G., *Brit. J. Cancer* **31,** 405 (1975).
12. Brightwell, J., and Heppleston, A. G., *Brit. J. Cancer* **35,** 433 (1977).
13. Witschi, H. P., and Lock, S., *Toxicol. Appl. Pharmacol.* **50,** 391 (1979).
14. Ullrich, R. L., Jernigan, M. C., and Adams, L. M., *Rad. Res.* **80,** 464 (1979).
15. Tomatis, L., The Value of Long Term Testing for the Implementation of Primary Prevention, in *Human Risk Assessment* (Book C), *Origins of Human Cancer,* Hiatt, H. H., Watson, J. D., and Winsten, J. A., eds., Cold Spring Harbor, 1977, pp. 1339–1358.
16. Sunderman, F. W., Jr., *Fed. Proc.* **37,** 40 (1978).
17. McCann, J., Choi, E., Yamashi, E., and Ames, B. N. *Proc. Natl. Acad. Sci.* **72,** 5135 (1975).

Chapter 23

Tissue Genotoxic Effects

Methods

D. J. Koropatnick and J. J. Berman

Alkaline Sucrose Gradient Analysis of DNA Fragmentation and Repair

To assay DNA fragmentation, rodents are administered multiple injections of ^{3}H-Tdr at infancy, at which time virtually all cells are actively dividing. This ensures radioactive DNA labeling in all organs. Alternatively, intraperitoneal injections of adult mice may selectively label those tissues that constantly divide in the adult (e.g., bone marrow, intestinal mucosal epithelium) or those tissues that have been induced to divide (liver hepatocytes after partial hepatectomy or renal tubular epithelium after partial nephrectomy). Compounds may be introduced by a variety of methods, including force-feeding, subcutaneous or ip injection, or skin painting. After a short period of time (1–6 h is allowed for maximal DNA breakage), animals are sacrificed, tissues excised, and a preparation of intact nuclei made. Approximately 5×10^5 cells are layered into a lysing solution containing detergent and alkali, overlying a 5–20% alkaline sucrose gradient. The lysing process separates DNA into single strands that are separated in size according to the frequency of compound-induced single-strand breaks. Control cells (cells from untreated animals) are always run in parallel to determine the size of single DNA strands from untreated rats. The sucrose gradients are spun at 25,000 rpm for 30

313

min. Longer strands will sediment further than shorter (broken) strands. Sequential fractions are collected and DNA measured by liquid scintillation counting.

Readily assayed tissues are liver and kidney, since excellent isolated nuclei preparations are obtained by gentle squashing in buffer with subsequent removal of tissue by low-speed centrifugation. Nuclei preparations from other organs may be made using slightly more elaborate procedures (1).

By observing DNA sedimentation profiles in animals sacrificed at longer and longer intervals following compound administration, the gradual shift back toward the control profile is noticed as DNA is repaired (strands are repaired) and dead cells are replaced by new cell populations.

The Alkaline Elution Assay (4, 5)

The tissues used are radioactively labeled by methods identical to those outlined above. After exposure to chemicals, animals are sacrificed and tissues are rapidly removed and placed in cold buffer. Samples of treated and untreated (tissues from animals only exposed to solvent) tissues are removed at the same time to monitor toxicity. Tissues are minced and hand-homogenized in 20 mL of buffer, centrifuged at 1500 rpm for 2–4 min, and the pellet resuspended in 5–10 mL of buffer. A 0.2 mL aliquot of this suspension (containing approximately 0.5×10^6 cells) is used in the assay.

The procedure involves layering the cells on polyvinyl filters, lysing with an alkaline Sarkosyl solution, washing the cells with EDTA buffer, and eluting single-stranded DNA by pmuping 12–40 mL of alkaline eluting solution through the filter at a slow steady rate (5). The rate at which DNA molecules elute from the filter increases with decreasing strand length. Fractions are collected and DNA assayed by scintillation counting. The filter is lysed in acid, neutralized with alkali, and the amount of DNA retained is likewise determined. Care must be taken to use several control procedures. Assay conditions should be adjusted so that 85–90% of the control DNA is retained, and internal filter controls (cells containing ^{14}C-TdR-labeled DNA, irradiated by 150 rads) should be included if fluctuation of duplicate filters is encountered. More than one animal should be assayed, duplicate aliquots of each sample should be run, and constant temperature and a location that has a minimum of vibration should be used. A peristaltic pump of steady, low flow rate must be used (the eight channel Gilson Minipuls peristaltic pump with slow speed control module works well).

In order to evaluate the results, assays should be conducted at different concentrations of the chemical up to toxic doses, and the time course of repair should be followed. Increased elution observed only at toxic doses is considered to be a negative result. The shape of the eluting curve may give some indication of the nature of the DNA damage. Single-strand breaks give first-order elution, while accelerating elution suggests two or more events must occur before strand scission. Dose-related decreases in elution over controls suggest DNA crosslinks (5).

A limitation of both assays is the requirement for DNA labeling prior to treatment. This is a particularly vexing problem in tissues of heterogenous cell populations where the cells that incorporate the ^{3}H-TdR are not the primary target cells of the suspected compound. For instance, in the gut tissue, the cells that preferentially incorporate ^{3}H-Tdr are entering the postmitotic state, in which they can no longer undergo malignant transformation. Thus, the dividing crypt cells, which are likely carcinogen targets, present only a minor fraction of the labeled cells.

Several fluorometric methods have been proposed that would measure all cellular DNA without prelabeling. Particularly promising is the use of ethidium bromide, a dye that intercalates duplex DNA with a 25-fold enhancement of its fluorescence. Neutralization of the alkaline sucrose gradient or DNA elution fractions leads to the formation of duplex DNA by intramolecular hydrogen bonding that provides about 50% double-strandedness. DNA from virtually all cells, both dividing and nondividing, may be detected in this manner. To the alkaline fractions derived from alkaline sucrose gradients or eluted from filters, enough stock ethidium bromide fluorescing solution (42.3 g KH_2PO_4, 163.5 g K_2HPO_4, 0.093 g Na_2EDTA, 1.25 m ethidium bromide made up to 1 L with distilled water) was added to neutralize the sample. Fluorescence was read at an emission wavelength of 600 nm and an exciting wavelength of 525 nm within 1 min of addition of fluorescing solution.

Unscheduled DNA Synthesis (UDS)

Compounds are administered to the animal and specific tissues are sampled at different post-treatment intervals. The tissue samples are divided into small (less than 1 mm^3) pieces, incubated in minimal essential medium supplemented with fetal calf serum in the presence of ^{3}H-TdR for 3–5 h, and prepared for autoradiography. Cells will incorporate ^{3}H-TdR into DNA that is being repaired (i.e., to replace excised thymidine bases). In dividing cells, unscheduled (repair) DNA synthesis is obscured by scheduled (semiconservative) DNA synthesis. These cells can be easily recognized because of their extremely high level of ^{3}H incorporation. Incubation of cells in arginine-deficient medium (6) or in hydroxyurea (7) can be used to depress cell division.

DNA Adduct Analysis

DNA adduct analysis is conducted by injecting or force-feeding radioactive (^{3}H or ^{14}C) genotoxic compounds. The aminals are sacrificed at times ranging from 1 h to 1 wk. DNA is isolated from the organ of interest by phenol extraction, RNAase and protease incubation, chloroform/ isoamyl alcohol extraction, and alcohol precipitation. After hydrolysis of the DNA in acid, the adduct and non-adduct nucleotides can be separated by Sephadex or high pressure liquid chromatography.

Chromatid Aberrations

Tissues that have been used are bone marrow or embryonic liver cells. For the analysis of bone marrow cells, mice are injected with a single dose of chemical. At 12–16 h before sacrifice, the intra-orbital plexus is punctured to produce hematological anemia as a stimulus to produce sufficient mitoses. Colcemid is injected 1 h before sacrifice to arrest cells at metaphase. Animals are killed 24 h after chemical treatment. Bone marrow is prepared for histology by the method of Datta et al. (8). In order to observe chromosome aberrations in embryonic liver cells, mice may be treated with chemical by intraperitoneal (ip) injection, mated with females of the same strain, and the resulting 13-d fetus removed. The liver is excised and made into a cell suspension. Colcemid is added, and the cells prepared for histology by the method of Datta et al. (8).

Micronuclei Introduction

This protocol involves two ip injections of the chemical of interest at 70% of the LD_{50} into a mouse 24 h apart. Samples of polychromatic red cells from bone marrow are taken at 48, 72, and 96 h after the first injection (9). When positive results are obtained, a second test is performed with a single dose of 50% of the LD_{50}, and samples are taken at 30, 48, and 72 h. Bone marrow samples are prepared by the method of Schmid (10).

Sister Chromatid Exchange

This technique presently uses either peripheral lymphocytes, bone marrow, or spermatogonia (11). Male mice are administered hourly injections of bromodeoxyuridine (BrdU) for nine injections when studying bone marrow and 14 injections when studying germ cells. The chemical of interest is administered in a single ip injection 11–19 h after the last BrdU injection (for bone marrow) or 32 h after (for germ cells). Colcemid is injected, and cells are excised, dispersed, and swollen and mounted. They are stained with Hoechst and Giemsa by the method of Allen and Latt (11). Peripheral lymphocytes may be analyzed by the analogous procedure of Stetka and Wolff (12). Sister chromatids are examined for reciprocal exchanges.

Sperm Anomaly Test

Mice are injected daily with small volumes of chemical in appropriate vehicle for 5 d. Five weeks after the first injection, mice are sacrificed, epididymides excised, sperm suspensions prepared, and the average number of sperm per epididymis determined (13). Sperm aliquots are stained with Eosin-Y, smears made, and morphological anomalies noted (13). Agents are deemed positive inducers of abnormal sperm if two doses show significant elevations in abnormalities, and negative inducers if no increase in sperm abnormalities is seen up to doses that cause test animal lethality (14).

Specific Locus Mutations

Analysis of these mutations is based upon the possibility of detecting mutant cells directly in tissues obtained from test animals or in cells isolated from tissue and cultured outside the body. An example of such a test is the HGPRT assay for 6-thioguanine-resistant cells detectable in peripheral blood lymphocytes (15). In this case, white blood cells from the periphery are suspended in medium containing phaetohaemagglutinin to stimulate mitosis. 6-Thioguanine (6-TG), when added to cultures, will prevent mitosis in all but those cells containing the Lesch-Nyhan mutation for 6-TG resistance. Mitosis is measured by incorporation of ^{3}H-TdR. Present evidence indicates that the host selects against these re-

sistant lymphocytes, and persistence may be in the order of several
months only (16).

Alternatively, the granuloma pouch assay may be used (17). A subcutaneous air pouch in the test animal is stimulated to induce mitosis
(granulation tissue), the chemical of interest is administered, and animals
are killed, and granulation tissue is dissected, dispersed, and the mutation
frequency determined by observing clone frequency in medium containing 6-TG.

Induction of Resistant Preneoplastic Liver Cells (7)

This assay is carried out by force-feeding or ip injection of chemical 12 h
later, when the height of the mitotic wave is reached. The largest dose
given should be lower than the dose that causes death 4 wk after injection. After 2 wk, animals are placed on a diet containing 0.02%
2-acetylaminofluorene (2-AAF) for two weeks to select for foci-forming
cells. Halfway through the feeding period the animals receive a single
dose of carbon tetrachloride at a concentration of 2 mL/kg of body weight
in corn oil by esophageal intubation. At the end of the feeding period, the
rats are placed on a basal diet without 2-AAF for one week and then
killed. Livers are analyzed for cellular foci histochemically positive for
GGT activity (19).

In choosing an in vivo short-term test for the carcinogenic biohazard
of a compound, several factors must be taken into consideration. The cost
of the test, the length of time it requires, and the selection of organ(s) to
study must be considered. DNA adduct determination may be very costly
because of the high costs of labeled compounds. Also, the adducts that
can be easily studied are quite limited. The induction of resistant
hepatocytes may take months to achieve results as compared to days for
primary genotoxic effects. Tests that require actively dividing tissue (cytogenetic assays) and those that need quiescent tissue (unscheduled DNA
synthesis) may miss carcinogens that are specific for cell types not assayed in the particular procedure. Cumulative effects of a single compound and cooperative effects among different compounds may be considered (20, 21). Such effects may require a protocol in which the action
of one agent is modified by another (2).

References

1. Cox, R., Damjanov, I., Abanobi, S. E., and Sarma, D. S. R., *Cancer Res.*
   33, 2114 (1973).

2. Abanobi, S. E., Popp, J. A., Chang, S. K., Harrington, G. W., Lotlikar, P. D., Hadjiolov, D., Levitt, M., Rajalakshme, S., and Sarma, D. S. R., *J. Nat'l Cancer Inst.* **58**, 263 (1977).
3. Koropatnick, D. J., and Stich, H. F., *Int. J. Cancer* **17**, 765 (1976).
4. Kohn, K. W., and Grimek- Ewig, R. A., *Cancer Res.* **33**, 1849 (1973).
5. Swenberg, J. A., Utilization of the Alkaline Elution Assay as a Short Term Test for Chemical Carcinogens, in *Short Term Tests for Chemical Carcinogens,* H. F. Stich, R. H. C. San, eds., New York, Springer-Verlag, 1980.
6. Stich, H. F., Lam, P., Lo, L. W., Koropatnick, D. J., and San, R. H. C., *Can. J. of Genet. Cytol.* **17**, 471 (1975).
7. Cleaver, J. E., *Radiation Res.* **37**, 334 (1969)
8. Datta, P. K., Friger, H., and Schleiermacher, E., The Effect of Chemical Mutagens on the Mitotic Chromosomes of the Mouse in Vivo, in *Chemical Mutagenesis in Mammals and Man,* F. Vogel and G. Rohrborn eds., Springer-Verlag, New York, pp. 194–213, 1970.
9. Heddle, J. A., and Salamone, H. F., The Micronucleus Assay. 1. In Vivo, in *Short Term Tests for Chemical Carcinogens,* H. F. Stich, R. H. C. San, eds., New York, Springer-Verlag, 1980.
10. Schmid, W., *Mutation Res.* **31**, 9 (1975).
11. Allen, J. W., and Latt, S. A., *Chromosoma* **58**, 325 (1976).
12. Stetka, D. G., Wolff, S., *Mutation Res.* **41**, 333 (1976).
13. Wyrobek, A. J., and Bruce, W. R., The Induction of Sperm-Shape Abnormalities in Mice and Humans, in *Chemical Mutagens: Principles and Methods for Their Detection,* vol. 5, A. Hollaender and F. J. de Serres, eds., New York, Plenum Press, pp. 257–285, 1978.
14. Wyrobek, A. J., Methods for Human and Murine Sperm Assays, in *Short Term Tests for Chemical Carcinogens,* H. F. Stich, R. H. C. San, eds., New York, Springer-Verlag, 1980.
15. Strauss, G. H., and Albertini, R. J., *Mutation Res* **61**, 353 (1979).
16. Mendelsohn, M. L., Short Term Genetic Tests Extended to the Human, in *Short Term Tests for Chemical Carcinogens,* H. F. Stich, R. H. C. San, eds., New York, Springer-Verlag, 1980.
17. Maier, P., and Zbinden, G., *Science* **209**, 299 (1980).
18. Farber, E., and Tsuda, H.: Induction of a Resistant Preneoplastic Liver Cell as a New Principle for the Short Term Assay *In Vivo* for Carcinogens, in *Short Term Tests for Chemical Carcinogens,* H. F. Stich, R. H. C. San, eds., New York, Springer-Verlag, 1980.
19. Laishes, B. A., Ogawa, K., Roberts, E., and Farber, E., *J. Nat'l Cancer Inst.* **60**, 1009 (1978).
20. Rosin, M. P., and Stich, H. F., *J. Environ. Path. and Toxicology,* 1980 (in press).
21. Warren, P. M., and Stich, H. F., *Mutation Res.* **28**, 285 (1975).

Section F

Conduct of Carcinogen Bioassays

Chapter 24

Conduct of Carcinogen Bioassays

J. F. Douglas

The most critical facet of bioassay conduct is scientific management. This includes command of both resources and processes. Once the experimental design is finalized, a plethora of details necessary over the three-year period of laboratory work must be accomplished to assure that the study is technically accurate. This aspect of the bioassay supplements the scientific input needed for design, and the two somewhat different approaches again merge when unforeseen events arise. Regulatory agencies have recognized the need for bioassay management and formalized some of their concepts in the Good Laboratory Practices (GLP) regulations (1). The latter, along with the use of quality assurance techniques, the rendering of careful scientific judgments, the use of explicit and unambiguous protocols, and close adherence to high laboratory standards form the basis for a well-managed study.

The GLP are a set of interlocking procedures that have generally been followed by any quality-oriented facility. They specify details of operations and record-keeping, but do not pertain to scientific judgment. For example, the experimental design, choice of analytical techniques, and so on lie outside the GLPs. Table 1 itemizes the various sections of the Federal Code as promulgated by the Food and Drug Administration (FDA) for nonclinical laboratory studies. Essentially they discuss protocols, standard operating procedures, personnel, and data handling. Ad-

TABLE 1
Part 58—Good Laboratory Practice for Nonclinical
Laboratory Studies

Subpart A	General provisions
Subpart B	Organization and personnel
Subpart C	Facilities
Subpart D	Equipment
Subpart E	Testing facilities operation
Subpart F	Test and control articles
Subpart G	Protocol for and conduct of a nonclinical study
Subparts H and I	(Reserved)
Subpart J	Record and reports
Subpart K	Disqualification of testing facilities

herence to each section significantly increases the chance of a successful bioassay and signals an alert to problems as they arise. A brief general discussion of bioassay operation will be useful prior to a more detailed breakdown of the GLPs. Bioassay is a multidisciplinary operation requiring the integrated effort of at least eight different scientific backgrounds (Table 2). It is the function of the study director to coordinate this effort and effectively utilize the skills of each discipline as needed. Unfortunately, many laboratories are organized by scientific area rather than biological function, making this task difficult in practice. It requires dedication by laboratory management to ensure that bioassay team functions efficaciously across organizational lines and that the study director has the cooperation of individuals not directly reporting or responsible to him. This problem is probably the biggest single handicap to successful first-class experiments.

TABLE 2
Disciplines Necessary
for Bioassay

- Biochemist
- Chemist
- Industrial hygienist
- Information specialist
- Pathologist
- Statistician
- Toxicologist
- Veterinarian
  Laboratory animal specialist

TABLE 3
Problems in Bioassay Conduct

- Insufficient management dedication
- Inadequate facilities
- Personnel shortage
- Improperly trained personnel
- Poorly kept records
- Improper animal care
- Improper chemical storage, analysis, and dose preparation
- Improper dosage
- Not adhering to protocols or SOPs
- Poorly maintained equipment

The problems that arise in bioassay conduct can be summarized in Table 3.

Perhaps the classical case of toxicological studies that were declared invalid were those conducted at a midwestern laboratory; this experience greatly fostered the growth of the GLP. The FDA found numerous unacceptable laxities in performance, most of which have been listed in Table 3. In fact, a recent tabulation of studies declared invalid was compiled in the July, 1981 issue of *Scientific News*. In nine experimental categories, the degree of unacceptability varied from 29 to 100%. For bioassay, 17 out of 18 studies were declared invalid, or 94%, while all 34 other chronic rodent experiments evaluated were also found to be unacceptable.

The GLP components can be divided into two categories: (1) *resources,* including personnel, facilities, equipment test systems, chemicals, and management/administration; and (2) *processes,* consisting of study design, study conduct, documentation, and quality assurance. A brief part-by-part description of the GLP serves as a framework to illustrate appropriate bioassay conduct.

Subpart B. Organization and personnel for bioassay programs may be classified into four subsections—personnel, testing facility management, study director, and quality assurance unit. Personnel (58.29) requires staff for carcingenesis studies to be efficiently qualified by training and experience, to carry out effective and reliable work. Each individual should have an appropriate job description, protective clothing, and be familiar with required health precautions. Testing facility management (58.31) must necessarily have an understanding of the protocol and operations by critical staff members, including the study director, to be able to respond to GLP deviations whey they occur, integrate resources in a timely manner, and be prepared to follow appropriate procedures when the study director is replaced. The requirements for the Study Director (58.33) were written to assure proper training and experience by the SD necessary for the conduct and interpretation of the study and to follow the GLPs. The Quality Assurance Unit (QAU), Subpart 58, 35, is a required group who are responsible for monitoring each study to assure integrity and accuracy of data. This unit must be independent of personnel employed in the study. The QAU maintains master files and records pertaining to all experiments and performs periodic inspections (quarterly) including report review. Problems detected are reported to management and, where necessary, studies reinspected. QAU files including Standard Operating Procedures (SOPs), inspection reports, internal reports, etc., are maintained at one location and are available to federal inspection representatives.

Subpart C pertains to facilities. Section, 58.41, General, applies to the overall building in terms of suitable size, type of construction, location, and design for various functions. A recent symposium discussed appropriate facilities for bioassay studies (2). Animal Care Facilities describes quarantining, separation of hazardous studies, safe storage of animal waste, pesticide, and vermin-free areas, and separation of species and test group. The NTP bioassay program has developed a system where it is equitable to have both rats and mice on the same chemical in the same room. This is only permissible where the animals are produced by the same animal supplier, are raised in a barrier atmosphere, are specific pathogen-free, and contain a defined gut flora. Animal Supply Facilities (58.45) discusses the need for an adequate storage area, separate from the animals, that is free from infestation and has adequate refrigeration. Included in these categories are bedding, supplies, equipment, and feed.

An area often poorly designed and utilized is the subject of subpart 58.47, Facilities for Handling Test and Control Articles. Separate accommodations outside the animal holding facility are needed for receipt, storage, and mixing of the test article (chemical). Too often, inspection of laboratories reveals sloppy practices in these categories that can lead to worker and animal contamination. The control feed must be handled so that adequate facilities are available to prevent introduction of unwanted materials. Color-coded labeling should be stressed to prevent errors. For gavage, we often suggest different size bottles for different species to eliminate the possibility of error.

Subsection 58.49, Laboratory Operation Areas, stresses the need for separate facilities for necropsy, histology, radiography, and handling of biohazardous materials. The cleaning and maintenance of equipment, including sterilization when used, should be separated from other activities. General supplies also need their own storage space. Once specimens are obtained, they and any archival material should be stored in an easily retrieved fashion, but in a limited access area (58.51). Another separate space requirement is for administration and personnel (58.53). This includes adequate office, supervisory, locker, and appropriate lavatory-shower space.

The GLP discusses equipment in *Subpart D*. Subsection 58.61 refers to environmental controls and their adequacy to meet the protocol requirements, while 58.63 requires compliance with satisfactory maintenance and calibration of equipment. These steps include SOPs and written maintenance records.

Subpart E, Testing Facilities Operation, includes SOPs, reagents and solutions, and animal care. Subsection 58.81 mandates SOPs for all operations. Specific SOPs should be available in each area where that activity is performed. Each facility must maintain an historical file of all SOPs, including any revisions. Any deviation from an SOP requires documentation with appropriate authority signature. Reagents and Solutions (58.33) covers the common-sense practice of proper labeling of these items with reference to identity, concentration, storage requirement, and expiration date.

When monitoring a study, one should rigorously check to determine whether all personnel are familiar with the SOP for their particular area. An unacceptably high percentage of laboratory workers are not fully cognizant of their performance requirements, which leads to substandard test quality.

Animal Care (58.90) is a large topic covered by SOPs for housing, feeding, quarantine, and the handling care of animals. Specifications must be developed for diagnosis, treatment, and sacrifice of moribund animals. This is a critical area, since it is tempting for technicians to skimp on observations, particularly in the late afternoon, and on weekends and holidays. If care is not exercised, excessive cannibalism and tissue autolysis occurs only too readily. Procedures for cage, rack, and accessory cleaning and sanitation are mandated, as are analyses of food, water, and bedding.

Subpart F covers characterization, handling, and mixing of test and control articles. Subsection 58.105 refers to the identity, strength, and purity of test and control articles prior to study initiation. Stability must be verified throughout the experimental period, with appropriate labeling of each container. SOPs for receipt, storage, distribution, and identity of chemicals are cited in 58.107. Mixtures (58.113) require appropriate analytical verification for uniformity, concentration, and stability.

Protocol and study conduct comprise *Subpart G*. The protocol is extensively discussed in Subsection 58.120. This detailed account has sixteen subheadings and includes experimental procedures, records, and documented changes. Conduct of the Study (58.130) cites records, record changes, monitoring, specimen identity, record of gross pathology findings, and so on that are necessary to assure that the protocol was adhered to and that a permanent reference is available regarding the experimental actions.

Records and reports are covered in *Subpart J*. Reporting Study Results (58.185) in detail is covered in this section. Final reports include not only all data generated, but also the QAU statement on their findings for the raw information. Records, reports, specimens, and so on must be maintained in a central file for many years, depending upon the use of the study results.

In addition to the GLPs, which cover a quality assurance unit for correct records control, translation of data to notebooks, following protocols and SOPs, and so on, it is also useful to carry out special assurance measures in chemistry, safety, animal care, and histopathology to obtain reliable information. The following integrated quality assurance program and discipline management suggested for a carcinogen bioassay study includes the management and practices developed in the NTP bioassays.

The chemist is primarily concerned with analysis to ascertain the nature of the material under test. Chemical analyses concentrate on two areas: assay of the bulk chemical and assay of the mixture produced when the vehicle and chemical are mixed for dosing. The former includes receipt of the chemical, milling to prepare uniform size, and mixing to ensure homogeneity. The bulk compound is identified by standard analytical techniques, the purity is determined, and the number and possible nature of the impurities is evaluated. Since carcinogenicity studies require 3–4 yr storage, the conditions needed to ensure stability must also be determined for the starting material. Analysis of the chemical in the administering vehicle must be done at a level commensurate with the dosage regimen (if an MTD is used, there are several years before this level is determined), while storage conditions have to be elucidated for the chemical-vehicle mixture. A mixing protocol for homogeneity must be developed, as well as a program to periodically check for the concentration and uniformity of the mixture given to the animals.

Animal management includes the selection of quality rodents, the use of appropriate shipping and immediate pickup, caging and equipment in accordance with Institute of Laboratory Animal Resources (ILAR) standards (3), health monitoring during quarantine, use of sentinel animals during the course of the study to ensure health, appropriate animal treatment, i.e., gavage, changing of cages, racks, bedding, water, and observation of clinical signs. Areas that can cause problems are effective vermin control without experimental contamination, sufficient bedding to prevent adverse reactions with ammonia, unpolluted water, automatic watering systems, and disease prevention. The veterinarian should be a diplomate of the American College of Laboratory Animal Medicine (ACLAM).

Quality performance dictates healthy animals and quick detection of those that are sick or moribund. Ballpark figures for evaluation often used are that 80% of pretermination deaths are moribund sacrifices and the autolysis rate should not exceed 2%. Only animals free of specific pathogens should be allowed to enter a facility. These can be obtained from barrier-isolator production units where the rodents are given pathogen-free-defined flora. Strict SOPs for shipping, quarantine, handling, housing, and maintenance are necessary to keep animals in a healthy condition. Effective animal health monitoring, preferably semidaily examination and extensive weekly checks, all contribute to a successful animal care program.

Toxicologists have an overall responsibility for the study, particularly dosage regimens, dosage procedures, and clinical signs. The toxicologist should have sufficient knowledge of the other sciences to span any interdisciplinary gaps.

In conducting a bioassay, it must be presumed that the test chemical could be a carcinogen and therefore appropriate safety procedure should be employed. The starting point for this requirement, which is often poorly done, is to unequivocally place responsibility on a single qualified individual. Assurance should be given to the area of safety and health to protect both the workers and the outer environment. Occupational areas include an assessment of the potential hazard, appropriate medical surveillance, SOPs for safe handling of chemicals, SOPs for safe personnel practices, a monitoring program with schedule, safe work area practices, an emergency procedure if an accident occurs, employee training, and facilities design where applicable. A program to verify that laboratory personnel observe safety regulations with regard to clothing, showering, respirators, entrances, exits, and so on would be useful in this regard. In the environmental area, responsibility may be broader, with care being taken to prevent pollution by air, water, or solid waste. Air contamination can usually be prevented by the use of proper air flow patterns and air filters; water contamination by careful handling of carcinogen materials and, where necessary, dilution, while solid wastes should be disposed of by an efficient incinerator. Landfill only postpones the problem to a later date. Periodic surveys should be taken to measure the effectiveness of the safety program. Occasionally, a resource receovery procedure can be helpful.

Pathology is a critical discipline for the evaluation of toxicological and carcinogen bioassay results. The tumorogenic endpoint should be identified microscopically, and the success of any study is dependent on this last stage of the laboratory experiment. Requirements for a pathologist should be fairly stringent. He or she should have extensive rodent tumor experience and preferably be boarded as a member of the American College of Veterinary Pathologists. If a target develops at an organ site relatively unfamiliar to the viewing pathologist, it is advisable to have the slides reviewed by an expert at that particular site. Since histopathology is somewhat subjective, it is mandatory that a single pathologist read all the slides from one species, including interim deaths. Considerable error can accrue if this is not done. Another possible source of error is at necropsy. A capable pathologist should be responsible for both observation and selection of tissue sections. Since terminology differences can lead to minor misunderstandings of results, a systemized nomenclature, such a SNOP (4) or SNOMED (5) should be employed.

Quality assurance of the pathology associated with bioassay has been developed by the NTP bioassay program (6). It consists of three essential steps: (1) validation of tissue counts; (2) validation of the histopathology diagnosis, including all tumors and all target sites where there are statistically significant compound related lesions; and (3) random (~10%) review of diagnosis from all tissues. A detailed report should be prepared and, where necessary, agreement reached between the original viewing pathologist and the QA pathologist. Histopathology contains subjective elements and is in part an art, so that care should be exercised that differences are real and not mildly interpretative or semantic.

A carcinogen bioassay literally generates reams of data. Pathology alone on the chronic study in a two-species two-dose experiment evaluates almost 20,000 tissues. Thus, adequte provision must be made for retention, sorting, and retrieval of information. Most modern laboratories that run multiple studies have turned to computerization, since it is the only practical way to meet the requirements of good laboratory practices and provide ready access to data for analysis. Management and analysis systems can be built into the systems employed. For example, animal weights, dead animals, and so on can be programmed so that errors are identified immediately. Computerized statistical approaches to data evaluation are freqeuntly used, eliminating much of the time and effort required for this step. The Carcinogenesis Bioassay Data System, the National Center for Toxicological Research, the Toxicology Data Management System of the NTP, and several commercially available packages are examples of extensive data systems available for carcinogen bioassays.

Reporting of results is fairly routine for most laboratory experiments. Carcinogen bioassays, because of their more intricate and voluminous nature, require more care, preparation, and time for adequate documentation. Models for a reasonable comprehensive evaluation report are the Technical Report series generated from the NTP bioassay program (7). After the study is completed and reported, provision must be made under the GLPs regulation for storage of residual study materials. This includes archival material, slides, blocks, and wet tissues.

The sponsor of the carcinogen bioassay has the ultimate responsibility for assuring the quality and integrity of the study. In this regard, monitoring is as critical as design to obtain an acceptable bioassay. Guidelines on monitoring (8) have recently been published by NTP, and they should be useful in ensuring a successful experiment.

References

1. *Good Laboratory Practice Regulations,* Nonclinical Laboratory Studies, Food and Drug Administration, US Department of Health, Education and Welfare, Rockville, MD 20857.
2. *Proceedings of a Working Seminar on the Optimal Use of Facilities for Carcinogenicity/Toxicity Testing,* May 28–29, 1980, National Toxicology Program, Bethesda, MD 20205.
3. *Guide For the Care and Use of Laboratory Animals,* Institute of Laboratory Animal Resources of National Research Council, DHEW Publication No. (NIH) 73–23, US Department of Health, Education and Welfare, Revised 1972.
4. *Systematized Nomenclature of Pathology (SNOP),* College of American Pathologists, Chicago, Illinois, 1969.
5. *SNOMED—Systematized Nomenclature of Medicine,* College of American Pathologists, Skokie, Illinois, 1979.
6. Ward, J. M., Goodman, D. G., Griesemer, R. A., Hardisty, J. F., Schueler, R. L., Squire, R. A., and Strandberg, J. D., *J. Environ. Pathol. Toxicol.* **2,** 371 (1978).
7. *Technical Report Series of Bioassayed Chemicals,* National Cancer Institute/National Toxicology Program, NIH Publications, US Department of Health, Education and Welfare.
8. *Monitoring Guidelines For the Conduct of Carcinogen Bioassays,* National Toxicology Program Technical Report Series No. 218, NIH Publication No. 81–1774, US Department of Health and Human Services, June 1981.

INDEX

333